Pre-expanded
Perforator Flaps

Editors

LEE L.Q. PU
CHUNMEI WANG

CLINICS IN
PLASTIC SURGERY

www.plasticsurgery.theclinics.com

January 2017 • Volume 44 • Number 1

ELSEVIER

1600 John F. Kennedy Boulevard • Suite 1800 • Philadelphia, Pennsylvania, 19103-2899

http://www.theclinics.com

CLINICS IN PLASTIC SURGERY Volume 44, Number 1
January 2017 ISSN 0094-1298, ISBN-13: 978-0-323-48268-4

Editor: Jessica McCool
Developmental Editor: Donald Mumford

Clinics in Plastic Surgery (ISSN 0094-1298) is published quarterly by Elsevier Inc., 360 Park Avenue South, New York, NY 10010-1710. Months of issue are January, April, July, and October. Business and Editorial Offices: 1600 John F. Kennedy Blvd., Suite 1800, Philadelphia, PA 19103-2899. Periodicals postage paid at New York, NY and additional mailing offices. Subscription prices are $495.00 per year for US individuals, $825.00 per year for US institutions, $100.00 per year for US students and residents, $561.00 per year for Canadian individuals, $982.00 per year for Canadian institutions, $636.00 per year for international individuals, $982.00 per year for international institutions, and $305.00 per year for Canadian and foreign students/residents. To receive student/resident rate, orders must be accompanied by name of affiliated institution, date of term, and the *signature* of program/residency coordinator on institution letterhead. Orders will be billed at individual rate until proof of status is received. Foreign air speed delivery is included in all *Clinics* subscription prices. All prices are subject to change without notice. **POSTMASTER:** Send address changes to *Clinics in Plastic Surgery*, Elsevier Health Sciences Division, Subscription Customer Service, 3251 Riverport Lane, Maryland Heights, MO 63043. **Customer Service: 1-800-654-2452 (US and Canada). From outside of the United States and Canada, call 314-447-8871. Fax: 314-447-8029. E-mail: JournalsCustomerService-usa@elsevier.com (for print support); JournalsOnlineSupport-usa@ elsevier.com (for online support).**

Reprints. For copies of 100 or more of articles in this publication, please contact the Commercial Reprints Department, Elsevier Inc., 360 Park Avenue South, New York, New York 10010-1710. Tel.: +1-212-633-3874; Fax: +1-212-633-3820; E-mail: reprints@elsevier.com.

Clinics in Plastic Surgery is covered in *Current Contents, EMBASE/Excerpta Medica, Science Citation Index, MEDLINE/ PubMed (Index Medicus), ASCA, and ISI/BIOMED.*

Contributors

EDITORS

LEE L.Q. PU, MD, PhD, FACS
Professor of Surgery, Division of Plastic
Surgery, University of California Davis Medical
Center, Sacramento, California

CHUNMEI WANG, MD, PhD
Chair and Professor, Department of Plastic and
Aesthetic Surgery, Dongguan Kanghua
Hospital, Dongguan, Guangdong Province,
P.R. China

AUTHORS

JIAKE CHAI, MD, PhD
Chief, Professor, Burns Institute of PLA, The
First Affiliated Hospital of PLA General
Hospital, Beijing, P.R. China

BO CHEN, MD
Department of Plastic and Reconstructive
Surgery, Plastic Surgery Hospital, Peking
Union Medical College and Chinese Academy
of Medical Sciences, Beijing, P.R. China

BRITT COLEBUNDERS, MD
Department of Plastic and Reconstructive
Surgery, Ghent University Hospital, Gent,
Belgium

SALVATORE D'ARPA, MD, PhD
Department of Plastic and Reconstructive
Surgery, Ghent University Hospital, Gent,
Belgium

QIANG DING, MD
Department of Plastic and Reconstructive
Surgery, Plastic Surgery Hospital, Peking
Union Medical College and Chinese Academy
of Medical Sciences, Beijing, P.R. China

YONG FANG, MD, PhD
Professor, Department of Plastic and
Reconstructive Surgery, Shanghai Ninth
People's Hospital, Shanghai Jiao Tong
University School of Medicine, Shanghai,
P.R. China

SHAOQING FENG, MD, PhD
Department of Plastic and Reconstructive
Surgery, Shanghai Ninth People's Hospital,
Shanghai Jiao Tong University School of
Medicine, Shanghai, P.R. China

JIANHUA GAO, MD
Professor, Former Director, Department of
Plastic and Aesthetic Surgery, Nanfang
Hospital, Southern Medical University,
Guangzhou,
P.R. China

YASHAN GAO, MD
Department of Plastic and Reconstructive
Surgery, Shanghai Ninth People's Hospital,
Shanghai Jiao Tong University School of
Medicine, Shanghai, P.R. China

JAMES D. GOGGIN, MD
Division of Plastic Surgery, Baylor Scott &
White Health, Temple, Texas

BIN GU, MD
Professor, Department of Plastic and
Reconstructive Surgery, Shanghai Ninth
People's Hospital, Shanghai Jiao Tong
University School of Medicine, Shanghai,
P.R. China

HIROMITSU HAYASHI, MD, PhD
Department of Radiology, Nippon Medical
School, Tokyo, Japan

EMRE HOCAOĞLU, MD
Associate Professor, Department of Plastic
Reconstructive and Aesthetic Surgery, Istanbul
Faculty of Medicine, Istanbul University,
Istanbul, Turkey

HIKO HYAKUSOKU, MD
Former Chairman and Professor, Department
of Plastic and Aesthetic Surgery, Nippon
Medical School, Tokyo, Japan

PING JIANG, MD
Professor, Vice Director, Department of Plastic
and Aesthetic Surgery, Nanfang Hospital,
Southern Medical University, Guangzhou,
P.R. China

HUSEYIN KARAGOZ, MD, PhD
Associate Professor, Department of Plastic
and Reconstructive Surgery, Haydarpasa
Training Hospital, Gulhane Military Medical
Academy, Üsküdar, Istanbul, Turkey

BONG-SUNG KIM, MD
Department of Plastic and Reconstructive
Surgery, Hand Surgery - Burn Center,
University Hospital of the RWTH Aachen,
Aachen, Germany

YALCIN KULAHCI, MD
Associate Professor, Department of Hand and
Upper Extremity Surgery, Gulhane Military
Medical Academy, Etlik, Ankara, Turkey

DAVIDE LAZZERI, MD
Plastic Reconstructive and Aesthetic Surgery
Unit, Villa Salaria Clinic, Rome, Italy

HAIZHOU LI, MD
Department of Plastic and Reconstructive
Surgery, Shanghai Ninth People's Hospital,
Shanghai Jiao Tong University School of
Medicine, Shanghai, P.R. China

QINGFENG LI, MD, PhD
Chairman and Professor, Department of Plastic
and Reconstructive Surgery, Shanghai Ninth
People's Hospital, Shanghai Jiao Tong
University School of Medicine, Shanghai,
P.R. China

YUNJUN LIAO, MD
Lecturer, Department of Plastic and Aesthetic
Surgery, Nanfang Hospital, Southern Medical
University, Guangzhou, P.R. China

YUANBO LIU, MD
Professor, Department of Plastic and
Reconstructive Surgery, Plastic Surgery
Hospital, Peking Union Medical College and
Chinese Academy of Medical Sciences,
Beijing, P.R. China

FENG LU, MD
Professor, Vice Director, Department of Plastic
and Aesthetic Surgery, Nanfang Hospital,
Southern Medical University, Guangzhou,
P.R. China

YONG LUO, MD
Associate Professor, Department of Plastic
and Aesthetic Surgery, Nanfang Hospital,
Southern Medical University, Guangzhou,
P.R. China

SHARON E. MONSIVAIS, MD
Division of Plastic Surgery, Baylor Scott &
White Health, Temple, Texas

STAN MONSTREY, MD, PhD
Chairman and Professor, Department of Plastic
and Reconstructive Surgery, Ghent University
Hospital, Gent, Belgium

REI OGAWA, MD, PhD, FACS
Chairman and Professor, Department of
Plastic, Reconstructive, and Aesthetic Surgery,
Nippon Medical School, Tokyo, Japan

HIROYUKI OHI, MD
Hand & Microsurgery Center, Seirei
Hamamatsu General Hospital, Shizuoka,
Japan

SHIMPEI ONO, MD, PhD
Department of Plastic, Reconstructive, and
Aesthetic Surgery, Nippon Medical School,
Tokyo, Japan

NORBERT PALLUA, MD, PhD
Chairman and Professor, Department of Plastic
and Reconstructive Surgery, Hand Surgery -
Burn Center, University Hospital of the RWTH
Aachen, Aachen, Germany

LEE L.Q. PU, MD, PhD, FACS
Professor of Surgery, Division of Plastic
Surgery, University of California Davis Medical
Center, Sacramento, California

CIHAN SAHIN, MD
Plastic Surgeon, Department of Plastic and
Reconstructive Surgery, Haydarpasa Training
Hospital, Gulhane Military Medical Academy,
Üsküdar, Istanbul, Turkey

MICHEL H. SAINT-CYR, MD
Professor and Chief, Division of Plastic
Surgery, Baylor Scott & White Health, Temple,
Texas

HUIFENG SONG, MD, PhD
Chief and Professor, Division of Plastic
Reconstructive Surgery, Department of Burn &
Plastic Surgery, Burns Institute of PLA,
The First Affiliated Hospital of PLA General
Hospital, Beijing, P.R. China

PING SONG, MD
Division of Plastic Surgery, University of
California Davis Medical Center, Sacramento,
California

FILIP STILLAERT, MD
Department of Plastic and Reconstructive
Surgery, Ghent University Hospital, Gent,
Belgium

MAOLIN TANG, MD
Department of Anatomy, Wenzhou Medical
College, Wenzhou University-Town, Wenzhou,
Zhejiang, P.R. China

CHUNMEI WANG, MD, PhD
Chair and Professor, Department of Plastic and
Aesthetic Surgery, Dongguan Kanghua
Hospital, Dongguan, Guangdong Province,
P.R. China

NICHOLAS D. WEBSTER, MD
Division of Plastic Surgery, Baylor Scott &
White Health, Temple, Texas

STACY WONG, MD
Division of Plastic Surgery, Baylor Scott &
White Health, Temple, Texas

WENJING XI, MD
Department of Plastic and Reconstructive
Surgery, Shanghai Ninth People's Hospital,
Shanghai Jiao Tong University School of
Medicine, Shanghai, P.R. China

FENG XIE, MD, PhD
Associate Professor, Department of Plastic
and Reconstructive Surgery, Shanghai Ninth

People's Hospital, Shanghai Jiao Tong
University School of Medicine, Shanghai,
P.R. China

LUN YAN, MD
Department of Plastic and Aesthetic Surgery,
Dongguan Kanghua Hospital, Dongguan,
Guangdong Province, P.R. China

LUN YANG, MD
Department of Plastic and Aesthetic Surgery,
Dongguan Kanghua Hospital, Dongguan,
Guangdong Province, P.R. China

SIFEN YANG, MD
Department of Plastic and Aesthetic Surgery,
Dongguan Kanghua Hospital, Dongguan,
Guangdong Province, P.R. China

TAO ZAN, MD, PhD
Associate Professor, Department of Plastic and
Reconstructive Surgery, Shanghai Ninth
People's Hospital, Shanghai Jiao Tong
University School of Medicine, Shanghai,
P.R. China

MENGQING ZANG, MD
Department of Plastic and Reconstructive
Surgery, Plastic Surgery Hospital, Peking
Union Medical College and Chinese Academy
of Medical Sciences, Beijing, P.R. China

JIANHUA ZHANG, MD
Department of Plastic and Reconstructive
Surgery, Plastic Surgery Hospital, Peking
Union Medical College and Chinese Academy
of Medical Sciences, Beijing, P.R. China

JING ZHANG, MD
Guangzhou University of Chinese Medicine,
Guangzhou, Guangdong Province,
P.R. China

JUNYI ZHANG, MD
Department of Plastic and Cosmetic Surgery,
Beijing Tongren Hospital, Capital Medical
University, Beijing, P.R. China

YI XIN ZHANG, MD, PhD
Professor, Assistant Chief, Department of
Plastic and Reconstructive Surgery, Shanghai
Ninth People's Hospital, Shanghai Jiao Tong
University School of Medicine, Shanghai,
P.R. China

ZHENG ZHANG, MD
Department of Plastic and Reconstructive
Surgery, Shanghai Ninth People's Hospital,
Shanghai Jiao Tong University School of
Medicine, Shanghai, P.R. China

YU ZHOU, MD
Department of Plastic and Reconstructive
Surgery, Plastic Surgery Hospital, Peking
Union Medical College and Chinese Academy
of Medical Sciences, Beijing, P.R. China

SHAN ZHU, MD
Department of Plastic and Reconstructive
Surgery, Plastic Surgery Hospital, Peking
Union Medical College and Chinese Academy
of Medical Sciences, Beijing, P.R. China

FATIH ZOR, MD
Associate Professor, Department of Plastic,
Reconstructive, and Aesthetic Surgery,
Gulhane Military Medical Academy, Etlik,
Ankara, Turkey

Contents

Preface: Pre-expanded Perforator Flaps   xiii

Lee L.Q. Pu and Chunmei Wang

An Overview of Pre-expanded Perforator Flaps: Part 1, Current Concepts   1

Chunmei Wang, Sifen Yang, Jing Zhang, Lun Yan, Ping Song, Hiko Hyakusoku, and
Lee L.Q. Pu

> Pre-expanded perforator flaps, a combination of tissue expansion with perforator
> flaps, are emerging as another landmark of plastic surgery. This flap inherits the
> characteristics of both perforator flaps and expanded flaps, making it a highly
> versatile option in reconstructive surgery. However, the definition of the pre-
> expanded perforator flap and the impact of pre-expansion on the superficial
> angio-architecture remain controversial. In this article, the authors review current
> concepts including the mechanism of expansion and the resultant changes in the
> angio-architecture. The authors also review the previous studies and classifications
> of pre-expanded perforator flaps.

An Overview of Pre-expanded Perforator Flaps: Part 2, Clinical Applications   13

Chunmei Wang, Jing Zhang, Hiko Hyakusoku, Ping Song, and Lee L.Q. Pu

> Pre-expanded perforator flaps have several advantages over their traditional coun-
> terparts owing to the thin, more pliable nature, larger size, and minimum morbidity of
> the donor site. Recently, plastic surgeons have begun to use pre-expanded perfo-
> rator flaps to reconstruct defects of almost the entire body, including the cervicofa-
> cial region, axilla, trunk, and extremities resulting from scar, congenital melanocytic
> nevi, hemangiomas, and neurofibromas. Such a versatile flap is especially appro-
> priate for face and neck resurfacing, which requires more optimal functional and
> cosmetic outcomes.

Imaging Studies for Preoperative Planning of Perforator Flaps: An Overview   21

Shimpei Ono, Hiromitsu Hayashi, Hiroyuki Ohi, and Rei Ogawa

> The vascular anatomy of perforators varies between individuals; thus, accurate pre-
> operative assessment of perforators is essential for safely planning perforator flaps.
> Perforator computed tomographic angiography (P-CTA) with multidetector-row
> computed tomography (MDCT) is one of the best available methods to precisely
> reveal the 3-dimensional anatomic details of perforators. The aim of this article is
> to describe the authors' experience using P-CTA with MDCT for detecting the perfo-
> rating vessel preoperatively and a step-by-step approach to harvest perforator flaps
> based on this technique. This article also provides a comprehensive review of liter-
> ature on other preoperative assessment tools of perforators.

Pre-expanded Super-Thin Skin Perforator Flaps   31

Chunmei Wang, Sifen Yang, and Lee L.Q. Pu

> Patients with severe postburn scar contractures underwent reconstruction of skin
> defects after scar excision with pre-expanded super-thin skin perforator flaps sup-
> plied primarily by perforators via the "bridging effect" from the branches of the adja-
> cent arteries as 2-stage procedures. Pre-expansion is an innovative technique and

may improve the anastomoses between subdermal vascular plexuses and extend the supplying area of these vessels to the flap. Such a flap becomes super thin, but with a prefabricated blood supply it can be used for reconstruction of skin defects of the face, neck, or other body part with improved functional and cosmetic outcomes.

Pre-expanded Transverse Cervical Artery Perforator Flap   41

Huifeng Song and Jiake Chai

The face and neck are important areas for function and appearance. High-quality skin flaps should be used to reconstruct defects in the cervicofacial region. This article introduces the pre-expanded transverse cervical artery perforator flap, which can be used for cervicofacial reconstruction after burns, trauma, and tumor resection with excellent results. This perforator flap is one of the best options for cervicofacial reconstruction in terms of color and texture match, and has fewer flap complications. With regard to the expanded flap, the donor site can be sutured directly leaving only an inconspicuous linear scar.

Pre-expanded Supraclavicular Artery Perforator Flap   49

Norbert Pallua and Bong-Sung Kim

The supraclavicular artery perforator (SAP) flap is a versatile flap for the reconstruction of head and neck defects. Recently, the authors have modified the SAP flap by using an anterior branch of the transverse cervical artery. The anterior SAP flap allows the harvest of a tissue island in the deltopectoral fossa, which is even thinner, is more pliable, and shows a superior color match to the face and neck compared with the original SAP flap. Pre-expansion increases flap size considerably, enabling the coverage of extended defects without the need of microsurgery.

Pre-expanded Internal Mammary Artery Perforator Flap   65

Stacy Wong, James D. Goggin, Nicholas D. Webster, and Michel H. Saint-Cyr

Internal mammary artery (IMA)-based pedicled perforator flaps can be used to reconstruct defects of the neck and anterior chest wall. Pre-expansion causes a possible delay phenomenon, improves flap survival, and decreases donor site morbidity. It also increases the area that can be covered. Pre-expanding can allow for perforator flaps that require a shorter arc of rotation. The pre-expanded internal mammary artery perforator (IMAP) flap is an excellent option for patients who have undergone multiple failed reconstructions and require large amounts of soft tissue while lacking other donor sites.

Pre-expanded Intercostal Perforator Super-Thin Skin Flap   73

Yunjun Liao, Yong Luo, Feng Lu, Hiko Hyakusoku, Jianhua Gao, and Ping Jiang

 Video content accompanies this article at http://www.plasticsurgery.theclinics.com.

This article introduces pre-expanded super-thin intercostal perforator flaps, particularly the flap that has a perforator from the first to second intercostal spaces. The key techniques, advantages and disadvantages, and complications and management of this flap are described. At present, the thinnest possible flap is achieved by thinning the pre-expanded flap that has a perforator from the first to second intercostal spaces. It is used to reconstruct large defects on the face and neck, thus restoring function and cosmetic appearance.

Pre-expanded Thoracodorsal Artery Perforator Flap 91

Yalcin Kulahci, Cihan Sahin, Huseyin Karagoz, and Fatih Zor

> The size of the thoracodorsal artery perforator (TDAP) flap or pedicle, in general, may be found to be inadequate. Pre-expansion of the flap before harvest can be a solution to increase the size of the TDAP flap in such instances. The pre-expanded TDAP flap can be used to reconstruct large-sized defects with the advantage of primary closure of the donor site. This article presents details on the surgical technique and provides discussion of the authors' experiences.

Pre-expanded Paraumbilical Perforator Flap 99

Yuanbo Liu, Mengqing Zang, Shan Zhu, Bo Chen, and Qiang Ding

> The paraumbilical perforator flap is the first and the most famous perforator flap. Pre-expansion increases the flap dimension and reduces the flap thickness and donor site morbidities, making the paraumbilical perforator flap a more effective option for upper extremity reconstruction. Pre-expanded pedicled paraumbilical perforator flaps can achieve excellent function and aesthetic outcomes in patients with extensive scar contracture and giant melanocytic nevi in the upper extremity. Although this technique requires multiple procures, each operation is relatively simple and has a low complication rate, when properly planned and performed.

Pre-expanded Deep Inferior Epigastric Perforator Flap 109

Sharon E. Monsivais, Nicholas D. Webster, Stacy Wong, and Michel H. Saint-Cyr

> The deep inferior epigastric perforator (DIEP) flap can be used to cover large defects of the proximal lower extremity, abdominal wall, perineum, vulva, and buttock. Pre-expanding DIEP flaps cause a possible delay phenomenon improving vascularity, decrease donor site morbidity, and increase the area that can be covered. Pre-expansion requires staged procedures, has risk of extrusion and infection, causes temporary contour deformity during the expansion process, and requires a longer course. Pre-expanded DIEP flaps can be a useful flap with proper patient selection and planning.

Pre-expanded Brachial Artery Perforator Flap 117

Yuanbo Liu, Mengqing Zang, Maolin Tang, Shan Zhu, Jianhua Zhang, and Yu Zhou

> The medial upper arm flap is a time-honored yet ignored technique. It may be revitalized by combining the techniques of tissue expansion and perforator flap surgery. Pre-expansion increases flap dimension, remodels flap vasculature, and reduces donor site morbidities, making the medial arm flap a more effective option for various defect reconstructions. A pre-expanded brachial artery perforator flap achieves excellent functional and aesthetic outcomes in patients with soft tissue defects on the head and neck, axilla, chest wall, and upper extremity. Although this technique requires multiple procedures, each operation is relatively simple and has a low complication rate when properly performed.

Pre-expanded Anterolateral Thigh Perforator Flap for Phalloplasty 129

Salvatore D'Arpa, Britt Colebunders, Filip Stillaert, and Stan Monstrey

> The anterolateral thigh (ALT) perforator flap for phalloplasty is gaining popularity because it avoids the well-known scars of the radial forearm flap. However, scars

are not eliminated, just moved to a different location, the thigh, that can for some patients be of great sexual value. Preexpansion of the ALT flap allows primary donor site closure, thus avoiding not only the unsightly appearance of a skin grafted ALT donor site, but also the skin graft donor site scar. Preoperative perforator location by means of computed tomography angiography allows safe expander placement through 2 small remote incisions.

Pre-expanded Free Perforator Flaps

143

Emre Hocaoğlu

 Video content accompanies this article at http://www.plasticsurgery.theclinics.com.

Pre-expanded perforator flaps are the most recent technical way to shape tissue for exact needs. Reconstruction with pre-expanded free perforator flaps has proven successful in terms of obtaining more extensive, more pliable, and thinner flaps that have increased vascularity, and also causing less donor site morbidity. In this article the author's experience with the clinical application of such flaps and the relevant published literature are reviewed.

Pre-expanded Bipedicled Supratrochlear Perforator Flap for Simultaneous Reconstruction of the Nasal and Upper Lip Defects

153

Shaoqing Feng, Zheng Zhang, Wenjing Xi, Davide Lazzeri, Yong Fang, and Yi Xin Zhang

The double "S" principle should be followed for facial reconstruction: the *"similarity"* of the donor site to the defect area and the reconstruction should be based on the different *"subunits"* of the face. In this article the pre-expanded, bipedicled supratrochlear perforator flap method is described, which is used for the resurfacing of both nasal and upper lip defects. This method can provide 2 independent flaps with sufficient tissue from 1 single donor site, resurfacing the nasal and upper lip units separately and providing an unparalleled color and texture match and ideal reconstructive result.

Pre-expanded, Prefabricated Monoblock Perforator Flap for Total Facial Resurfacing

163

Tao Zan, Yashan Gao, Haizhou Li, Bin Gu, Feng Xie, and Qingfeng Li

In this article, we present the pre-expanded, prefabricated supercharged cervicothoracic monoblock perforator flap for total or subtotal facial resurfacing. This technique can be a reliable reconstruction option for extensive facial skin defect with undamaged muscles and deep structures, which could provide excellent aesthetic and functional outcomes with acceptable complications. Our approach may replace a conventional "skin-only" face allotransplantation in selected patients.

Pre-expanded and Prefabricated Abdominal Superthin Skin Perforator Flap for Total Hand Resurfacing

171

Chunmei Wang, Junyi Zhang, Sifen Yang, Ping Song, Lun Yang, and Lee L.Q. Pu

Reconstruction of the postburn hand remains a challenge for surgeons. For cosmetic and functional requirements, the desired flap should be thin enough to ensure the flexibility of the hand. Conventional perforator flaps serve as a viable option when reconstructing the postburn hand to regain functionality. However, limitations include the discrepancy in tissue thickness and the difficulty with donor site closure. Thus, a pre-expanded superthin skin perforator flap can be an ideal choice for postburn hand reconstruction, with the trade-off being a longer treatment course (3–4 months), but with results that satisfy both patients and their surgeons.

Future Perspectives of Pre-expanded Perforator Flaps 179

Lee L.Q. Pu and Chunmei Wang

Although clinical application of a pre-expanded perforator flap is primarily focused on face and neck reconstructions, such a flap has also been used to reconstruct defects in the trunk, extremities, or hands. With better understanding of the improved blood supply to the flap and the mechanism on the prefabrication of blood supply within the flap, the pre-expanded perforator flap will definitely play a more important role in reconstructive surgery and can be used in selected patients by many plastic surgeons worldwide with good reconstructive and cosmetic outcomes.

Index 185

CLINICS IN PLASTIC SURGERY

FORTHCOMING ISSUES

April 2017
Microsurgery: Global Perspectives
Jin Bo Tang and Michel Saint-Cyr, *Editors*

July 2017
Burn Care: Rescue, Resuscitation, and Resurfacing
C. Scott Hultman and Michael W. Neumeister, *Editors*

RECENT ISSUES

October 2016
Free Tissue Transfer to Head and Neck: Lessons Learned from Unfavorable Results
Fu-Chan Wei and Nidal Farhan AL Deek, *Editors*

July 2016
Minimally Invasive Rejuvenation of the Face and Neck
Kenneth O. Rothaus, *Editor*

April 2016
Complications in Breast Reduction
Dennis C. Hammond, *Editor*

ISSUE OF RELATED INTEREST

Facial Plastic Surgery Clinics of North America, Volume 24, Issue 3 (August 2016)
Facial Reconstructive Controversies
Mark K. Wax, *Editor*
Available at: http://www.facialplastic.theclinics.com/

Preface

Pre-expanded Perforator Flaps

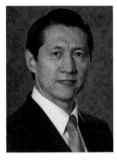
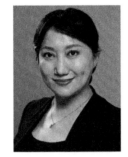

Lee L.Q. Pu, MD, PhD, FACS   Chunmei Wang, MD, PhD

Editors

Perforator flap surgery has indeed revolutionized reconstructive plastic surgery. With accurate knowledge of the perforator anatomy, plastic surgeons now can not only raise the skin and subcutaneous tissue as a flap but also spare the muscle for various reconstructions. With more advanced knowledge in perforator anatomy and also imaging studies to identify perforators, a known perforator flap can even be evolved to an unknown freestyle perforator flap as long as a reliable perforator can be identified and can be surgically dissected out. Therefore, advances in perforator flap surgery have definitively improved the outcome of reconstructions with less donor site morbidities.

Tissue expansion is a known technique and has commonly been used mainly for breast reconstructions and scalp reconstructions in North America. Its clinical application would not only minimize donor site morbidities but also improve vascularity within the pre-expanded tissue. The combination of tissue expansion and perforator flap surgery is a relatively new concept and has not fully been recognized as a valid and effective option for reconstructions among plastic surgeons worldwide.

Pre-expanded perforator flap is an innovative approach in plastic surgery that has been used primarily by plastic surgeons to reconstruct various skin defects after release of burn scar contracture. It starts with identification of perforators first and then placement of an expander between two or more identified perforators. After a series of tissue expansions, a pre-expanded perforator flap can be developed with enhanced blood supply within

the flap and has almost no donor site morbidities except a scar. Such a technique can produce a thin or superthin skin flap for reconstruction of a defect in the face, neck, extremities, and hands. It can also provide an adequate amount of flap tissue for organ reconstruction. Although a minimum of a two-stage procedure may be needed, the flap generated by this technique can be used to reconstruct various defects with "like-for-like" tissue and improved overall outcome.

A pre-expanded perforator flap can be designed as a pedicle or free perforator flap. It can become a primary reconstructive option for burn scar reconstruction in various parts of the body. It can definitely become a valid option selected by plastic surgeons to reconstruct various soft tissue defects and achieve unparalleled outcomes compared with some of the traditional techniques used in the past. Most importantly, a pre-expanded perforator flap offers an effective option for reconstruction with well-vascularized flap and minimal donor site morbidity.

This current issue represents an international effort by many renowned plastic surgeons from P.R. China, United States, Turkey, Germany, and Japan, who have made contributions to pre-expanded perforator flaps. The issue starts with an overview of current concepts in pre-expanded perforator flaps followed by an overview of clinical applications for the pre-expanded perforator flap. Imaging studies for perforator flaps are also nicely reviewed. It then includes an article on pre-expanded superthin skin perforator flaps, followed by articles on pre-expanded transverse cervical

Clin Plastic Surg 44 (2017) xiii–xiv
http://dx.doi.org/10.1016/j.cps.2016.10.001
0094-1298/17/© 2016 Published by Elsevier Inc.

perforator flap, supraclavicular perforator flap, internal mammary perforator flap, intercostal perforator flap, thoracodorsal perforator flap, para-umbilical perforator flap, deep inferior epigastric perforator flap, brachial perforator flap, and anterolateral thigh perforator flap. An article on pre-expanded free perforator flaps is also included. In addition, pre-expanded and prefabricated perforator flaps for total nasal, face, and hand resurfacing are also presented in this issue. The last article provides an overview of future perspectives from the two editors for pre-expanded perforator flaps. The reader can discover the innovations from each article as well as the different approaches among experts from different centers or countries.

We would like to express our heartfelt gratitude to all of the contributors for their expertise, dedication, and responsibility to produce such a world-class monograph in plastic surgery. It is certainly our privilege to work with these respected authors in the exciting field of reconstructive plastic surgery. We would also like to express our appre-ciation to the publication team of Elsevier, who has put this remarkable issue together with the highest possible standard. We sincerely hope that you will enjoy reading this special issue of *Clinics in Plastic Surgery* and find it useful to improve your knowledge and skill in reconstructive plastic surgery.

Lee L.Q. Pu, MD, PhD, FACS
Division of Plastic Surgery
University of California Davis Medical Center
2221 Stockton Boulevard, Suite 2123
Sacramento, CA 95817, USA

Chunmei Wang, MD, PhD
Department of Plastic and Aesthetic Surgery
Dongguan Kanghua Hospital
1000 Donguan Avenue
Dongguan, Guangdong Province, P.R. China
523080

E-mail addresses:
llpu@ucdavis.edu (L.L.Q. Pu)
chunmei22@hotmail.com (C.M. Wang)

An Overview of Pre-expanded Perforator Flaps: Part 1, Current Concepts

Chunmei Wang, MD, PhD[a],*, Sifen Yang, MD[a],
Jing Zhang, MD[b], Lun Yan, MD[a], Ping Song, MD[c],
Hiko Hyakusoku, MD[d], Lee L.Q. Pu, MD, PhD[c],*

KEYWORDS

- Pre-expansion • Pre-fabrication • Pre-expanded perforator flaps • Perforator flaps • Skin flaps

KEY POINTS

- Through previous studies on basic anatomy and prior clinical experience, pre-expanded perforator flaps have become a focus of ongoing research in plastic surgery because of advantages of both perforator flap and tissue expansion.
- The expansion process not only equals a flap delay procedure but also increases and enlarges the capillary vascular anastomosis, thereby increasing perfusion of the flap.
- Pre-expansion enables choke anastomoses to reform into real anastomoses, allowing a single perforator to carry 2 or more adjacent angiosomes, thereby increasing the flap survival area.
- Because of the different soft tissue planes that can be expanded, each with their respective blood supply, pre-expanded perforator flaps can repair soft tissue defects of various thicknesses.

INTRODUCTION

Tissue expansion has allowed plastic surgeons to recruit greater amounts of soft tissue for repairing various defects throughout the body. This technique has proved invaluable in plastic surgery and can be seen as a reconstructive milestone in the history of plastic surgery.

When Neumen[1] first reported the clinical application of rubber balloons as an implant in the 1950s, he used the term "skin expansion," describing the concept that "skin and subcutaneous tissue are capable of being expanded and it is possible to achieve such expansion in regions where it may be needed for clinical use."[1]

However, the first modern clinical application of the soft tissue expansion technique did not emerge until Radovan[2] applied the technique for breast reconstruction in 1976. In the same period of time, Zhang and Jin[3] first used tissue expanders underneath the skin to reconstruct postburn malformations and achieved good clinical outcome in P.R. China in 1985. Vistnes[4] thought highly of tissue expansion and its astounding results and equated such a technique to microsurgery as one of the landmark techniques in reconstructive surgery. Since then, there has been a tremendous growth of basic science research on the biochemistry, biomechanics, hemodynamics, and molecular biology of tissue expansion. Studies have paid

[a] Department of Plastic and Aesthetic Surgery, Dongguan Kanghua Hospital, 1000 Donguan Avenue, Dongguan, Guangdong Province 523080, P.R. China; [b] Guangzhou University of Chinese Medicine, Guangzhou, Guangdong Province, P.R. China; [c] Division of Plastic Surgery, University of California Davis Medical Center, Sacramento, CA, USA; [d] Department of Plastic and Aesthetic Surgery, Nippon Medical School, Tokyo, Japan
* Corresponding author.
E-mail addresses: chunmei22@hotmail.com; llpu@ucdavis.edu

Clin Plastic Surg 44 (2017) 1–11
http://dx.doi.org/10.1016/j.cps.2016.09.008

especially close attention to investigating changes in the regional angio-architecture and survival of the donor tissues after flap expansion. Based on these studies, tissue expansion techniques have developed to include expanded random flaps, expanded axial flaps, and expanded free flaps.

The clinical application of the perforator flap by Kroll and Rosenfield[5] showed reduction in donor site deformity with obvious improvements in the repair. These changes transitioned soft tissue flaps from crude to refined. Tissue reconstruction no longer needed to simply cover the defect. Plastic surgeons gradually could restore both form and function. The *"Gent" Consensus on Perforator Flap Terminology: Preliminary Definitions*[6] was published by a group of internationally renowned plastic surgeons in 2003. This article acknowledged the impact of perforator flaps and the increasing value within the international plastic surgery community.

Along with such profound studies on perforators, the combination of the tissue expansion technique with perforator flaps coincidentally emerged at the right time. Tsai[7] first used such an innovative technique in reconstruction after the release of burn scar contracture. As the combination of tissue expansion with perforator flaps had been applied by plastic surgeons worldwide for various clinical applications, this marked the naissance of the pre-expanded perforator flap.

In this article, the authors review the changes to the superficial vascular system after tissue expansion and the proposed mechanism as well as the clinical values and classifications of the pre-expanded perforator flap, based on the updated knowledge on perforator flaps and tissue expansions.

UPDATED KNOWLEDGE ON PERFORATOR FLAPS

In 1987, Taylor and Palmer[8] used radiographic investigations and dye injections in several fresh cadavers to study the anatomic territory of source arteries in the skin and deep tissues; 374 major perforators were identified resulting in the concept of angiosomes.

Taylor and Palmer's[8] angiosome theory indicated that the superficial vessels do not end in the cutaneous layer of tissue but rather form a vascular network across the body. Between adjacent angiosomes are 2 types of anastomosis: true vessels and choke vessels (**Fig. 1**). In between each territory are choke zones that serve as a dividing line. The traditional axial flap (including the perforator flap) is equivalent to having one dominant vessel supplying the vascular flap. A random-based flap consists of several small, nondominant vascular plexuses that supply the

flap. However, it has been shown that the vascular territory of axial-based flaps is often supplemented by adjacent smaller, nondominant vascular perforators. This finding supports the concept that the safe *clinical* territory of a cutaneous perforator extends beyond the *anatomic* territory of that perforator to include the *anatomic* territory of the next adjacent cutaneous perforator, situated radially in any direction. Based on Taylor and Palmer's[8] studies, the flap survival area depends on the spacing between the territories of each perforator flap. The dominant flap can expand into neighboring nondominant territory flap areas because of the changes of the choke vessels between the perforator territory flaps developing into true vessel anastomosis (**Fig. 2**).

Expanding on the angiosomes theory, Saint-Cyr and colleagues[9] further extend the angiosome theory to the term *perforasome* based on their anatomic studies in 2009. This theory states each perforator holds a unique vascular territory. The most important idea is that each perforasome is linked with adjacent perforasomes by means of 2 main mechanisms that include both direct and indirect linking vessels, the large vessels named direct linking vessels and indirect linking vessels linking perforasomes through the subdermal plexus. Meanwhile, mass vascularity of a perforator found adjacent to an articulation is directed away from that same articulation, whereas perforators found at a midpoint between 2 articulations or at the midpoint in the trunk have a multidirectional flow distribution. Therefore, perforasomes have the following characteristics: adjacent perforating branches of the blood supply to the region have connections through direct and indirect links and through different directions of communication between the different branches (**Fig. 3**).

Taylor and colleagues[10] performed angiography on human skin to better describe the vascular architecture. The arteries were studied in detail, according to the system proposed by the vascular territories concept. (Angiosomes were to define the characteristics and laws of stereoscopic 3-dimensional [3D] distribution of blood vessels.) Statistics of the perforating skin vessels of the average human body revealed average diameters of 0.5 mm or greater; 374 identified vessels can be distributed to form nearly 40 perforator vessel flaps. These vascular findings (referred vascular distribution areas) promote a novel approach to identifying potentially new flap donor sites. It also paves the way for a new generation of surgical procedures based on perforator flaps and promotes improvements in the traditional way flap reconstruction is performed. In 2008, Tang and colleagues[11] proposed an application of

Three Territory Flap

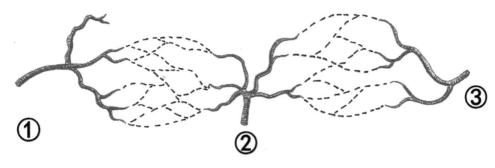

Elevated Flap

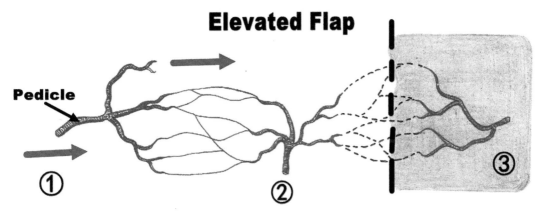

Elevated after delay or expansion

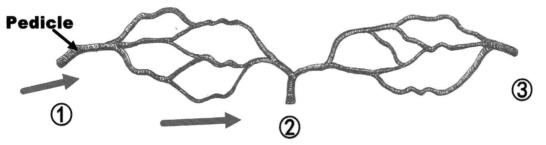

Fig. 1. Three vessels (1, 2, and 3) do not communicate directly, leaving 2 choke zones between each angiosome (*top*). One choke zone can be opened by increasing number of vessels and enlargement of caliber for existing vessels (*middle*). However, 2 choke zones can be opened with the same mechanism after delay or expansion (*bottom*).

3D-Doctor, Mimics, Amira, and other 3D reconstruction software that could be succeeded traditional computed tomography (CT)–guided imaging of perforator flaps by way of 3D visualization.[12,13] Over the same period, Masia and colleagues[14] and Alonso-Burgos and colleagues[15] reported using CT-guided 3D imaging software in preoperative planning for deep inferior epigastric artery perforator flap reconstruction. These novel surgical planning tools have further accelerated

perforator flaps into the digital era, allowing for enhanced visualization of the surgical anatomy with direct translation for clinical application of perforator flap design.

CONTEMPORARY CONCEPTS OF PRE-EXPANDED PERFORATOR FLAPS

Kroll and Rosenfield[5] first introduced the perforator in 1988.[5] Soon after, Koshima and Soeda[16]

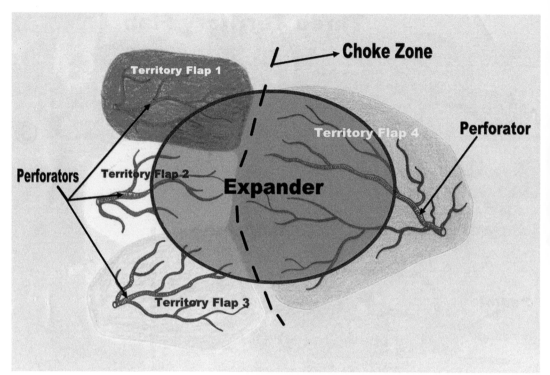

Fig. 2. There are 4 angiosomes in this picture. An expander is suggested to be placed to the area between perforators so that maximal amount of vascular rearrangement and neovascularization can be accomplished after expansion.

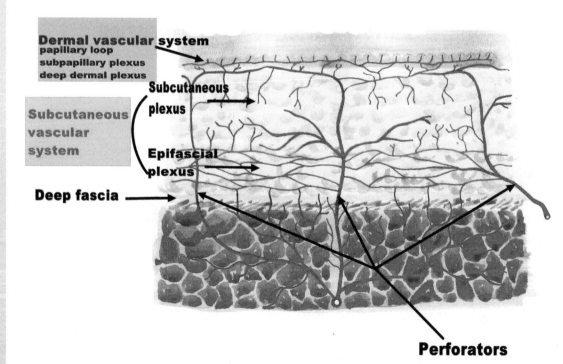

Fig. 3. There are direct linking vessels with large caliber communicating between 2 perforators on the epifascial plexus and abundant indirect linking vessels with small caliber on the dermal vascular system. Perforators also give off oblique and vertical branches to the subdermal plexus.

described the rectus abdominis musculocutaneous perforator flap in 1989. Since the late 1980s, perforator flaps have become widely used in breast reconstruction. However, there was confusion regarding perforator flaps in definition and nomenclature; this caused difficulties when surgeons attempted to communicate their results or surgical techniques. In 2003, the Gent consensus was reached, creating standardized definitions and agreed rules on terminology and nomenclature regarding perforator flaps.[6] Thus, a perforator flap is defined as a flap that only consists of skin and/or subcutaneous fat. The vessels that proved blood supply to the flap are isolated perforators.

Sensibly then, the pre-expanded perforator flap refers to the creation of a perforator flap that has greater soft tissue coverage by using the technique of tissue expansion. Expanders are placed in the subcutaneous layer and under the perforator in order to recruit skin and/or soft tissue overlying the flap. Current clinical applications of pre-expanded flaps include expanded local flap, expanded axial flap, expanded free flap, expanded superthin flap, and expanded prefabricated flap.[17–25] Although all these flaps are applied as perforator flaps, their classification remains ambiguous. However, for a pre-expanded perforator flap, the effect of tissue expansion on improvement of blood supply to the flap is more important than its classification.

PREVIOUS STUDIES ON PRE-EXPANDED SKIN FLAPS
Comparison of Flap Expansion with Flap Delay

In the early literature, most investigators regarded the effect caused by tissue expansion as analogous to the delay phenomenon.[26] However, current evidence shows that the result of expansion may surpass the delay phenomenon. Some studies indicate that expansion can also increase the ratio of length to width in random-pattern skin flaps as a result of the augmentation of blood vessels and the enlargement of vessel caliber along the long axis of the flap.[27] Saxby[28] also found that the survival lengths of expanded flaps were approximately 50% greater than those of delayed controls.

The delay phenomenon in expanded flaps occurs with changes of the vascular structure in the dermal layer. Leighton and colleagues[29] found that the superficial vascular networks enlarge following expansion. The study described prominent neovascularization within the papillary dermis and capsular layers during expansion of their musculocutaneous flaps. Furthermore, microscopic observations of expanded skin revealed increases in capillary count and significant increases in capillary blood flow within the dermal blood vessels. Although their studies focused on axial flaps, the vasculature is the same in perforator flaps. Therefore, pre-expanded perforator flaps can be used to cover any soft tissue defect without the need of muscle transplantation or reinnervation.

Different Ways of Tissue Expansion

Different ways of tissue expansion induce different patterns of angiogenesis. Marks and colleagues[30] found that rapid expansion led to augmentation of capillary blood flow in expanded skin and enhanced preservation of capillary flow. Moreover, repeated rapid expansion may be better than rapid expansion. Liu and colleagues[31] found that repeated rapid expansions can effectively improve vascular density in expanded skin flaps and is superior to rapid expansion or conventional expansion technique. Thus, the researchers recommended repeated rapid expansion because of its efficacy in promoting vascularization of the flap and the added benefit of shortening the period of treatment needed. Moreover, they recommended a 4-week period after expansion so as to increase the area of expanded skin. Zeng and colleagues[32] also substantiated these recommendations by performing biomechanical studies. However, based on the authors' clinical experience, they think that normal expansion techniques can also achieve an ideal result when developing superthin skin perforator flaps.

Role of Formed Capsule

The capsule that forms around the expander during tissue expansion remains a controversial topic, specifically, whether it should be excised or not during the subsequent procedure. One study shows that the immediate retraction rate reduces greatly after capsule excision.[32] Thus, the biomechanics of the expanded tissue can better approximate normal skin. However, Yang[33] argues that it is necessary to keep the capsule when elevating the flap because vessel density between expanded skin and expanded capsule is conspicuous. Therefore, the associated capsule plays a crucial role in improving the survival rate of expanded skin flaps; the authors routinely keep the capsule with the flap while elevating a pre-expanded superthin skin perforator flap because the capsule developed during the initial expansion may play a role to improve survival of the distal flap for reconstruction.

Cross-Area of Blood Supply

In the authors' experimental study[34] on mini-pigs in 2005, using angiography to study the deep iliac circumflex artery and superior epigastric artery, their research showed that in the tissue expansion group, target vessels are fully perfused with abundant anastomoses of considerable size and caliber. This finding is compared with the delay group, which had relatively less anastomoses, smaller calibers, and smaller territory perfused, compared with the control group, with hardly any visualized target vessels. The flap survival rate in the expanded group was significantly higher than the control group in experiment A. The survival rate in the expanded group was also significantly higher than the delay group in experiment B (**Fig. 4**).

In 2010, Sun and colleagues[35] found that after expansion of perforator flaps in rabbits, vessel diameter enlarged and there were marked proliferation of vascular networks and increased blood flow. Larger size of the flap can be elevated with less chance to develop flap necrosis and overall a thinner flap. Expansion can stimulate the development of choke anastomoses into real anastomoses. This development makes the blood supply within the crossing area more reliable, bridges 2 neighboring axial vessels, and improves flap survival.[3] The mechanism of this bridging effect during expansion includes the following: (1) The expansion procedure is also a delay procedure. (2) Expansion can lead to neovascularization and dilation of existing vessel caliber with resultant improvement in skin perfusion.[4] Expansion can ameliorate venous drainage. The probable mechanism involves valvular incompetence and the opening of communicating veins bypassing the valves.[5] The research into bridging effects of expansion on axial pattern flaps with overlapping vascular supply and the probable mechanisms can provide some guidance for the clinical application and development of axial-based flaps with crossing area supply.

The bridging effect during the soft tissue expansion relates to the neovascularization between the neighboring axial vessels with enlargement of choke anastomosis into real anastomosis. Angiography studies have shown that the caliber of the anastomosis was big enough to assist in perfusion and drainage. One perforator can perfuse its own territory and its adjacent perforators' territories through these enhanced direct anastomoses. Thus, pre-expanded perforator flaps can be safely used clinically for indicated reconstructions.

Although the animal experiments have demonstrated that the bridging effect can allow for a larger flap with improvement in survival outcome, it still has not been well confirmed in humans. The changes in venous drainage during expansion are still poorly studied. Further studies are still needed to better understand how the cross-area of blood supply is developed among perforators after expansion of an axial skin flap.

The clinical significances based on all the aforementioned studies are summarized in the following:

1. During tissue expansion, the blood flow of the flap is redistributed and augmented. The expanded flap inherits a robust vasculature with fewer operative complications and ultimately improved survival.
2. Animal experiments have established the model for the axial flap with crossing areas of perfusion, which establishes the clinical basis and provides new ideas for the traditional axial flap.
3. The bridging effect during expansion allows for recruitment of neighboring vessels. This recruitment results in the axial flap supplying a larger and more reliable surface area for which to use in reconstruction
4. During expansion, validated and confirmed changes occur within associated vascular anastomosis between neighboring vessels. This can replace the need for microvascular anastomosis, thus, simplifying the surgery and reducing the risk.

CLASSIFICATIONS OF THE PRE-EXPANDED PERFORATOR FLAP

Nakajima and colleagues[36] reported that the vascular structure of a flap from superficial to deep is divided into the dermal vascular system, subcutaneous vascular system, muscular vascular system, and septocutaneous system. A perforator that supplies the skin travels just under the dermis and divides into branches to form the subdermal plexus. It then travels within the deep dermis, joins other subdermal plexuses, and forms the deep dermal plexus. The deep dermal plexus then divides into several branches in the dermis papillary layer to form subpapillary plexus. The subpapillary plexus then forms the dermis papillary capillary network. The dermis papillary capillary network, subpapillary plexus, and deep dermal plexus form the dermal vascular system (see **Fig. 3**).

The subcutaneous adipofascial tissue is made up of 2 adipofascial layers. The superficial layer formed a solid structure and is thought to protect against external forces and, thus, is named the protective adipofascial system (PAFS). The deep layer formed a mobile layer thought to lubricate musculoskeletal movement, and this adipofascial system formed by the mobile structure is named

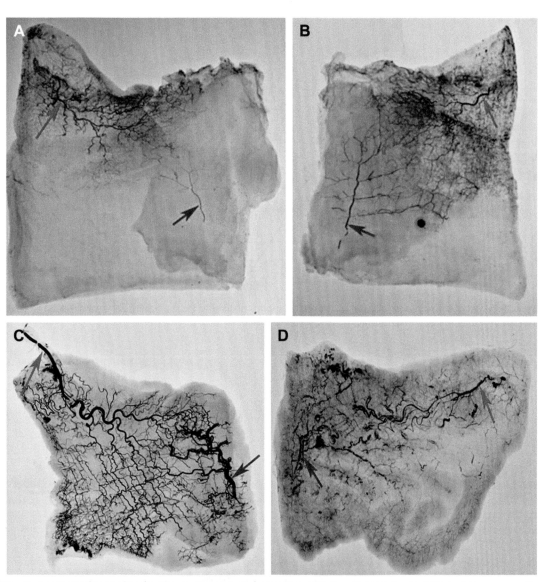

Fig. 4. Angiographic studies from experiment *A* and experiment *B*. *Experiment A* was designed to compare the expansion group with the control group. Each flap was randomly selected on its own control from the contralateral side in each animal. Angiographic analysis and gross survival observation were performed. *Experiment B* was designed to compare the expansion group with the delay group. Each flap was randomly selected on own its control from the contralateral side in each animal. Angiographic analysis and gross survival observation were performed. Red arrow: the deep iliac circumflex artery. Blue arrow: the superior epigastric artery. (*A*) The control group in experiment *A*. There were less anastomoses between the deep iliac circumflex artery and the superior epigastric artery in control group with insufficiency visualization. (*B*) The expansion group in experiment *A*. Abundant anastomoses with large caliber between the deep iliac circumflex artery and the superior epigastric artery with greater visualization. (*C*) The expansion group in experiment *B*. Rich anastomosis between 2 arteries, abdominal artery developed clearly. (*D*) The delay group in experiment *B*. Two arteries can be visible with poor enhancement, and the anastomoses were not abundant and with small caliber.

the lubricant adipofascial system (LAFS)[36] (**Fig. 5**). However, each region contains various fat fascial structures depending on its location on the body (**Fig. 6**).

According to Nakajima's theory of layered blood supply by vessels, Surgeons can place the expanders into 3 different subcutaneous layers with different blood supply systems respectively. To obtain different thicknesses of each flap after expansion, the authors categorize the pre-expanded flap as full-thickness perforator flaps (carrying the epifascial plexus and full layer of fat

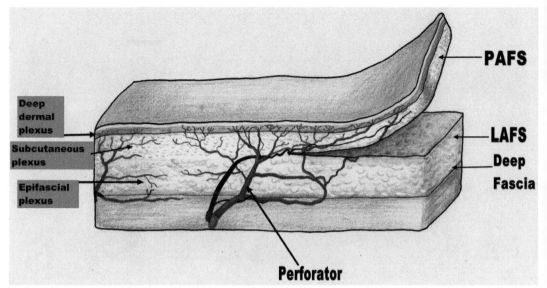

Fig. 5. Two disfigured adipofascial layers in the subcutaneous tissue. PAFS is the superficial layer; LAFS is the deep layer.

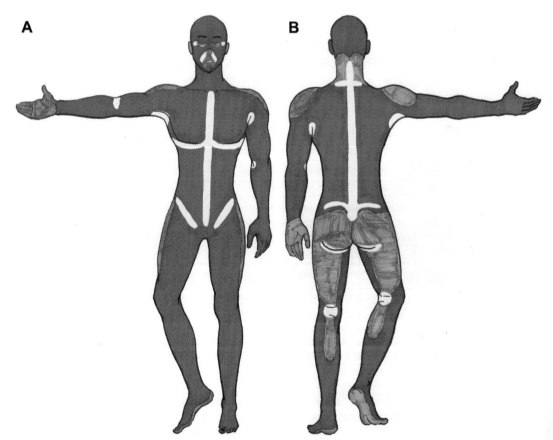

Fig. 6. (A, B) Different distributions of the fat layer in the body. Red: Fat layer contains both PAFS and LAFS. Blue: Fat layer contains only PAFS. Yellow: Fat layer adheres to the deep fascia and bones.

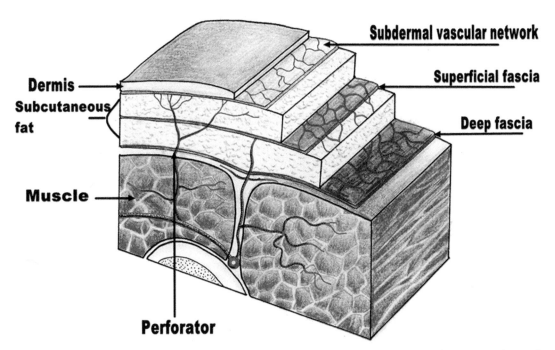

Fig. 7. The perforator flap contains a different layer of fat has its blood supply respectively. An expander can be placed under the subdermal vascular plexus, between superficial and deep fasciae, or the deep fascia for a pre-expanded perforator flap.

tissue), thin perforator flaps (carrying the subcutaneous plexus and partial layer of fat tissue), or superthin perforator flaps (carrying only the dermal vascular system and minimal layer of fat tissue) (**Fig. 7**). This categorization allows for flap versatility in order to use the like-with-like principle and cover defects of various depths with optimal function and appearance.

The expander can be placed in a various layer of subcutaneous fatty tissue and each corresponds blood supply system theoretically functioning independent of each other. However, as the clinical value of pre-expanded perforator flaps increases, further investigation into the mechanism of change within each superficial microvasculature system, during and after expansion, should be required.

The authors found that the superthin perforator flap with postflap elevation defatting results in the best aesthetic appearance without compromising adequate coverage and function in special regions, such as the face and neck as well as on the dorsum of the hands.[23] Because these specific regions have a minimal fat layer with thin surface contours, the authors harvest the superficial layer but keep the LAFS later down in the recipient site. By incorporating only the PAFS with our superthin flap, the defect can be reconstructed to regain its former contour in addition to the appropriate amount of soft tissue coverage. The authors recommend these pre-expanded superthin skin perforator flaps, when adhering to the like-for-like principle, are used to reconstruct defects in those aesthetically sensitive regions.

SUMMARY

Through previous studies on basic anatomy and prior clinical experience, pre-expanded perforator flaps have become a focus of ongoing research in plastic surgery because of advantages of both perforator and expansion technologies. On one hand, the expansion process is not only equivalent to a delay process flap but also increases and enlarges the capillary vascular anastomosis, thereby increasing perfusion of the flap. Furthermore, pre-expansion enables the choke anastomoses to form into real anastomoses, allowing a single perforator to carry 2 or more adjacent angiosomes, thereby increasing the flap survival area. Pre-expanded perforator flaps of varying thicknesses, with their respective blood supply, can be used to restore the appropriate amount of soft tissue coverage. However, how to shorten the expansion period, accurately locate the course and territory of perforators, and what maximum size the expanded perforator flap can achieve remain for future investigations.

REFERENCES

1. Neumann C. The expansion of an area of skin by progressive distention of a subcutaneous balloon; use of the method for securing skin for subtotal reconstruction of the ear. Plast Reconstr Surg 1957;19:124–30.

2. Radovan C. Breast reconstruction after mastectomy using the temporary expander. Plast Reconstr Surg 1982;69(2):195–208.

3. Zhang D, Jin Y. Application of soft-tissue expansion in post-burn reconstruction (with 10 10 cases). Zhonghua Shao Shang Wai Ke Za Zhi 1985;4:242–3.

4. Vistnes L. Invited discussion to: Radovan C: tissue expansion in soft-tissue reconstruction. Plast Reconstr Surg 1984;74:491.

5. Kroll SS, Rosenfield L. Perforator-based flaps for low posterior midline defects. Plast Reconstr Surg 1988; 81(4):561–6.

6. Blondeel PN, Van Landuyt KH, Monstrey SJ, et al. The "Gent" consensus on perforator flap terminology: preliminary definitions. Plast Reconstr Surg 2003;112(5): 1378–83 [quiz: 1383, 1516; discussion: 1384–7].

7. Tsai FC. A new method: perforator-based tissue expansion for a preexpanded free cutaneous perforator flap. Burns 2003;29(8):845–8.

8. Taylor GI, Palmer JH. The vascular territories (angiosomes) of the body: experimental study and clinical applications. Br J Plast Surg 1987;40:113–41.

9. Saint-Cyr M, Wong C, Schaverien M, et al. The perforasome theory: vascular anatomy and clinical implications. Plast Reconstr Surg 2009;124:1529–44.

10. Taylor GI, Corlett RJ, Dhar SC, et al. The anatomical (angiosome) and clinical territories of cutaneous perforating arteries: development of the concept and designing safe flaps. Plast Reconstr Surg 2011;127(4):1447–59.

11. Tang M, Yin Z, Morris SF. A pilot study on three-dimensional visualization of perforator flaps by using angiography in cadavers. Plast Reconstr Surg 2008; 122(2):429–37.

12. Zhi-hao Z, Yan-bing LI, Jin MEI, et al. A pilot study on 3D visualization of vessels using lead oxide and angiography. Chin J Clini Anato 2006;24(3):255–8.

13. Zhang Y, Li Y, Tang M. Application of digitalization and virtual reality in transplantation with anterolateral thigh flap. Chin J Orthop Trauma 2006;8(6):501–4.

14. Masia J, Clavero JA, Larranaga JR. Multidetector-row computed tomography in the planning of abdominal perforator flaps. J Plast Reconstr Aesthet Surg 2006;59(6):594–9.

15. Alonso-Burgos A, Garcia-Tutor E, Bastarrika G. Preoperative planning of deep inferior epigastric artery perforator flap reconstruction with multislice-CT angiography: imaging findings and initial experience. J Plast Reconstr Aesthet Surg 2006;59(6): 585–93.

16. Koshima I, Soeda S. Inferior epigastric artery skin flaps without rectus abdominis muscle. Br J Plast Surg 1989;42(6):645–8.

17. Ai YF. Planning of a local flap of expanded scalp for repair of alopecia cicatrisata. Zhonghua Wai Ke Za Zhi 1989;27(9):558–60, 575.

18. Zhang PH, Huang XY, Ren LC, et al. Repair of nose and adjacent tissue defect deformities after burn. Zhonghua Shao Shang Za Zhi 2009;25(6):419–21.

19. Huang YX, Zhan XH, Fan JC, et al. Repair of scars in submaxillary region using expanded forehead axial flaps with fascia pedicles carrying bilateral frontal branches of superficial temporal artery and vein. Zhonghua Shao Shang Za Zhi 2010;26(4):251–5.

20. Song B, Xiao B, Liu C, et al. Neck burn reconstruction with pre-expanded scapular free flaps. Burns 2015;41(3):624–30.

21. Kakibuchi M, Asada Y, Kobayashi S. Expanded free scalp flap. Br J Plast Surg 1996;49(7):468–70.

22. Lu F, Gao JH, Ogawa R, et al. Preexpanded distant "super-thin" intercostal perforator flaps for facial reconstruction without the need for microsurgery. J Plast Reconstr Aesthet Surg 2006;59(11):1203–8.

23. Wang C, Zhang J, Yang S, et al. The clinical application of preexpanded and prefabricated super-thin skin perforator flap for reconstruction of post-burn neck contracture. Ann Plast Surg 2016;77(Suppl 1):S49–52.

24. Zhang L, Yang Q, Jiang H, et al. Reconstruction of complex facial defects using cervical expanded flap prefabricated by temporoparietal fascia flap. J Craniofac Surg 2015;26(6):e472–5.

25. The HN, Kloeppel M, Staudenmaier R, et al. Neovascularization in prefabricated flaps using a tissue expander and an implanted arteriovenous pedicle. Microsurgery 2005;25(3):213–9.

26. Callegari PR, Taylor GI, Caddy CM, et al. An anatomic review of the delay phenomenon: I. Experimental studies. Plast Reconstr Surg 1992;89(3): 397–407 [discussion: 417–8].

27. Zhou XT. Effects of tissue expansion on the ratio of length to width of random-pattern skin flaps. Zhonghua Wai Ke Za Zhi 1989;27(7):417–8, 445.

28. Saxby PJ. Survival of island flaps after tissue expansion: a pig model. Plast Reconstr Surg 1988;81(1): 30–4.

29. Leighton WD, Russell RC, Feller AM, et al. Experimental pretransfer expansion of free-flap donor sites: II. Physiology, histology, and clinical correlation. Plast Reconstr Surg 1988;82(1):76–87.

30. Marks MW, Burney RE, Mackenzie JR, et al. Enhanced capillary blood flow in rapidly expanded random pattern flaps. J Trauma 1986;26(10):913–5.

31. Liu G, Chang J, Shi P, et al. The impact of different skin expansion on vascularization degree in flap and its clinical significance. Med Philosophy 2012; 7:49–52.

32. Zeng Y, Yang J, Xu C, et al. Comparison of skin biomechanical properties in vitro according to different expanded methods. Chin J Biom Engi 2003;6:559–63.

33. Yang Y. Experimental investigation and clinical application of expanded capsule angioarchitecture. Beijing, China: Peking Union Medical College Press; 2006. p. 4.

34. Zhang J, Wang C, Gui L, et al. Bridging effect of expansion prefabrication on crossing area supply axial pattern flap in pigs. Zhongguo Xiu Fu Chong Jian Wai Ke Za Zhi 2008;22(5):554–7 [in Chinese].

35. Sun W, Zhao Y, Shang Z, et al. The experimental study and clinical application of the morphologic structural changes of expanded perforator flaps. Anhui Medi J 2010;5:411–4.

36. Nakajima H, Imanishi N, Minabe T, et al. Anatomical study of subcutaneous adipofascial tissue: a concept of the protective adipofascial system (PAFS) and lubricant adipofascial system (LAFS). Scand J Plast Reconstr Surg Hand Surg 2004;38(5):261–6.

An Overview of Pre-expanded Perforator Flaps: Part 2, Clinical Applications

Chunmei Wang, MD, PhD[a],*, Jing Zhang, MD[b],
Hiko Hyakusoku, MD[c], Ping Song, MD[d],
Lee L.Q. Pu, MD, PhD[e],*

KEYWORDS

- Pre-expanded perforator flap • Tissue expansion • Perforator flaps • Reconstruction
- Clinical application

KEY POINTS

- Along with the development of the flap and comprehension of the vascular anatomy, pre-expanded perforator flaps are a versatile option for reconstructive surgery.
- With the advantage of offering thinner, more pliable tissue as well as the primary closure of the donor site with minimal morbidity, pre-expanded perforator flaps can be used to reconstruct defects of the whole body.
- Several principles should be recognized and adhered to in order to ensure the success of the procedure when performing the pre-expanded perforator flap.
- Guidelines for the procedural approach are summarized to assist the surgeon in better performing such a reconstruction.

INTRODUCTION

Major challenges for soft tissue reconstruction include the lack of adequate skin coverage to allow for both a functional recovery and esthetically acceptable contour. Clinicians have developed multiple variations of flaps; from random pattern flaps to axial based flaps to modification of the axial flap into perforator flaps, all in attempt to overcome such difficulties. Presently, the combination of tissue expansion with perforator flaps has now created the pre-expanded perforator flap that is becoming a better option in reconstructive surgery.

Neumann[1] first described the tissue expansion technique in 1957. With the aid of tissue expansion, surgeons can harvest additional soft tissues to cover targeted defects. This technique became rapidly and widely applied in reconstructive surgery, as it offered a flap with similar color and texture without the morbidity at the donor site. At the same time, plastic surgeons gained progressive understanding of the superficial soft tissue vascular anatomy. In 1988, deriving from the axial pattern flap, the first perforator flap was performed clinically by Kroll and Rosenfield.[2] As such, perforator flaps have become well known for their thinner and more pliable nature. Subsequently in 2003, Tsai[3] used the concept of tissue expansion and perforator flaps to prefabricate a free anterolateral

[a] Department of Plastic and Aesthetic Surgery, Dongguan Kanghua Hospital, 1000 Donguan Avenue, Dongguan, Guangdong Province 523080, P.R. China; [b] Guangzhou University of Chinese Medicine, Guangzhou, Guangdong Province, P.R. China; [c] Department of Plastic and Aesthetic Surgery, Nippon Medical School, Tokyo, Japan; [d] Division of Plastic Surgery, University of California Davis Medical Center, Sacramento, CA, USA; [e] Division of Plastic Surgery, University of California Davis Medical Center, 2221 Stockton Boulevard, Suite 2123, Sacramento, CA 95817, USA
* Corresponding author.
E-mail addresses: chunmei22@hotmail.com; llpu@ucdavis.edu

Clin Plastic Surg 44 (2017) 13–20
http://dx.doi.org/10.1016/j.cps.2016.09.007

thigh flap for resurfacing of larger postburn cervical contractures. This was the first introduction of a pre-expanded perforator flap. Since then, pre-expanded perforator flaps have received more and more attention in the field of reconstructive surgery, especially in Asia.

PREVIOUSLY PUBLISHED WORKS

At present, with the results of such an excellent flap, surgeons as well as patients support the benefits of pre-expanded perforator flaps to obtain improved functional and cosmetic outcomes. The pre-expanded perforator flap has been used to reconstruct defects of the face, neck, axilla, breast, trunk, and the upper and lower extremities.

The flap is able to be used for extremity resurfacing with primary closure of the donor site. Hocaoğlu and colleagues[4] demonstrated the utilization of free pre-expanded lateral circumflex femoral artery perforator flaps in an aesthetic and functional reconstruction of severe postburn hand deformity. Pre-expanded oblique perforator-based paraumbilical flaps were described for resurfacing of the upper limb with maximal size measuring 30 × 14 cm by Zang and colleagues.[5] Hallock[6] applied the expansion technique and methodology of Wei and Mardini[7] for free-style free flaps to 2 burn patients with unstable lower extremity scars and achieved adequate reconstruction as well as simultaneous primary donor site closure with avoidance of a skin graft. Wang and Wang[8] applied an expanded thoracoacromial artery perforator flap measuring 19 × 11 cm for a 53-year-old man with upper and lower lip ectropion. Other surgeons have used this technique for axillary as well as abdominal contracture reconstruction. Kulahci and colleagues[9] used pre-expanded pedicled thoracodorsal artery perforator flaps for postburn axillary contracture reconstruction. Cheng and Saint-Cyr[10] applied pre-expanded pedicled right deep inferior epigastric perforator flaps in conjunction with a pre-expanded left contralateral superficial inferior epigastric artery flap, for staged reconstruction of a large abdominal scar with meshed split-thickness skin graft. Additionally, pre-expanded flaps also can be applied in perineum reconstruction. Dong and colleagues[11] performed a pre-expanded free scapular flap to reconstruct the penis of a patient with electrical burn who had loss of his genitals.

Furthermore, pre-expanded perforator flaps can be a popular technique when it comes to cervicofacial reconstruction. There are several kinds of pre-expanded perforator flaps that have been performed by various surgeons around the globe. We compare these different flaps to show the variation among them in **Table 1**.

As compared earlier in this article, pre-expanded perforator flaps can be used in different varieties. According to the distance between the defect and the flap, pre-expanded perforator flaps can be divided by proximity into local flaps, adjacent flaps, and distant flaps, and according to how the flap is transferred, they are divided into pedicled and free flaps. However, there remains uncertainty as to how to choose the best flap to achieve an ideal outcome. The principles of this procedure are discussed as follows.

PREOPERATIVE EVALUATION
How to Select the Donor Site?

One must first understand the principle "replace like with like." Consideration must be given to the color and texture of both donor site and recipient site when designing the flap. Thus, the local flap could be the best initial choice, whereas adjacent flaps come second followed by distal flaps last.

Furthermore, it is vital to choose an appropriate perforator to supply the flap. A named and constant perforator is usually selected to be the target vessel for nourishing the flap. However, a small-caliber perforator can suffice if the dimensions of the flap are appropriately chosen to avoid excessive size. To avoid twisting or kinking of the flap pedicle, adequate dissection should be performed to ensure sufficient length of the pedicle. In addition, it is important to choose a donor site that camouflages the resultant donor site scar if possible.

How to Evaluate the Recipient Site?

According to reconstructive surgery principles, we must evaluate the size and shape of the recipient site. Usually, most reconstructions involve skin and subcutaneous tissue. If a skin defect only, the ideal flap needs to be as thin as possible, whereas if the defect includes skin, subcutaneous fat, muscle, or even nerve and bone, composite flaps play an important role in reconstructing such complicated defects.

One example is reconstruction of the face and neck. The skin overlying this region is both elastic and thin, with a compact subcutaneous fat layer adherent over the muscles of facial expression. This is what provides the countless variations and nuances behind human facial expression. In addition, this region also contains many important sensory-stereo organs, such as the eyes, nose, mouth, and ears, giving the face its own unique construction. It is important to rebuild these multiple components with an adequate flap. In this way,

Li and colleagues[18] applied an innovative pre-expanded, prefabricated monoblock perforator flap for total facial resurfacing and reconstruction of stereo organs. As to reconstructing the fine nature of facial expression with improved contouring, Wang and colleagues[12] used a pre-expanded super-thin perforator flap to reconstruct the facial subunits to achieve improved functional and cosmetic outcome.

How to Identify and Locate the Perforator?

It is crucial to select and locate the appropriate perforators for a pre-expanded perforator flap design because of the unique vascular nature of perforators. At present, many methods including unidirectional handheld Doppler, color duplex ultrasound, and computed tomography angiography, are used to locate the perforators. Because of its accessibility, and economic and noninvasive nature, unidirectional handheld Doppler is widely used for preoperative preparation. However, with aid of multi-detector row computed tomography, (MDCT)[19] clinicians can identify the perforators visually and more precisely in multiple dimensions, thus making it more helpful when planning expander placement.

OPERATIVE TECHNIQUES
First Stage

Incision
A mini incision[20] perpendicular to the axis of the expander is made within the donor site. This allows the expansion stress vector to be perpendicular to the incision, reducing the tension over the incision. This technique also allows for more rapid tissue expansion, allowing initial saline fill intraoperatively as well as to reduce the chance for capsule formation within 1 week. In addition, a mini incision can reduce the risk of wound infection and expander exposure.

Placement of expander
It is critical to harvest extra skin with expansion for the second-stage operation. Thus, careful planning with regard to expander placement should be considered. First, one must understand that the combination of tissue expansion with a perforator flap will result in changes to the underlying vascular anatomy, allowing for harvest of a larger skin flap.[21,22] Studies have shown[23] that during the process of expansion, the choke vessels between perforators develop into more reliable vessels if the expander is placed at the choke zone. So, from the authors' perspective based on the literature and our clinical experience, we suggest expander placement in the choke zone between perforators.

Furthermore, based on the principle of replacing "like with like," so as to obtain an ideal flap, surgeons should select the placement of the expander as described: Place the expander adjacent to the deep fascia if a thick flap containing fat tissue is needed. Place the expander between the superficial and deep fasciae so that an injury to the subcutaneous plexus can be avoided if only a portion of fat within the flap is needed. Otherwise, place the expander under the subdermal vascular plexus if a super-thin flap, only containing the subdermal plexus, is desired. Such a thin and pliable pre-expanded super-thin perforator skin flap is a good option to resurface the face, neck, and hands.

Creation of the pocket
Take a pre-expanded super-thin perforator flap, for example. To protect the subdermal vascular plexus, tumescent anesthesia is suggested to be performed before creating the pocket for the expander. The pocket can then be created by either sharp or blunt dissection, depending on the surgeon's preference, as long as the subdermal vascular plexus is protected from injury.

Expansion
The expansion phase before raising the perforator flap not only improves the transferable flap size but also the vascularity and safety of the flap, with reduced donor site morbidity. The expander is filled with saline to approximately 20% intraoperatively. The first postoperative expansion begins as soon as the suction drain is removed. Then the expander should be filled with saline at frequent intervals so as to prevent capsule contracture. This process is contingent on the pressure of the expanded flap.

Second Stage

1. Identify and locate the perforator again preoperatively by MDCT or Doppler to avoid injuring the perforator during the second operation.
2. After the pre-expanded perforator flap is elevated at the desired level, it can be transferred to cover the soft tissue defect or used in a stepwise reconstruction of the face and its various stereo organs.

All procedures for a 2-stage pre-expanded perforator flap reconstruction are summarized in **Fig. 1**.

SPECIAL CONSIDERATIONS
Pedicled Flap

Some surgeons develop a pedicled pre-expanded perforator flap without skeletonizing the pedicle.[17]

Table 1
Comparison of different flap selections for cervicofacial resurfacing

Type of Flap	Author	Key Points of the Procedure	Indication	Advantages	Disadvantages
Pre-expanded super-thin skin perforator flaps	Wang et al,[12] 2016	The tissue expander is placed between *adjacent perforators and underneath the subdermal vascular plexus to prefabricate a pre-expanded super-thin skin perforator flap. A minimum amount of fat should be kept to prevent the* subdermal vascular network and the perforator from injury when elevating the skin flap.	Topical use for the reconstruction of the face and neck.	Super-thin, large (skin flap). Improved functional and cosmetic outcome. No microsurgery. Easy to perform.	Cannot reconstruct stereo facial organs.
Pre-expanded anterior perforator of transverse cervical artery flap	Chen et al,[13] 2016	First procedure: the dissection is made *down to the deep fascia and the* expander is placed superficial *to the pectoral major muscle.* No need to dissect the vascular branches. Donor site closed directly or covered by split skin graft.		An option for covering large defects of the face and neck with primary closure of the donor site.	Too bulky; eliminates facial expression and contour.
Pre-expanded supraclavicular artery perforator flap	Pallua & von Heimburg,[14] 2002	Tissue expander initially implanted under *the supraclavicular flap.* After expansion, the flap is elevated *subfascial as an island flap or a pedicled flap with skin tube.*			
Pre-expanded cervico-acromial fasciocutaneous flap	Yang et al,[15] 2014	The expander implanted under the deep *fascia of the cervico-acromion region. No vascular pedicle isolation* was performed in stage 1. Skin, subcutaneous tissue, and fascia were elevated en bloc with the axial running supraclavicular vessels when flap transferred to the defect.			
Pre-expanded thoracodorsal artery perforator-based flap	Wang et al,[16] 2014	One or 2 expanders were implanted into pockets *dissected under the deep fascia* through *8-cm incision.* After expansion, the flap was transferred to reconstruct the neck by end-to-end anastomosis of the thoracodorsal artery and its incorporated veins to the facial artery and facial veins.			Microsurgery, time-consuming. Bulky when resurfacing the cervicofacial regions.

Pre-expanded internal mammary artery pedicle perforator flap	Saint-Cyr, et al,[17] 2009	The second intercostal *internal mammary perforator pedicle flap* was harvested in the suprafascial plane, above the pectoral fascia, without skeletonizing the pedicle. Then transposed the pedicled flap into the defect while a *thoracodorsal artery perforator free flap* was used to resurface the right lateral portion of the neck.	Large defects of head or neck.	Combined pedicled flap with free flap to cover relatively large defects.	Difficult techniques, involves microsurgery.
Pre-expanded, prefabricated monoblock perforator flap for total facial resurfacing	Li et al,[18] 2014	1. The descending branch of the lateral circumflex femoral artery is dissected to anastomose to the superior thyroid artery or the facial artery and their venae comitantes as a vascular carrier. 2. The vascular carrier is inset into the pocket created in the cervicothoracic region. 3. Tissue expander is placed beneath the vascular carrier. 4. Tissue overexpansion assisted by stem cells. 5. Several cosmetic surgeries are needed. 6. Post care: airway nursing care and enteral nutrition are needed.	Total facial resurfacing and organ reconstruction.	Good aesthetic outcome with uniform coverage and delicate features. Resurfacing with a monoblock can reconstruct various components simultaneously.	Difficult technique. Multiple procedures. Complicated postprocedure care.

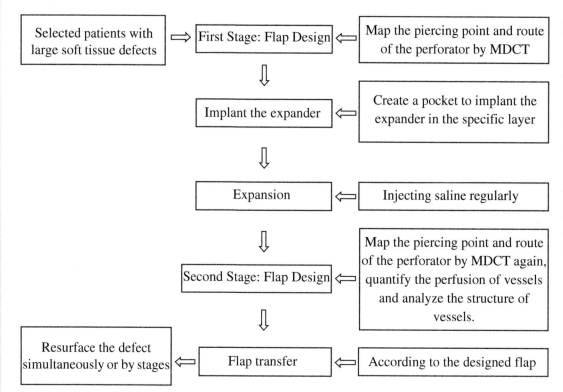

Fig. 1. The procedural algorithm to a 2-stage pre-expanded perforator flap.

To avoid the pedicle from folding on itself, the vascular pedicle isolation is performed concurrently with island flap dissection.[15] Sometimes, the pedicle is developed with a skin tube that is dissected to cover another defect in the pedicle division procedure.[14]

Free Flap

Like traditional free flaps, the pre-expanded perforator flap is elevated from the donor site preserving at least 2 perforators. All branches of the source artery are ligated on their course and the nerve is protected.[16] Then the flap is transferred to the recipient site to be anastomosed to an appropriate recipient artery or vein in end-to-end or end-to-site fashion.[24]

Super-Thin Flap

Two kinds of procedures for super-thin flaps have been described here. The first was demonstrated by Wang and colleagues.[12] The expander was implanted under the subdermal vascular plexus to develop a pre-expanded perforator flap that did not need to be thinned by excision of capsule or fat in the second stage. The second was demonstrated by Lu and colleagues.[25] The expander was placed under the designed

perforator flap in a subfascial plane during the first stage. Then in the second stage, flap elevation and transfer along with excision of the capsule was performed. Blood supply to the distal flap may be compromised in this way because the newly formed capsule also contains new blood vessels that supply the flap.

Fabricated Flap

Fabricated flaps are usually used for facial resurfacing. Before expansion, the surgeon must harvest a fascial free flap with an associated named vessel to be placed into the pocket that has been dissected with a named perforator above. Next, the vascular carrier is anastomosed to the 2 designated vessels. After expansion, the fabricated flap can be transferred to cover the defect by anastomosing the perforator to the other artery or vein if necessary.[26]

POSTOPERATIVE MANAGEMENT

Staged procedures such as these can be associated with complications, including hematoma, infection, implant failure, exposure, and flap ischemia or congestion. However, by knowing the preemptive operative interventions, pre-expanded perforator flaps can be more practical and safe.

After First Stage

To prevent hematoma and seroma formation, it is necessary that the operative areas must be drained with suction drains during both stages.

Additionally, surgeons should focus on infection prevention. If infection cannot be controlled, inflammation could lead to flap ulceration and pain. If this occurs, the expander should be removed or washout and reimplantation should be performed. We recommend the use of perioperative antibiotics. During the process of expansion, capsule contracture can be prevented or reduced by rapid expansion rather than expansion at regular intervals. This also avoids the capsule from limiting the degree of tissue expansion. However, too rapid of expansion will expose the flap to the risk of ulceration and expander exposure as a result of overthinning. Li and colleagues[18] apply autologous stem cells for their patients who suffer from flap ulceration and expander exposure.

After Second Stage

Local hemodynamic disorders can be an intractable complication in the second stage. Hemodynamic disorders include insufficient arterial perfusion and venous outflow obstruction. Issues with venous congestion occur more often than issues with arterial inflow. Either injury of the vas of vein during the flap dissection or the twisting or kinking of the flap pedicle can lead to venous flow obstruction. It is vital to recognize these flap-threatening complications. Clinical examination and monitoring are crucial in these scenarios. One reliable finding is change in flap color. The surgeon can identify that pallor means insufficient arterial perfusion, whereas petechia points to venous flow obstruction. In addition, obvious flap engorgement also indicates venous flow obstruction. The use of medications may improve the symptoms in the early period. If distal flap ischemia or venous congestion becomes obvious and not reversible, the portion of the flap can be thinned further and compression can be added to ensure this part of the flap survival as a skin graft. However, once flap necrosis occurs, debridement is unavoidable. Skin grafting is advocated to be performed in worst-case conditions.

SUMMARY

Since the first description of the pre-expanded perforator flap, advancements in several aspects of this technique have led to its increasing popularity all over the world. Although not without its own challenges, the procedure becomes popular because of its ability to offer a larger, thinner, more pliable skin flap to reconstruct most superficial defects without the usual donor site morbidities. However, because this novel flap is still in its infancy, a general consensus has not yet been reached by most plastic surgeons. As a flap that combines the reliability of a perforator flap with the techniques of tissue expansion, the pre-expanded perforator flap has the potential to become a workhorse procedure in the field of reconstructive plastic surgery. However, the technique behind this novel flap continues to be refined, and as our knowledge grows with respect to perforator vessel anatomy, the pre-expanded perforator flap may become a workhorse for certain kinds of reconstructions with a promising outcome.

REFERENCES

1. Neumann C. The expansion of an area of skin by progressive distention of a subcutaneous balloon; use of the method for securing skin for subtotal reconstruction of the ear. Plant Reconstr Surg 1957;19:124–30.
2. Kroll SS, Rosenfield L. Perforator-based flaps for low posterior midline defects. Plast Reconstr Surg 1988;81(4):561–6.
3. Tsai FC. A new method: perforator-based tissue expansion for a preexpanded free cutaneous perforator flap. Burns 2003;29(8):845–8.
4. Hocaoglu E, Arinci A, Berkoz O, et al. Free pre-expanded lateral circumflex femoral artery perforator flap for extensive resurfacing and reconstruction of the hand. J Plast Reconstr Aesthet Surg 2013;66(12):1788–91.
5. Zang M, Zhu S, Song B, et al. Reconstruction of extensive upper extremity defects using pre-expanded oblique perforator-based paraumbilical flaps. Burns 2012;38(6):917–23.
6. Hallock GG. The preexpanded anterolateral thigh free flap. Ann Plast Surg 2004;53(2):170–3.
7. Wei FC, Mardini S. Free-style free flaps. Plast Reconstr Surg 2004;114(4):910–6.
8. Wang Q, Wang J. Expanded thoracoacromial artery perforator flap for reconstruction of full-perioral scar contracture. J Craniofac Surg 2015;26(2):506–8.
9. Kulahci Y, Sever C, Uygur F, et al. Pre-expanded pedicled thoracodorsal artery perforator flap for postburn axillary contracture reconstruction. Microsurgery 2011;31(1):26–31.
10. Cheng A, Saint-Cyr M. Use of a pre-expanded "propeller" deep inferior epigastric perforator (DIEP) flap

for a large abdominal wall defect. J Plast Reconstr Aesthet Surg 2013;66(6):851–4.

11. Dong L, Dong Y, He L, et al. Penile reconstruction by preexpanded free scapular flap in severely burned patient. Ann Plast Surg 2014;73(Suppl 1):S27–30.

12. Wang C, Zhang J, Yang S, et al. The clinical application of preexpanded and prefabricated super-thin skin perforator flap for reconstruction of post-burn neck contracture. Ann Plast Surg 2016; 77(Suppl 1):S49–52.

13. Chen B, Song H, Xu M, et al. Reconstruction of cica-contracture on the face and neck with skin flap and expanded skin flap pedicled by anterior branch of transverse cervical artery. J Craniomaxillofac Surg 2016;44(9):1280–6.

14. Pallua N, von Heimburg D. Pre-expanded ultra-thin supraclavicular flaps for (full-) face reconstruction with reduced donor-site morbidity and without the need for microsurgery. Plast Reconstr Surg 2005; 115(7):1837–44 [discussion: 1845–7].

15. Yang Z, Hu C, Li Y, et al. Pre-expanded cervico-acromial fasciocutaneous flap based on the supraclavicular artery for resurfacing post-burn neck scar contractures. Ann Plast Surg 2014; 73(Suppl 1):S92–8.

16. Wang AW, Zhang WF, Liang F, et al. Pre-expanded thoracodorsal artery perforator-based flaps for repair of severe scarring in cervicofacial regions. J Reconstr Microsurg 2014;30(8):539–46.

17. Saint-Cyr M, Schaverien M, Rohrich RJ. Preexpanded second intercostal space internal mammary artery pedicle perforator flap: case report and anatomical study. Plast Reconstr Surg 2009;123(6): 1659–64.

18. Li Q, Zan T, Li H, et al. Flap prefabrication and stem cell-assisted tissue expansion: how we acquire a monoblock flap for full face resurfacing. J Craniofac Surg 2014;25(1):21–5.

19. Yang SF, Wang CM, Ono S, et al. The value of multi-detector row computed tomography angiography for preoperative planning of freestyle pedicled perforator flaps. Ann Plast Surg 2016. [Epub ahead of print].

20. Wang CM, Nie JY. Clinical study of vertical mini-incision and tension-reduced suture in the skin tissue expansion. J Plast Reconstr Surg 2005;2(03): 35–7.

21. Coskunfirat OK, Oksar HS, Ozgentas HE. Effect of the delay phenomenon in the rat single-perforator-based abdominal skin flap model. Ann Plast Surg 2000;45(1):42–7.

22. Ghali S, Butler PE, Tepper OM, et al. Vascular delay revisited. Plast Reconstr Surg 2007;119(6):1735–44.

23. Mei J, Yin Z, Zhang J, et al. A mini pig model for visualization of perforator flap by using angiography and MIMICS. Surg Radiol Anat 2010;32(5):477–84.

24. Acarturk TO. Aesthetic reconstruction of the post-burn neck contracture with a preexpanded antero-lateral thigh free flap. J Craniofac Surg 2014;25(1): e23–6.

25. Lu F, Gao JH, Ogawa R, et al. Preexpanded distant "super-thin" intercostal perforator flaps for facial reconstruction without the need for microsurgery. J Plast Reconstr Aesthet Surg 2006;59(11):1203–8.

26. Topalan M, Guven E, Demirtas Y. Hemifacial resurfacing with prefabricated induced expanded supra-clavicular skin flap. Plast Reconstr Surg 2010; 125(5):1429–38.

Imaging Studies for Preoperative Planning of Perforator Flaps: An Overview

Shimpei Ono, MD, PhD[a],*, Hiromitsu Hayashi, MD, PhD[b],
Hiroyuki Ohi, MD[c], Rei Ogawa, MD, PhD[a]

KEYWORDS

- MDCT • Perforator flap • Propeller flap • CT angiography • Suprafascial perforator directionality

KEY POINTS

- For safely planning perforator flaps, accurate preoperative assessment of perforators is recommended because their vascular anatomy varies between individuals.
- To assist in preoperative perforator assessment, perforator computed tomographic angiography (P-CTA) with multidetector-row computed tomography is currently one of the best available methods.
- The location of reliable perforators and their subcutaneous course between the deep fascia and skin, known as suprafascial perforator directionality, can be accurately determined preoperatively using P-CTA.
- Using P-CTA, surgeons can share 3-dimensional information of the perforator's location, diameter, and course, in relation to other anatomic structures preoperatively in a short time, which can shorten operative time and improve operative outcomes.

INTRODUCTION

Perforator flaps have been gaining popularity over the last decade in the reconstructive surgery field. Advances in perforator-flaps transfer techniques allow harvesting of thin, pliable, and well-vascularized cutaneous flaps with minimal donor site morbidity as a consequence of the preservation of innervation, vascularization, and functionality of the underlying donor muscle. Perforator flaps are usually harvested as island flaps separated from all the surrounding skin and nourished by only one or 2 perforators arising from the deep major artery (**Fig. 1**). Vascular anatomy of perforators varies between individuals; therefore, accurate preoperative determination of the location of reliable perforators and their subcutaneous course between the deep fascia and skin is important for safely planning perforator flaps.

To assist in preoperative perforator assessment, perforator computed tomographic angiography (P-CTA) with multidetector-row computed tomography (MDCT) has been developed to reveal the anatomic details of individual flap perforators.[1] MDCT differs from traditional computed tomography (CT) in that the scanner array has multiple detector rows in the scanning direction as opposed to just one detector row in traditional CT, allowing for acquisition of more than one image per

Funding Sources: None.
Conflict of Interest: None.
[a] Department of Plastic, Reconstructive, and Aesthetic Surgery, Nippon Medical School, 1-1-5 Sendagi, Bunkyo-ku, Tokyo 113-8603, Japan; [b] Department of Radiology, Nippon Medical School, 1-1-5 Sendagi, Bunkyo-ku, Tokyo 113-8603, Japan; [c] Hand & Microsurgery Center, Seirei Hamamatsu General Hospital, 2-12-12 Sumiyoshi, Naka-ku, Hamamatsu-shi, Shizuoka 430-0906, Japan
* Corresponding author. Department of Plastic, Reconstructive, and Aesthetic Surgery, Nippon Medical School, 1-1-5 Sendagi, Bunkyo-ku, Tokyo 113-8603, Japan.
E-mail address: s-ono@nms.ac.jp

plasticsurgery.theclinics.com

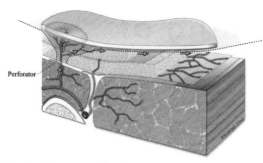

Fig. 1. The course of perforators. Red cross: the point where the perforator penetrates the deep fascia. Pink arrows: vascular flow from the perforator to the subdermal vascular network.

revolution of the x-ray detector tube around the patients. Thus, MDCT provides several thin-sliced CT images obtained in a short time. Compared with the product image provided by traditional single-detector-row CT, the higher number of thin-sliced CT images from MDCT provides increased spatial resolution in the resulting product image allowing for a multiplanar evaluation of perforators and 3-dimensional images of the perforating vessels.

The aim of this report is to describe the authors' experience using P-CTA with MDCT in detecting the perforators preoperatively and a step-by-step approach to harvest perforator flaps based on this technique.

STEP-BY-STEP APPROACH TO HARVEST OF PERFORATOR FLAPS
Case Presentation

A 37-year-old male truck driver presented with a pilonidal sinus in the sacrococcygeal region (**Fig. 2**). The patient had symptoms of the disease with multiple recurrent abscesses and spontaneous drainage for more than 5 years. A perforator-based propeller flap vascularized by the superior gluteal artery perforator (SGAP) was planned to cover the

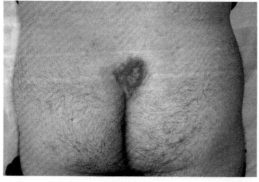

Fig. 2. A pilonidal sinus in the sacrococcygeal region.

defect after the pilonidal sinus resection. Perforator-based propeller flap, a type of pedicled perforator flaps, is an island flap in which flap movement is achieved by rotation around its vascular (perforator) axis (**Fig. 3**).[2,3] The perforator axis itself is stationary, and flap movement is achieved by rotation around this perforator. It has been so called because it is like a propeller in which the blades rotate around a fixed axis.[2]

Perforator computed tomographic angiography

Because a perforator-based propeller flap is usually nourished by one or 2 perforators, preoperative assessment of candidate perforators is an important step in designing the flap. In this case, the SGAP was selected as the flap's pedicle. P-CTA analyses used 64-row MDCT (Light Speed VCT; GE Healthcare, Waukesha, WI) and were performed by a team including plastic surgeons, radiologists, and radiology technicians (**Fig. 4**). Scan parameters are summarized in **Table 1**.[4] The patient was scanned in a prone position similar to the operative positioning in which the normal contours of the buttock fat are not distorted by the pressure of lying against a flat surface. The scan range was limited by the superior border of the iliac bone to the gluteal fold to include tissues that will be used intraoperatively. The scan was performed with a rotation speed of 0.4 seconds per rotation, detectors coverage of 40 mm, and a detector configuration of 0.625 mm and 64 rows. This acquisition protocol allowed for a table speed of 137.5 mm/s and a scan time of less than 10 seconds for CTA.

For CTA, axial images of 0.625-mm thickness were reconstructed with an interval of 0.3 mm overlapping technique (eg, a 50% overlap means that half of the current image slab is covered by the preceding image and the other half by trailing image. Each point in the scanned volume is contained in exactly two reconstructed images. This would improve quality of MPR and volume images) and transferred to a workstation (Advantage Workstation; GE Healthcare, Chicago, IL) in the department of radiology or to a personal computer (Macintosh OSX; Apple Inc, Cupertino, CA) having an open-source digital imaging and communications in medicine (DICOM) image viewer software (OsiriX software; Pixmeo, Geneva, Switzerland) installed on it. The CTA images were reconstructed using maximum-intensity projection and volume-rendering techniques (**Fig. 5**).

Selection of perforator
A couple of candidate perforators suitable to act as the pedicle of a flap were easily identified around the defects in the reconstructed images.

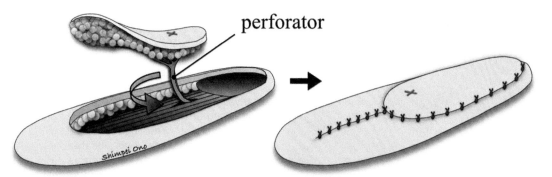

perforator

Fig. 3. A perforator-based propeller flap. Red cross: the point where the perforator penetrates the deep fascia.

Selection of a proper perforator is based on 2 criteria. The first is the perforator's location. If 2 perforators of almost the same diameters can be found around the defect, the closer perforator to the defect is preferred because using the closer perforator minimizes the flap size, resulting in less vascular complications at the flap end. The second criterion is the perforator's size. A measurement tool can measure the diameter of perforators. If 2 perforators are located at almost the same distances from a defect, the perforator with the larger diameter should be selected. A perforator greater than 1.0 mm in diameter is reliable for vascularity as a flap pedicle perforator.

Assessment of 3-dimensional course of perforators

The location where the selected perforator penetrates the deep fascia of the gluteus maximus muscle was indicated by a solid yellow circle in the image (**Fig. 6**). The distance from the circle to important anatomic landmarks, such as the midline or the prominence of the bone, can be measured, allowing the authors to draw marks on the patient's skin and making the flap design easier. In addition, by using the multiplanar reconstruction view (**Fig. 7**), the course of the suprafascial perforator branches was traced on the

computer. This directionality between the deep fascia and skin is known as suprafascial perforator directionality (SPD), and including it in perforator-flaps' design is considered a key indicator of

Table 1 **Multidetector-row computed tomography scan parameters**	
Parameter	
Scanner	64-slice MDCT scanner (LightSpeed VCT; GE Healthcare, Milwaukee, WI)
Detector configuration	64-row × 0.625-mm slice thickness
Detector coverage	40 mm
Helical detector pitch	0.516–0.984
Gantry rotation speed	0.4 s/rot
Tube potential	120 kVp
Tube current	600 mA (dose modulation)
Contrast	Iopamidol 370 mgI/mL (Iopamiron 370, Bayer Yakuhin Ltd, Osaka, Japan)
Volume	BW × (0.8–1.0) mL + Physiological saline 20 mL
Injection rate	BW × (0.08–0.1) mL/s (upper limit: 5 mL/s)
Bolus tracking method	SmartPrep
Initiation of CT scanning	Increase of >150 HU at aorta or the parent artery from which perforators emerge
Image reconstruction	0.3-mm overlapping axial images

Abbreviations: BW, body weight; HU, Hounsfield units; mgI, mg Iodine.

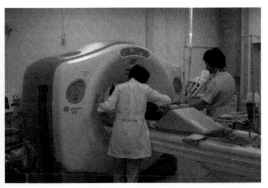

Fig. 4. The CT room with a radiologist and radiology technician.

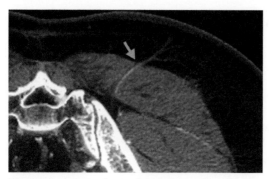

Fig. 5. Blue arrow shows the superior gluteal artery perforator.

reliable flap harvesting.[5] The authors' previous study revealed that many small branches diverge from the suprafascial perforator branch itself and reach the subdermal vascular network to nourish the overlying dermis (**Fig. 8**). SPD length was measured by using the software's measurement tool.

Flap design

The detected point where a perforator penetrates the deep fascia on the computer was marked on the patient's skin. At that time, information about the distance from midline to the perforator was used, which was measured previously (**Fig. 9**). An SGAP-based propeller flap was designed including a perforator as flap pedicle and the SPD along the flap's long axis. The distance from the pedicle to the flap's distal end (*A* in **Fig. 10**) should be slightly longer, approximately 10% to 20%, than the length from the pedicle to the defect's distal edge (*B* in **Fig. 10**) to avoid closure with excessive tension on the flap's edges during suturing.

Flap elevation

Flap elevation was performed under magnification loupes (2.5–4.0 ×) or microscopes with microsurgical instruments and technique. The initial incision

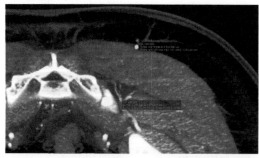

Fig. 6. The solid yellow circle indicates the point where the perforator penetrates the deep fascia of the gluteus maximus muscle.

was made along one lateral border of the flap. It is preferable to do a subfascial dissection initially because it is easier. With increasing experience, a suprafascial dissection will allow a thinner flap to be raised. One should be careful not to injure a suprafascial perforator branch detected preoperatively when thinning the flap. The flap was carefully raised until the previously marked perforator was visualized. The perforator identified by P-CTA preoperatively was located accurately intraoperatively without any errors (**Fig. 11**). Consequently, it was not required to change the flap design intraoperatively. After identifying the reliable perforator visually, an additional incision was made circumferentially to harvest the flap as an island flap.

Flap rotation and inset

Before the flap is rotated into the defect, it is important to allow for flap perfusion and for the spasm in the vessels to relax for at least 10 to 15 minutes. The extent of dissection of the perforator depends on the degree of flap rotation required. The perforator is dissected to the point at which the flap can be rotated easily into the defect by carefully dividing any fibrous strands along the pedicle that impede this rotation. After rotating the flap, its pedicle should be checked for twisting or stretching. If any limitation exists, the pedicle should be further dissected into the muscle by keeping a sufficient pedicle length to relieve torsion on the pedicle, thereby allowing for adequate circulation. Preoperative P-CTA can help surgeons to safely dissect the pedicle into muscle. In the authors' case, the SGAP flap was rotated 135° clockwise without any vascular complications (**Fig. 12**). The donor defect after flap transfer was closed linearly, and a suction drain was securely placed well away from the pedicle.

DISCUSSION

The choice of preoperative assessment tools in the planning of perforator flaps is still a controversial topic in reconstructive surgery. There are 4 main tools that can be used to assess perforators preoperatively: handheld acoustic Doppler sonography (ADS), color duplex sonography (CDS), P-CTA with MDCT, and magnetic resonance angiography (MRA). Characteristics of these 4 tools are summarized in **Table 2**.

Handheld Acoustic Doppler Sonography

ADS is widely used because it is easy to operate, relatively inexpensive, portable, and available intraoperatively (**Fig. 13**). However, it has been reported that ADS is less accurate in identifying

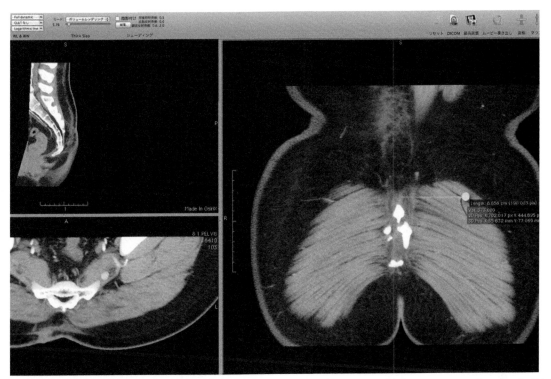

Fig. 7. The course of the suprafascial perforator branches can be traced by using multiplanar reconstruction view (*solid yellow circle* indicates the point where the perforator penetrates the deep fascia of the gluteus maximus muscle).

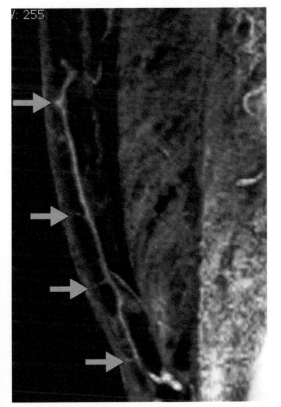

perforators preoperatively compared with CDS[6–8] and P-CTA[9–12] because the Doppler probe (8 MHz) can only detect vessels located up to 20 mm from the skin surface. If the skin and subcutaneous tissue are thick, detecting the point where perforators penetrate the deep fascia is difficult.[6] Therefore, ADS tends to generate false positives; this is exaggerated in thin patients and reversed in obese patients.[13] Another reason is that ADS

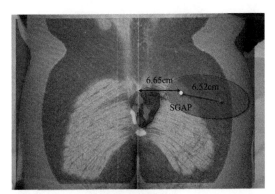

Fig. 9. An SGAP-based propeller flap (*red ellipse*) is designed including the perforator (*solid yellow circle*) as a pedicle and the SPD (*pink arrow*; its length is 6.52 cm). The blue area indicates the area affected by the pilonidal sinus. The distance from the midline to the perforator (*double-headed black arrow*) is 6.65 cm.

Fig. 8. Many small branches (*blue arrows*) diverged from a suprafascial perforator branch reaching to the subdermal vascular network.

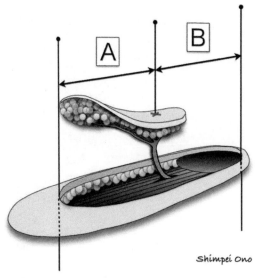

Fig. 10. Distance A (from perforator to the distal end of the flap) is slightly longer than distance B (from perforator to the distal edge of the defect). Red cross: the point where the perforator penetrates the deep fascia.

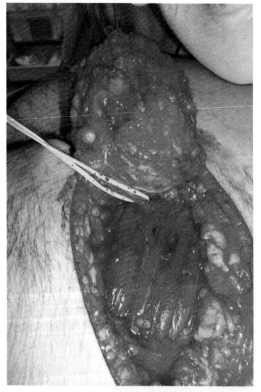

Fig. 11. Intraoperative photograph showing that the perforator identified preoperatively was located accurately during the operation without errors.

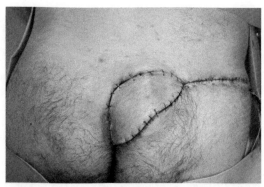

Fig. 12. Postoperative photograph. The flap was rotated 135° and the donor site was closed linearly.

cannot visualize vessels; thus, an examiner never knows for certain which vessels ADS detects. ADS may detect perforators that are too small to sustain a perforator flap; it is also too unspecific because of the background noise from vessels in the vicinity. ADS is recognized as less accurate in detecting perforators, but the authors prefer to use it in clinical practice. In addition to the advantages described earlier, ADS is useful as a screening for mapping perforators in free-style flaps' planning[14] and as a complementary tool to P-CTA or MRA. Furthermore, ADS can be available intraoperatively by using a sterilized probe or a probe cover to check the pulsation of a perforator during the operation.[6] When searching for perforators with ADS, signals that are pulsatile, loud, and high pitched can be consistently detected by the probe.[15] It has been suggested to vary the amount of pressure and angle applied with the probe to the skin surface. Prominent Doppler signal usually means the existence of a reliable perforator. With little experience, one can differentiate between Doppler signals from the main vessel versus those from perforators. The sound made by the main vessel will still be heard when the probe is moved proximally or distally, whereas the sound from a perforator is heard only at one location. Additionally, the sound from the main vessel is louder than that from the perforator.[16]

Color Duplex Sonography

To overcome the disadvantages of ADS, CDS was developed as a noninvasive perforators' mapping device; it began to be used widely from the beginning of the 1990s.[8,17–19] The use of CDS spread rapidly because it provided more visual information about vessels compared with ADS. It could reveal not only the position of a perforator but also measure its diameter, course, and blood flow. The

Table 2
Characteristics of preoperative assessment tools in the planning of perforator flaps

Preoperative Planning Tools	ADS	CDS	P-CTA	MRA
Portability	Excellent	Good	Not portable	Not portable
Cost/examination ($)	None or low	Moderate (200)	Relatively high (400)	High (600)
Invasiveness	None	None	Injection of IV contrast	Injection of IV contrast
Operator dependence	Yes	Yes	No	No
Reproducibility	+	+	+++	++
Learning curve	Little	Significant	No	No
Accuracy of perforator detection	High false positive[a]	Relatively high	High	High
Hemodynamic information of perforator	No	Yes	No	No
Time to image acquisition	Depends on operator ($\approx$10 min)	Depends on operator ($\approx$30 min)	Short (<30 s)	Long (20 min)
Resolution (minimal detectable perforator caliber)	No image	0.5 mm	0.3–0.5 mm	1.0 mm
3D view	No image	No	Yes	Yes
Contrast material	–	–	+	+ (Safer risk profiles, eg, gadolinium)
Ionizing radiation exposure	–	–	+	–
Contraindications	None	None	Metal implants[b] Allergy to the contrast agent Renal insufficiency	

Abbreviations: 3D, 3 dimensional; IV, intravenous.
[a] A false positive rate is exaggerated in thin patients and reversed in obese patients.[13]
[b] Perforators may not be clearly determined because of the artifacts of metal implants.

major advantage of CDS compared with other assessment tools is its ability to provide hemodynamic information, such as flow velocity and pulsatility with time. However, there are several

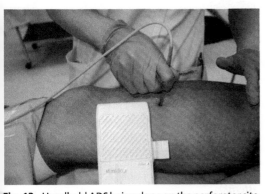

Fig. 13. Handheld ADS being done on the perforator site.

disadvantages for this imaging tool. First, its uses are limited by the fact that it is relatively time consuming, taking approximately 30 minutes, and requires a skilled examiner who has knowledge of perforators' anatomy (see **Table 2**). Secondly, it is less reproducible because of its real-life dynamics[20] and does not allow for sharing of the 3-dimensional vascular images between surgeons. Thirdly, CDS can only provide the perforator's information in a limited area. CDS is very sensitive to the perforators in the superficial tissue layer, whereas it is less sensitive in deeper tissues because of the intermittent image capture. Furthermore, it does not provide the whole structural information about the perforator and adjacent anatomic landmarks in one image. Therefore, the authors recommend that the use of CDS should be limited to selected cases, such as patients with metal implants, allergy to the contrast agent, or renal insufficiency.

Perforator Computed Tomographic Angiography

As described earlier, advancements in CT technology made it possible to reveal small perforators as narrow as 0.3 to 0.5 mm in diameter. Several investigators have reported the clinical usefulness of P-CTA with MDCT for preoperative detection of perforators.[4,9,21–25] P-CTA with MDCT can provide surgeons with detailed 3-dimensional images of vessels, including the perforator's location, diameter, and course, with its relation to other anatomic structures. Surgeons can share the images preoperatively in a short time, which can shorten operative time and improve operative outcomes.[26] Based on studies investigating abdominal perforators, P-CTA with MDCT enables the precise assessment of perforators, with a high sensitivity (96%–100%) and specificity (95%–100%).[9,10,25] In 3 studies comparing CDS with P-CTA, all the investigators[23,27,28] concluded that P-CTA was superior to CDS with regard to its accuracy in identifying perforators. The authors' past study, for assessing usefulness of preoperative P-CTA for 16 propeller flaps, revealed similar results.[4] All perforators identified by P-CTA preoperatively were accurately located during the operation without any errors. The distance between the estimated preoperative positions and the actual intraoperative positions were within 1 cm, and there were no false positives or negatives. Furthermore, in all cases but one, the operations finished on or before the scheduled time. On average, the actual operative time was 23% less than the scheduled time.

On the contrary, Feng and colleagues[28] reported that CDS is more accurate than P-CTA in the preoperative mapping of perforators in the lower extremity. This finding is based on 2 anatomic characteristics of the lower extremity: the relatively thin subcutaneous tissue and its tubelike 3-dimensional structure. Because P-CTA can provide a clearer perforator image based on sharp distinction between the density of the contrasted perforator (white) and fat tissue (black) in areas with less fat tissue, such as the lower extremity, it is not accurate enough in areas rich in fat tissue, such as the abdomen. They also mentioned that the rotation of the lower extremity could cause displacement of the skin surface from the deep tissue, leading to more errors in locating perforators by P-CTA. The authors agree that detection of perforators by P-CTA requires more careful observation of images in patients and anatomic sites with less fat tissue; however, P-CTA can provide detailed information about the perforator course in the deeper tissue layers

and the surrounding anatomic landmarks (**Fig. 14**). Furthermore, by taking P-CTA exactly on the same as the position in the operating room, we can minimize the displacement of detected perforators during operations.

Major disadvantages of P-CTA are the exposure to ionizing radiation and the use of potentially nephrotoxic contrast agent.[9] Moreover, metal components, such as an internal fixation plate or external fixator around target perforators, compromise the accuracy of their detection secondary to artifacts.

Magnetic Resonance Angiography

Contrast-enhanced MRA has been developed recently for identifying the 3-dimensional anatomy of perforators with an accuracy approaching that of P-CTA. MRA is advantageous over P-CTA as it works with magnetism instead of radiation and can be performed with a noniodinated contrast medium, making it a safer examination for patients. Implanted metal devices or pacemakers are contraindications for MRA. Rozen and colleagues[29,30] reported in their 2 studies comparing

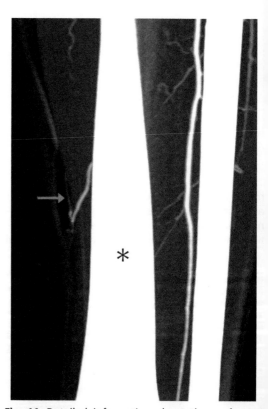

Fig. 14. Detailed information about the perforator course even in sites with less fat tissue (lower leg). Blue arrow: the posterior tibial artery perforator. Tibia (*asterisk*).

MRA with P-CTA that the depiction of smaller perforators, less than 1.0 mm, was less accurate with MRA. In conclusion, P-CTA is currently superior to MRA regarding accuracy in detecting smaller perforators; nevertheless, MRA has a future potential to become as accurate as CTA because it does not require radiation or iodinated contrast medium.

SUMMARY

A comprehensive literature review shows that P-CTA with MDCT is highly accurate in identifying and mapping perforators preoperatively, although it uses radiation and contrast medium. Three-dimensional images of perforators and their surrounding anatomy allow easy interpretation by surgeons and can shorten the operative time improving the operative outcomes. Further studies are required to properly assess the role of P-CTA regarding costs and impact on patient outcomes.

REFERENCES

1. Ono S, Ogawa R, Hayashi H, et al. Multidetector-row computed tomography (MDCT) analysis of the supra-fascial perforator directionality (SPD) of the occipital artery perforator (OAP). J Plast Reconstr Aesthet Surg 2010;63:1602–7.
2. Hyakusoku H, Yamamoto T, Fumiiri M. The propeller flap method. Br J Plast Surg 1991;44:53–4.
3. Teo TC. The propeller flap concept. Clin Plast Surg 2010;37:615–26.
4. Ono S, Chung KC, Hayashi H, et al. Application of multidetector-row computed tomography in propeller flap planning. Plast Reconstr Surg 2011;127:703–11.
5. Ono S, Ogawa R, Hayashi H, et al. How large a pedicled perforator flap can be harvested? Plast Reconstr Surg 2012;130:195e–6e.
6. Yu P, Youssef A. Efficacy of the handheld Doppler in preoperative identification of the cutaneous perforators in the anterolateral thigh flap. Plast Reconstr Surg 2006;118:928–35.
7. Khan UD, Miller JG. Reliability of handheld Doppler in planning local perforator-based flaps for extremities. Aesthetic Plast Surg 2007;31:521–5.
8. Tsukino A, Kurachi K, Inamiya T, et al. Preoperative color Doppler assessment in planning of anterolateral thigh flaps. Plast Reconstr Surg 2004;113:241–6.
9. Masia J, Clavero JA, Larrañaga JR, et al. Multidetector-row computed tomography in the planning of abdominal perforator flaps. J Plast Reconstr Aesthet Surg 2006;59:594–9.
10. Alonso-Burgos A, García-Tutor E, Bastarrika G, et al. Preoperative planning of deep inferior epigastric artery perforator flap reconstruction with multislice-CT angiography: imaging findings and initial experience. J Plast Reconstr Aesthet Surg 2006;59:585–93.
11. Puri V, Mahendru S, Rana R. Posterior interosseous artery flap, fasciosubcutaneous pedicle technique: a study of 25 cases. J Plast Reconstr Aesthet Surg 2007;60:1331–7.
12. Rozen WM, Phillips TJ, Ashton MW, et al. Preoperative imaging for DIEA perforator flaps: a comparative study of computed tomographic angiography and Doppler ultrasound. Plast Reconstr Surg 2008;121:9–16.
13. Shaw RJ, Batstone MD, Blackburn TK, et al. Preoperative Doppler assessment of perforator anatomy in the anterolateral thigh flap. Br J Oral Maxillofac Surg 2010;48:419–22.
14. Chang CC, Wong CH, Wei FC. Free-style free flap. Injury 2008;39:S57–61.
15. Wallace CG, Kao HK, Jeng SF, et al. Free-style flaps: a further step forward for perforator flap surgery. Plast Reconstr Surg 2009;124:e419–26.
16. Ono S, Sebastin SJ, Yazaki N, et al. Clinical applications of perforator based propeller flaps in upper limb soft tissue reconstruction. J Hand Surg Am 2011;36:853–63.
17. Rand RP, Cramer MM, Strandness DE Jr. Color-flow duplex scanning in the preoperative assessment of TRAM flap perforators: a report of 32 consecutive patients. Plast Reconstr Surg 1994;93:453–9.
18. Chang BW, Luethke R, Berg WA, et al. Two-dimensional color Doppler imaging for precision preoperative mapping and size determination of TRAM flap perforators. Plast Reconstr Surg 1994;93:197–200.
19. Hallock GG. Evaluation of fasciocutaneous perforators using color duplex imaging. Plast Reconstr Surg 1994;94:644–51.
20. Smit JM, Dimopoulou A, Liss AG, et al. Preoperative CT angiography reduces surgery time in perforator flap reconstruction. J Plast Reconstr Aesthet Surg 2009;62:1112–7.
21. Masia J, Larranaga J, Clavero JA, et al. The value of the multidetector row computed tomography for the preoperative planning of deep inferior epigastric artery perforator flap: our experience in 162 cases. Ann Plast Surg 2008;60:29–36.
22. Rozen WM, Ashton MW, Stella DL, et al. The accuracy of computed tomographic angiography for mapping the perforators of the deep inferior epigastric artery: a blinded, prospective cohort study. Plast Reconstr Surg 2008;122:1003–9.
23. Badiul PO, Sliesarenko SV. Multidetector-row computed tomographic angiography in the planning of the local perforator flaps. Plast Reconstr Surg Glob Open 2015;22:e516.
24. Yang SF, Wang CM, Ono S, et al. The value of multidetector row computed tomography angiography for preoperative planning of freestyle pedicled perforator flaps. Ann Plast Surg 2016. [Epub ahead of print].

25. Rosson GD, Williams CG, Fishman EK, et al. 3D CT angiography of abdominal wall vascular perforators to plan DIEAP flaps. Microsurgery 2007;27:641–6.

26. Uppal RS, Casaer B, Van Landuyt K, et al. The efficacy of preoperative mapping of perforators in reducing operative times and complications in perforator flap breast reconstruction. J Plast Reconstr Aesthet Surg 2009;62:859–64.

27. Imai R, Matsumura H, Tanaka K, et al. Comparison of Doppler sonography and multidetector-row computed tomography in the imaging findings of the deep inferior epigastric perforator artery. Ann Plast Surg 2008;61:94–8.

28. Feng S, Min P, Grassetti L, et al. A prospective head-to-head comparison of color Doppler ultrasound and computed tomographic angiography in the preoperative planning of lower extremity perforator flaps. Plast Reconstr Surg 2016;137:335–47.

29. Rozen WM, Stella DL, Bowden J, et al. Advances in the pre-operative planning of deep inferior epigastric artery perforator flaps: magnetic resonance angiography. Microsurgery 2009;29:119–23.

30. Rozen WM, Ashton MW, Stella DL, et al. Magnetic resonance angiography and computed tomographic angiography for free fibular flap transfer. J Reconstr Microsurg 2008;24:457–8.

Pre-expanded Super-Thin Skin Perforator Flaps

Chunmei Wang, MD, PhD[a], Sifen Yang, MD[a], Lee L.Q. Pu, MD, PhD[b],*

KEYWORDS

- Pre-expansion • Pre-fabrication • Super-thin flaps • Perforator flaps • Skin flaps
- Crossing-area blood supply

KEY POINTS

- The ideal skin flap should be large enough for adequate coverage but thin enough to match the regional anatomy of each particular anatomic area.
- A super-thin skin perforator flap is created via pre-expansion during the first stage operation.
- A tissue expander is placed essentially under the subdermal vascular plexuses based on the location of identified 2 or more adjacent perforators.
- Our preferred technique can create a large super-thin skin flap that has prefabricated blood supply.
- The flap can be used to reconstruct a large surface skin defect with a "like-for-like" tissue.

INTRODUCTION

Perforator flaps were first described by Koshima and Soeda in 1989. They are adipocutaneous flaps within which blood is circulated through a cutaneous perforator artery and its vena commitae. Since then, perforator flaps have been used widely by many plastic surgeons to reconstruct varies soft tissue defects with good success.[1–3]

Reconstruction of a large superficial open area in the face, body, or extremity area with a "like-for-like tissue" is an ongoing challenge for plastic surgeons. The ideal skin flap should be large enough for adequate coverage but thin enough to match the regional anatomy of each particular anatomic area. This may be especially true for the face, neck, and hand or finger, where there is a need for such a supper-thin skin for reconstruction. Our group's innovative approach to reconstruct extensive postburn surface scar contracture is based on the theory of "bridging" of the neighboring axial pattern flap.[4] We combine this theory with pre-expansion to acquire the desired large flap that has "prefabricated" blood supply so that such a flap can be used to reconstruct a large surface skin defect with a "like-for-like" tissue for a more desirable outcome.

Super-thin flaps, by their definition, are primarily thinned to the layer where the subdermal vascular network (subdermal plexus) can be seen through the minimal fat layer.[5] Over the last 10 years, super-thin skin perforator flaps have been used widely by these authors to reconstruct various defects after release of postburn face, neck, or hand scar contracture with a good success. A super-thin skin perforator flap is created via pre-expansion during the first stage operation where a tissue expander is placed essentially under the subdermal vascular plexuses based on the location of identified 2 or more adjacent perforators. In this article, we introduce our preferred pre-expanded super-thin skin perforator flap and its clinical application for reconstruction of large

---

[a] Department of Plastic and Aesthetic Surgery, Dongguan Kanghua Hospital, 1000 Donguan Avenue, Dongguan 523080, Guangdong Province, P.R. China; [b] Division of Plastic Surgery, University of California Davis Medical Center, 2221 Stockton Boulevard, Suite 2123, Sacramento, CA 95817, USA
* Corresponding author.
E-mail address: llpu@ucdavis.edu

Clin Plastic Surg 44 (2017) 31–40
http://dx.doi.org/10.1016/j.cps.2016.08.008
0094-1298/17/© 2016 Elsevier Inc. All rights reserved.

skin defect after release of postburn scar contracture in the face, neck, or other part of body.

TREATMENT GOALS AND PLANNED OUTCOMES

In the past, the pre-expanded random skin flap is designed with a wide pedicle. However, the flap could not cross the midline of the face or neck and survive well without an adequate length of the pedicle. During the pre-expansion of the skin perforator flap, we believe the diameter of adjacent communicating branches increases. Because more perfusion occurs through these communicating branches, it is possible that the blood from the subcutaneous perforators of 1 supplying artery can flow into other perforators through the communicating branches. Thus, the flap can be designed significantly larger with a narrower pedicle as long as the perforator is not injured. With this narrower pedicle, the flap can be rotated easily. Again, the color, character, and thickness of the pre-expanded flap are more able to mimic the normal skin of the face, neck, or other part of the body.

During pre-expansion, the "bridging effect" can merge 2 neighboring axial flaps into 1 larger cross-area flap. The advantages of this flap are not only its larger size and thinner contour, but also its ease of rotation and malleability. Thus, this kind of pre-expanded super-thin skin perforator flap can be used to reconstruct a large skin defect after release of the massive postburn cicatrix without significant donor site deformity. It may have an essential role in reconstructing a large face or neck defect, a region where both aesthetic appearance and functional result are required. Therefore, with the application of our preferred pre-expanded super-thin skin perforator flap for indicated reconstructions, patients may have more optimal reconstructive and aesthetic outcome with "like-for-like" tissue but minimal donor site scarring and other morbidity.

PREOPERATIVE PLANNING AND PREPARATION

The mechanism to improve pre-expanded flap survival is thought to be the "bridging effect" through prefabrication of the blood supply within the flap. First, pre-expansion of the flap can change choke anastomoses into real anastomoses and bridge 2 neighboring axial vessels (**Fig. 1**). Second, the perfusion of the flap may be improved by neovascularization and dilation of vessel's caliber during the pre-expansion from adjacent perforators (**Fig. 2**). Importantly, the positive effect of pre-expansion on the blood supply of a crossing area to the flap has been confirmed experimentally in our previous study and, thus, pre-expansion of a perforator skin flap can be applied clinically with possibly good success.[6]

To identify perforators as part of the preoperative planning for creation of super-thin skin

Pre-Fabrication of Blood Supply Within Expanded Skin Flap

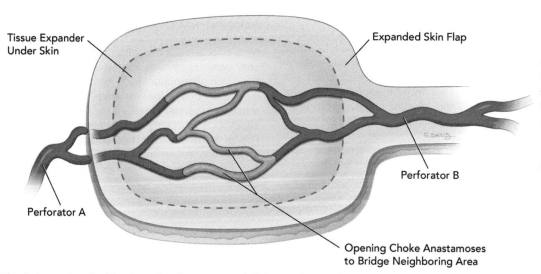

Fig. 1. Improving the blood supply of a pre-expanded skin perforator flap. The "bridging effect" through opening of choke anastomoses between 2 neighboring area has been considered as one primary mechanism for pre-fabrication of the blood supply within the flap. (*From* Wang CM, Pu LLQ. Pre-expanded super-thin skin perforator flap. QMP's Plastic Surgery Pulse News 2016;8:1 A Featured Article Focus on Flap; with permission.)

Pre-Fabrication of Blood Supply Within Expanded Skin Flap

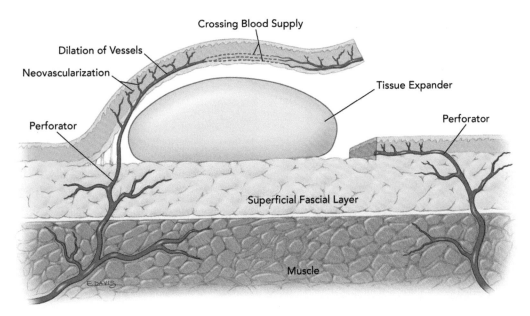

Fig. 2. Improving the blood supply of a pre-expanded skin perforator flap. The crossing area's blood supply through dilation of the existing vessels and/or neovascularization between 2 neighboring areas has been considered as another primary mechanism for prefabrication of the blood supply within the flap. (*From* Wang CM, Pu LLQ. Pre-expanded super-thin skin perforator flap. QMP's Plastic Surgery Pulse News 2016;8:1 A Featured Article Focus on Flap; with permission.)

perforator flap, we prefer to use multidetector row computed tomography (MDCT) angiography to map perforators in a region of the body. For a pre-expanded skin perforator flap, when a dominant perforator over the flap can be identified, the flap can be made extra long, as long as the distal tip of the flap receives adequate blood supply. Therefore, we recommend MDCT angiography as a routine preoperative test for all pre-expanded pedicled perforator flaps. It allows more appropriate preoperative selection of a sizable perforator with the shortest intramuscular and suprafascial course leading to safer and easier flap dissection. MDCT angiography can certainly play an important role in a safe design of any free-style pedicled perforator flaps.[7]

PATIENT POSITIONING

Patients in general are placed in a supine position for most of our procedures. Less often, they may be placed in a prone or lateral decubitus position for the procedure, depending on where the donor site or reconstructive site of the flap.

PROCEDURAL APPROACH

Our preferred approach includes 2-stage operative procedures for each patient during about a 3-month period. The first stage procedure involves the placement of a tissue expander based on the location of adjacent perforators to prefabricate a pre-expanded super-thin skin perforator flap in a selected donor site. The second-stage procedure involves the removal of the tissue expander, elevation of the super-thin skin flap, inset of the flap, and closure of the donor site.

At the first stage, a super-thin skin flap is designed based on at least 2 perforators with crossing area of blood supply from adjacent vessels depend on the area where the tissue expander is placed (**Fig. 3**). All vessels or perforators are detected by MDCT and then confirmed by an intraoperative Doppler study.

The expander is placed under the subdermal vascular plexuses (subdermal vascular network) according to the preoperative design. A minimum amount of fat should be kept with the elevated skin flap to prevent the subdermal vascular network and the perforator from injury (**Fig. 4**).

At the second stage, usually about 3 months after the first stage procedure, the preoperative MDCT is used to identify the pedicle of the flap based on the perforators from the adjacent vessels. The shape and size of the flap is designed to match the potential skin defect (**Fig. 5**).

A large super-thin skin perforator flap with crossing area's blood supply is elevated after the

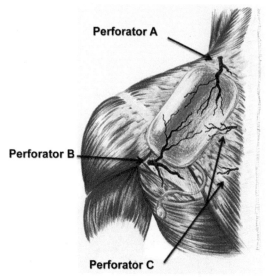

Fig. 3. Example of our preoperative design. A properly sized tissue expander is placed among perforators of the 3 feeding vessels. The development of crossing area's blood supply is the key to ensure the adequate circulation of the flap. This can be considered as "prefabrication" of blood supply to the flap through pre-expansion with proper location for placement of an expander. (*From* Wang CM, Zhang JY, Yang SF, et al. The clinical application of pre-expanded and pre-fabricated super-thin skin perforator flap for reconstruction of post-burn neck contracture. Ann Plast Surg 2016;77(Suppl 1):S50; with permission.)

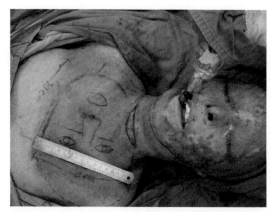

Fig. 5. During the second-stage procedure, the shape and size of the pre-expanded flap should be designed to match the potential skin defect (in the face for this patient).

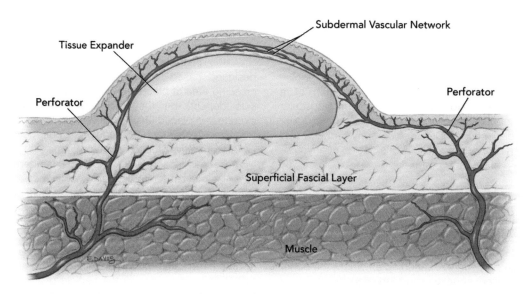

Fig. 4. A tissue expander should be placed within the subcutaneous fascia layer. It is placed under the subdermal vascular network adjacent to at least 2 perforators of several feeding vessels to the flap. The development of crossing area's blood supply is the key to ensure the adequate blood supply to the flap. (*From* Wang CM, Pu LLQ. Pre-expanded super-thin skin perforator flap. QMP's Plastic Surgery Pulse News 2016;8:1 A Featured Article Focus on Flap; with permission.)

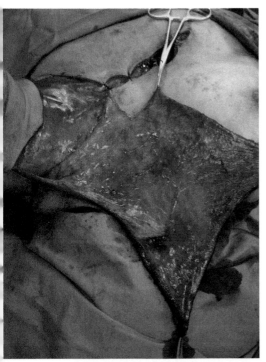

Fig. 6. A large pre-expanded super-thin skin perforator flap is elevated after removal of the expander. The crossing blood vessels within the flap are clearly visible after expansion.

removal of the expander (Fig. 6). The flap is then transposed to cover the skin defect of the face, neck, or other part of the body and the donor site is closed primarily without tension (Fig. 7).

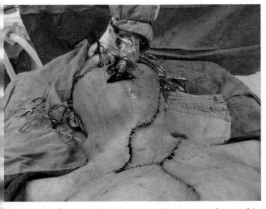

Fig. 7. The flap can be transposed to cover a large skin defect (of the face for this patient) and the donor site can be closed primarily.

POTENTIAL COMPLICATIONS AND THEIR MANAGEMENT

Just like any skin flaps, complications related to flap rotation and advancement include partial or total flap loss owing to distal flap ischemia, twisting or kinking of the flap pedicle, compression of the distal flap, hematoma or seroma under the flap, delayed flap healing, or flap site or flap donor site scarring. The overall management of these complications is the same as other skin flaps. In general, a well-designed, well-executed flap surgery with proper postoperative care minimizes the incidence of those flap-related complications.

POSTPROCEDURAL CARE

Flap monitoring is done clinically after the expanded flap is transferred to the planned reconstructed site. If the distal portion of the flap shows the sign of venous congestion, one should check if the pedicle of the flap has been twisted or kinking.

Drains from the expander site are usually taken out on postoperative day 3 to 5 when the drainage from each drain is less than 15 mL/d. Expansion is usually begun at 3 to 5 days after surgery with normal saline added weekly. Compression dressing may be necessary at the distal part of the flap. The dressing is changed every 2 days. Patients are usually discharged on postoperative day 4 to 6.

REHABILITATION AND RECOVERY

Appropriate physical therapy may be necessary to aid rehabilitation of the patient after pre-expanded super-thin skin perforator flap reconstruction. All patients are asked to use silicone gel sheet in both donor and recipient sites for 6 months to prevent hypertrophic scar formation.

OUTCOMES

Based on our greater than 10-year experience with more than 300 clinical cases, all super-thin skin perforator flaps were transferred successfully to reconstruct the large face, neck, or hand defect with satisfactory healing of the skin wound. A satisfactory appearance in the flap site and regain of function after such a flap reconstruction was seen in almost all patients. All patients had improved appearance of their face, neck, or hand contour and range of motion at postoperative clinic visits. In addition, there was no deformity or morbidity at the donor site. Primary closure was accomplished in all patients.

CASE DEMONSTRATIONS
Case 1

A 28-year-old Chinese woman developed significant burn scar contracture in her middle and low face after previous skin grafting for treatment of facial burn about 24 years ago. (A) She was offered to a 2-stage soft tissue reconstruction with a pre-expanded super-thin skin perforator flap from her neck. Two tissue expanders were placed under her anterior neck skin based on the location of identified perforators in the area during the first-stage operation and were subsequently fully expanded. (B, C) At about 3 months during the second stage operation, burn scars over her entire low face and portion of the middle face were completely excised (D) and the skin defect of her face was reconstructed with a large pre-expanded super-thin skin perforator flap. (E) The flap was transferred successfully to cover her facial wound without any complications. She has been followed for more than 1 year with a well-healed flap and good functional and cosmetic outcomes (F).

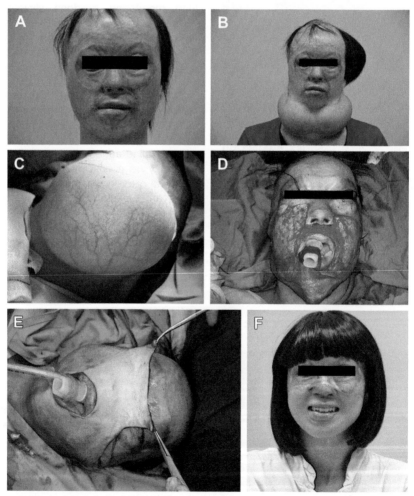

Case 1: (A) Preoperative photograph showing severe middle and lower face scar contracture in this patient. (B) Two tissue expanders were placed under her anterior neck skin based on the perforators in the areas and were subsequently fully expanded. (C) Three months after fully expansion, newly developed vessels within the flap from the perforators were easily visible under the light. (D) Burn scars over her entire low face and portion of the middle face were excised. (E) The skin defect was reconstructed with the large pre-expanded super-thin skin perforator flap. (F) The reconstructive result at the 6-month follow-up.

Case 2

A 29-year-old Chinese man developed a severe cervical contracture after an extensive lower face, neck, shoulder, chest, and upper extremity burn. (A) Because he has no good flap donor site from the anterior chest, 2 expanded "super-thin" skin perforator flaps were designed from each side of his back. Each flap was also based on the perforators' "pass-bridge" between the descending branch of the transverse cervical artery and the circumflex scapular artery. Two expanders were placed subcutaneously to each side of the back. (B, C) During a subsequent procedure, the left-sided flap with a 4-cm-wide pedicle was rotated to cover the neck defect and the right-sided flap was advanced to the front to cover the shoulder wound. (D, E) Closure of the donor site was free of tension. Good reconstructive outcome and functional improvement of the lower face and neck was achieved during follow-up. (F) No shrinking of the flap or hypertrophic scarring was observed after 2 years.

Case 3

A 29-year-old Chinese man developed significant burn scar contracture over his right forearm after previous skin grafting for burn injury. He had a significant limitation of his wrist movement. (A1, A2) He was offered to a 2-stage soft tissue reconstruction with a pre-expanded super-thin skin perforator flap from his abdomen. A tissue expander was placed under his right midabdominal skin based on the location of identified perforators in the area during the first stage operation and were subsequently fully expanded. (B, C) At 3 months during the second-stage operation, burn scars over his right forearm were completely excised. (D) The skin defect of the forearm was coved with a large pre-expanded super-thin skin perforator flap, and both pedicles of the flap were still connected and the flap donor site was approximated without difficulty. (E, F) Each pedicel of the flap was then divided 14 days later and the blood supply to the flap remained good. (G) His flap site healed nicely and the range of

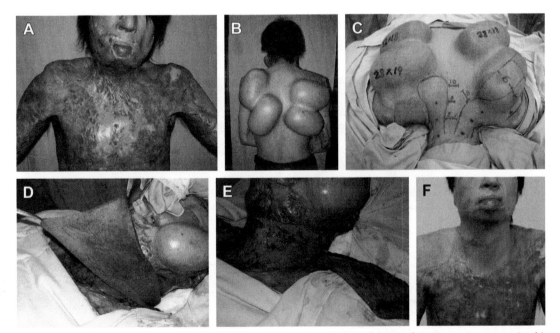

Case 2: (A) Preoperative photograph showing severe anterior neck and lower face scar contracture in this patient. (B) The upper expander on each side was placed under the subdermal vascular plexuses between the perforators in the areas. The lower expander on each side was placed to expand the skin for each flap donor site closure. (C) The surgical design during the second stage of the surgery. (D) The soft tissue defect after excision and release of face and neck scar contracture. (E) A large super-thin skin flap from the patient's left back was transposed to cover the neck soft tissue defect. (F) The reconstructive result at 6 months of follow-up. (From Wang CM, Zhang JY, Yang SF, et al. The clinical application of pre-expanded and pre-fabricated super-thin skin perforator flap for reconstruction of post-burn neck contracture. Ann Plast Surg 2016;77(Suppl 1):S51; with permission.)

Wang et al

motion over his right wrist was improved successfully. He had been followed for 8 months
with good functional and cosmetic outcomes
(*H1, H2*).

DISCUSSIONS

Super-thin flaps are primarily thinned to the layer
where the subdermal vascular network (subdermal
plexus) can be seen through the remaining layer of

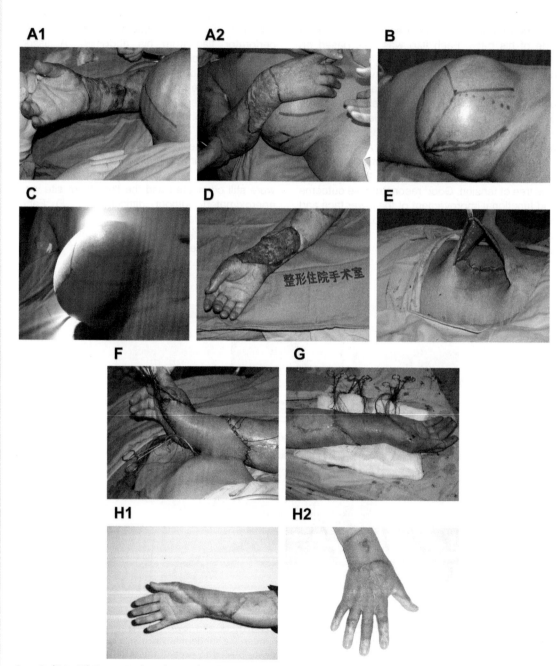

Case 3: (*A1, A2*) Preoperative photos showing scar contracture of the right forearm in this patient. (*B*) A tissue
expander was placed under his midabdominal skin based on the perforators in the area and was subsequently
fully expanded. (*C*) Three months after full expansion, newly developed vessels within the flap from the perforators were easily visible under the light. (*D*) Burn scar over his right forearm was excised. (*E, F*) The skin defect
of the forearm was completely coved with the large pre-expanded super-thin skin perforator flap. Both pedicles
of the flap were still connected. (*G*) Each pedicle of the flap was divided 14 later and the final inset of the flap
was completed. (*H1, H2*) The reconstructive result at 8 months follow-up.

fat. The study was carried out in our laboratory using a minipig model to explore the effects of tissue expansion on the anastomoses between different angiosomes and the survival of the flap with a cross-area's blood supply.[6] According to these experimental findings, we subsequently designed the pre-expanded super-thin skin perforator flaps with a possible cross area's blood supply as prefabrication of the flap for a large skin defect reconstruction (**Fig. 8**).

The mechanism to improve expanded flap survival is thought to be the "bridging effect" through prefabrication of the blood supply within the flap. First, pre-expansion of the flap can change choke anastomoses into real anastomoses and bridge 2 neighboring axial vessels (see **Fig. 1**). Second, the perfusion of the flap may be improved by neovascularization and dilation of vessel's caliber during the pre-expansion from adjacent perforators (see **Fig. 2**). Importantly, the positive effect of pre-expansion on the blood supply of a crossing area to the flap has been confirmed experimentally in our previous study[6] and, thus, pre-expansion of a perforator skin flap can be applied clinically with a possibly good success.[8–10]

In the early stage, the blood supply of the pre-expanded and prefabricated super-thin flap relies mainly on the pedicle. The local environment favors neovascularization and formation of increased perfusion between the flap and the base. The pedicle becomes less important as the flap gains more blood supply from the base. According to our clinical experience, this kind of pre-expanded super-thin skin perforator flap can tolerate initial ischemia well during flap elevation and transfer to the recipient site and therefore, such a flap can be used to reconstruct large face or neck soft tissue defect with improved color and characteristics of the flap in addition to the thinner nature of the flap.

During pre-expansion, the bridging effect can merge 2 neighboring axial flaps into 1 larger cross-area flap. The advantages of this flap are not only its larger size and thinner contour, but also its ease of rotation and malleability. This novel flap can be applied to restore the massive postburn cicatrix without donor site deformity. It may have an essential role in reconstructing a large face or neck defect, a region that both aesthetic appearance and functional result are required. During the pre-expansion, the flap is both delayed and supercharged, increasing its durability and survivability. In our opinion, the pre-expanded super-thin crossing flap is an ideal choice for

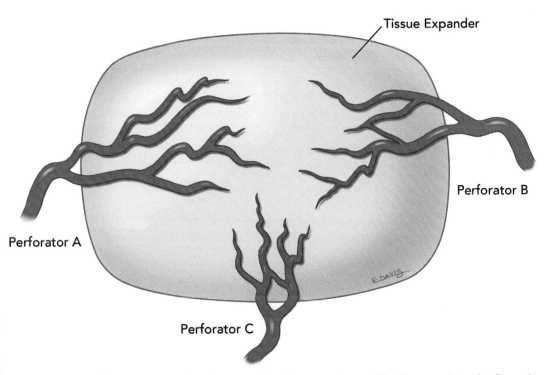

Fig. 8. Placement of a tissue expander adjacent to 3 perforators of several feeding vessels to the flap. After expansion, the crossing area's blood supply can be developed to improve circulation of the flap. (*From* Wang CM, Pu LLQ. Pre-expanded super-thin skin perforator flap. QMP's Plastic Surgery Pulse News 2016;8:1 A Featured Article Focus on Flap; with permission.)

reconstructing massive defects after complete excision of burn hypertrophic scars that can minimize contractures and deformities.

The major advantages of the flap are to reconstruct large skin defect with like-for-like but super-thin tissue from adjacent areas of the body for an optimal reconstruction with potential better outcome, avoid other extensive or complex reconstructive procedures such as free tissue transfer, and minimize donor site deformity or morbidity after primary closure. The disadvantages of the flap are the duration of the treatment is relatively longer and multiple procedures are needed to complete such a reconstruction. In addition, the method for detecting and mapping out the perforators is often needed for the success of such a flap reconstruction.

SUMMARY

The pre-expansion of a super-thin skin perforator flap can possibly improve the anastomoses between neighboring subdermal vascular plexuses and extend the supplying area of these vessels to the flap. This method may provide a favorable super-thin skin flap that can effectively be used for reconstructing a large surface skin defect with good cosmetic and functional outcomes. Such a kind of flap reconstruction can be performed by plastic surgeons with some skills for perforator flap dissection and should be added to their armamentarium for appropriately chosen patients.

REFERENCES

1. Kochima I, Soeda S. Inferior epigastric artery skin flap without rectus abdominis muscle. Br J Plast Surg 1989;42:645–8.

2. Saint-Cyr M, Schaverien MV, Rohrich RJ. Perforator flaps: history, controversies, physiology, anatomy, and use in reconstruction. Plast Reconstr Surg 2009;123:132e–45e.

3. Wei FC, Jain V, Celik N, et al. Have we found an ideal soft-tissue flap? An experience with 672 anterolateral thigh flaps. Plast Reconstr Surg 2002;109: 2219–26.

4. Wang CM, Yang SF, Fan JC, et al. Clinical application of prefabricated super-thin perforator flaps after expansion in the reconstruction of facial and cervical scar. Chin J Plast Surg 2015;31:4–9 [in Chinese].

5. Hyakusoku H, Gao JH. The "super-thin" flap. Br J Plast Surg 1994;47:457–64.

6. Zhang J, Gui L, Mei J, et al. A radioanatomic study of minipig skin flap model. Chin J Clin Anat 2007; 5:502–6.

7. Yang SF, Wang CM, Ono S, et al. The value of multi-detector row computed tomography angiography for preoperative planning of freestyle pedicled perforator flaps. Ann Plast Surg 2016. [Epub ahead of print].

8. Ogawa R, Hyakusoku H, Murakami M, et al. An anatomical and clinical study of the dorsal intercostal cutaneous perforators - its application to free microvascular augmented subdermal vascular network (ma-SVN) flaps. Br J Plast Surg 2002;55: 396–401.

9. Ogawa R, Hyakusoku H, Murakami M, et al. Clinical and basic research on occipito-cervico-dorsal flaps -including a study of the anatomical territories of dorsal trunk vessels-. Plast Reconstr Surg 2004;113: 1923–33.

10. Chin T, Ogawa R, Murakami M, et al. An anatomical study and clinical cases of "super-thin flaps" with transverse cervical perforator. Br J Plast Surg 2005;58:550–5.

Pre-expanded Transverse Cervical Artery Perforator Flap

Huifeng Song, MD, PhD[a],*, Jiake Chai, MD, PhD[b]

KEYWORDS

- Perforator flap • Transverse cervical artery • Pre-expansion • Face reconstruction
- Neck reconstruction

KEY POINTS

- High-quality and thin skin flaps should be used to reconstruct defects in the cervicofacial region.
- The transverse cervical artery perforator flap is useful for reconstruction of cervicofacial defects because it has good color and texture match, and minimal flap complications.
- This pre-expanded perforator flap is one of the best options for cervicofacial reconstruction, producing excellent result with only an inconspicuous linear scar on the donor site after being sutured directly.

INTRODUCTION

Deformed appearance and impaired function in the face and neck region necessitate appropriate and high-quality reconstructive tissue. Microsurgical techniques using distant free flaps are time consuming and costly. Local flaps (eg, pectoralis major, deltopectoral flaps) are bulky. With an excellent color and contour match for this application, the supraclavicular island flap (SIF) should be considered, and is pedicled by the supraclavicular artery, a branch of the transverse cervical artery (TCA). The inconspicuous scar is located on the donor site at the shoulder. The arteria cervicalis superficialis, first illustrated by Toldt,[1] originates from the thyrocervical trunk. The first clinical application of a shoulder flap was described by Kazanjian and Converse.[2]

The supraclavicular artery flap has a long history. The original report was by Lamberty[3] for neck reconstruction in 1979. A vessel named the supraclavicular artery was reported in 1983.[4] Pallua studied the anatomy of this flap and examined the vascularity of what is now known as the SIF. Then Pallua and colleagues[5] reported the SIF used for mentosternal contracture and tumor defect from 1997 to 2000,[6] and for postburn head and neck reconstruction in 2005.[7] From 2006 to 2012, a larger number of reports focused on SIF used in noma deficits, the mandibular region, postburn head and neck reconstruction, tracheocutaneous fistulas, posterolateral skull base repair, and so forth.[8–16] Free flaps were also used.[17–19] The results were not always satisfactory because of inadequate skin match or a patchwork facial appearance.

The supraclavicular angiosome is supplied by a constant and reliable vascular pedicle, which allows safe pedicled flap transfer. There are several main branches extending forward that dominate the blood supply for the supraclavicular and chest

Disclosure: The authors have nothing to disclose.
[a] Division of Plastic Reconstructive Surgery, Department of Burn & Plastic Surgery, Burns Institute of PLA, The First Affiliated Hospital of PLA General Hospital, 51 Fucheng Road, Haidian District, Beijing 100048, P.R. China;
[b] Burns Institute of PLA, The First Affiliated Hospital of PLA General Hospital, 51 Fucheng Road, Haidian District, Beijing 100048, P.R. China
* Corresponding author.
E-mail address: song_huifeng@126.com

wall regions, so it is termed the anterior branch flap. A fairly constant anterior cutaneous branch and main skin artery arise from the TCA perforator and can guarantee reconstructive success. The area of the flap can reach the chest wall, but not in the area near the shoulder. In accordance with the perforating point located on the supraclavicular region, the transverse cervical arteries perforator (TCAP) flap can be rotated and advanced much more easily than other flaps. Moreover, a pre-expanded TCAP flap can be designed. With the help of the expanded flaps, not only can the face and cervical sites be covered but also the donor area can be closed directly. This article introduces use of the TCAP flap and the pre-expanded TCAP flap.

TREATMENT GOALS AND PLANNED OUTCOMES

The pre-expanded TCAP flap is a better choice for the reconstruction of lesions and deformities on the middle and lower face, and the cervical region with a perfect match in color, elasticity, texture, and thickness. It also can be used for the repair of wounds on the lateral and posterior neck, and shoulders. In our experience, this perforator flap is very safe and has few complications. All the reconstructive cases have had satisfactory results in terms of appearance and functional recovery, especially because there have been no complaints of secondary deformities at the donor sites, which can be sutured directly after expansion leaving only linear scars.

PREOPERATIVE PLANNING AND PREPARATION

Before the operation, the perforator site of the TCA should be detected and determined by Doppler ultrasonography. The flap is designed according to the dimensions of the defect. However, severe scar contractures become larger than was estimated following the release. By referring to the unaffected region, a corresponding flap should be outlined. To some extent, a slightly larger flap is mapped. Depending on the actual and potential defects, a larger filling expander is placed at the first stage. If the defect is much larger, bilateral pre-expanded TCAP flaps could be designed to repair or reconstruct the a defect.

PATIENT POSITIONING

During the operation, patients are maintained in a supine position with the head positioned backward. The arms are kept away from the body,

ideally at 80° to 85° to reduce the chance of neurologic injury.

PROCEDURAL APPROACH

During the first stage, the pre-expanded region is marked. In order to avoid possible damage to the large supplying vessels, Doppler is performed preoperatively to identify the perforator site of TCA and the main anterior branches (**Fig. 1**A). The vertical incision is made lateral to the expander pocket area. The dissection is made down to the deep fascia. The expander is placed superficial to the major pectoral muscle. The rectangular expander is placed in the pocket and the filling valve is immobilized. The expander inflation is begun 10 days later when the stitches are removed. With saline added 2 times a week, the duration averages 3 months.

During the second procedure, when the perforator site of TCA is reconfirmed by the Doppler probe, the dimensions and boundary of the flap, including the identified branch and the pedicle, are outlined and marked (**Fig. 1**B). The pedicle is located at the sternocleidomastoid trailing edge, 1.8 cm above clavicle, the front is the trapezius's leading edge, the lateral edge is 2 to 3 cm from the acromion, the inner circle is the middle of the sternum, and the lower border is 3 to 4 cm below the nipple. The largest size of the flap is 13 × 22 cm. With the head in a tilted position and normally leaning to the side that has the largest area of tissue defect, the pattern is cut open again along the operative scar from the first procedure. The expander is taken out, the scar is excised, and its surrounding contracture is released. There is no need to dissect the perforator vessel. Care should be taken to preserve the perforator and branches, which not only provide sufficient blood supply but also are elevated with free or minimal tension. The incision is made along the marked line, down to the deep fascia layer (**Fig. 1**C). The route of the vessels that enter the flap is identified definitely in the clavicle region. The perforator branches originating from TCA are separated carefully. Tissue that includes vein and nerve surrounding the pedicle should be preserved (**Fig. 1**D). When the island flap is entirely raised, turned, and easily rotated by 180° or more to the recipient site, the donor site is closed directly or covered by split skin graft (**Fig. 1**E and F).

POTENTIAL COMPLICATIONS AND THEIR MANAGEMENT

The potential complications include bleeding, hematoma, infection, injected fluid leaking, expander

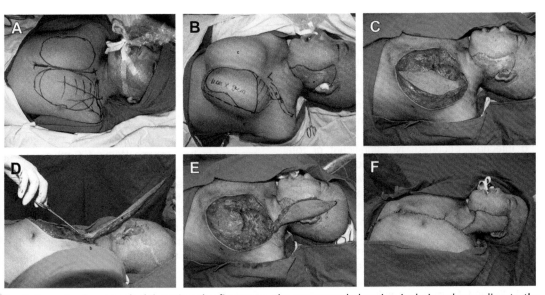

Fig. 1. Procedural approach. (*A*) During the first stage, the pre-expanded region is designed according to the defect and the donor site, then the expansion is followed. (*B*) After the expansion, the pre-expanded TCAP flap is designed in the second stage, in which the TCAP artery is detected using a Doppler ultrasonography blood stream detector. Two 400-mL to 600-mL expanders are embedded under the deep fascia on the chest. In this photo the TCAP flap design from the second-stage operation after the expansion process is finished (a, clavicle; b, the middle point of the clavicle; c, the pre-expanded TCAP flaps; d, the nipple; e, the scar). (*C–F*) The pre-expanded TCAP flap is formed from the deep fascia layer and transferred to the recipient site on the face and neck. (*D*) The expanders are taken out and the TCAP flaps are elevated at the deep fascia level. There are 2 methods for using the TCAP flaps. One is the unilateral TCAP flap to reconstruct the face and neck, in which the donor site is repaired and the other pre-expanded skin flap advanced. The second method is to use bilateral pre-expanded TCAP flaps to reconstruct the face and neck. The donor sites are sutured directly. This photo shows the first method. (a, The pre-expanded TCAP flap; b, TCA Perforator). (*F*) The unilateral TCAP flap is transferred to reconstruct the face and neck, and the donor site is repaired by advancing the other pre-expanded skin flap.

rupture, blood circulation disorders, necrosis of expanded skin or flap, hypertrophic scar, or cicacontracture. Some key suggestions are as follows: although the postoperative mark is performed according to a fixed projection, Doppler is also indispensable. The flap is advocated to be raised in the deep fascia level to avoid, as far as possible, damage to arteries. Care should be taken when approaching the pedicle. However, meticulously separating circumjacent tissue may be fatal to flap survival. Emplaced below the deep fascia, the vessels are certain to be included in the dilated flap. With a long period of expansion, more vessels are developed. The flap may be delayed before the second operation, although this has not happened at our center. The complications discussed earlier are rare under carefully designed and managed perioperative care. The flaps survived completely in all of our patients.

POSTPROCEDURAL CARE

Patients are examined on the first postoperative day of the flap transposition to check for excessive

pain, bleeding, hematoma, infection, and blood circulation in the flap. Patients are seen on the seventh postoperative day, the Steri-Strips are removed, and, if no problems have occurred, the patient is seen again at 1 month, 6 months, and 1 year postoperatively.

REHABILITATION AND RECOVERY

After the surgery, scar rehabilitation should be emphasized, especially for patients with scar physique. Some patients receive Z-plasty of the incisional scar at 6 months postoperatively. Functional exercises are needed for the recovery of facial organs and neck.

OUTCOMES

Between May 2008 and December 2011, 7 male and 3 female patients with a mean age of 32 years underwent reconstructive operations with the TCAP in our center. Ten cases involved severe burn and trauma in the facial and/or cervical area. The basic criteria for selecting patients were (1) no significant damage in the donor area, especially the anterior perforator areas; (2) female patients should be aware, and should accept, that there will be scarring on the breasts after the operation. A summary of these patients is shown in **Table 1**. The mean follow-up was 6 months. The size of the TCAP flap ranged between 5 × 8 cm and 13 × 22 cm. No failed flap necrosis or venous congestion was encountered in any of the flaps. No common complications, such as hematoma and infection, occurred. No significant or total flap loss of flap coverage was encountered in the group. In 4 cases no expanders were used, but in the other cases 1 or 2 expanders were used. The donor sites healed primarily with no complications. Plastic material was used to minimize incidence of flap contracture after the operations. All patients were told to wear it as long as possible. Moreover, functional exercise was also an influential factor in the postoperative result. Satisfactory aesthetic and functional results were achieved overall. However, only 1 woman complained about the conspicuous scars on the 2 bilateral breasts immediately after the operation. The unsatisfactory scars matured and became unclear 26 months after surgery. Other patients did not complain about the donor regions, although linear scarring or split skin was seen on the chest wall. The satisfaction rate was about 90%. The flap improved gradually to become a well-matched donor to the adjacent tissue.

CASE DEMONSTRATIONS
Case 1

A 53-year-old man had an ulcer scar in the left neck and mandibular region that was causing severe pruritus. A TCAP flap of 14 × 12 cm was designed, and the defect was totally reconstructed. Because of the long period of expansion that was needed, an expander was not approved by the patient. The donor site was covered by split skin flap. The result 8 months later was encouraging later (**Fig. 2**).

Case 2

A 38-year-old woman's quality of life was severely impaired by burn trauma. With a 400-mL expander positioned on each side, and injected with 1200-mL each side, the pre-expanded TCAP flaps were extended to cover the middle of the face. Using a preoperatively designed flap of 21 × 13 cm, the defect was repaired satisfactorily. The patient was content with the facial and neck appearance and accepted the bilateral scar on the breast (**Fig. 3**).

Case 3

A 44-year-old woman with a bilateral face burn was operated on using 2 rectangle expanders for about 4 months before expansion with about 1000 mL of saline in each side. With preoperatively designed flap of 22 × 10 cm for each TCAP flap, the wound was covered fully. Satisfactory results were obtained, and there was no complaint about mammary scarring (**Fig. 4**).

DISCUSSION

Face and neck reconstruction is very important after burn, trauma, tumor, and so forth, in which appearance and function are very important. Although many free flaps have previously been reported, the adjacent pedicled skin flap is still the primary option for the reconstruction of the face

Table 1
Patient summary

ID	Age (y)	Location	Side Used for Flap	Flap Size (cm)	Survival
327141	53	Left face and neck	Left	14 × 12	TS
327087	45	Left face and neck	Left	15 × 14	TS
324468	8	Neck	Left (E)	12 × 8 (E)	TS
328833	44	Bilateral face and neck	Bilateral (E)	22 × 10^1 (E)	TS
329331	38	Bilateral face and neck	Bilateral (E)	21 × 13^2 (E)	TS
379203	57	Neck	Left (E)	13 × 12 (E)	TS
337646	22	Right face and neck	Right (E)	24 × 12 (E)	TS
323594	10	Neck and chest wall	Left	20 × 15	TS
341721	19	Left neck	Left	13 × 11	TS
344505	13	Chin and neck	Right	13 × 10	TS

22 × 10^1 and 21 × 13^2 represents each expanded flap size, not 2 expanded flap sizes in total.
   Abbreviations: E, expander (as used in the first operation); ID, identification number; TS, total survive.

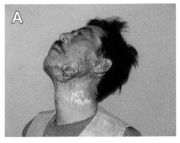
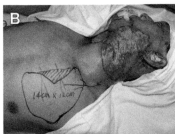
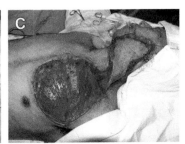
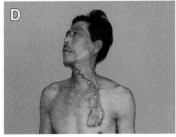

Fig. 2. A 53-year-old man's with an ulcer scar in the left neck and mandibular region (A). A flap size of 14 × 12 cm was designed and the scar was excised completely (B). The defect was completely reconstructed and the donor site was repaired with a skin graft (C). The result 8 months later was encouraging (D).

and neck, because it provides a better match in color, elasticity, and texture. Lamberty and colleagues[3] originally reported the supraclavicular artery flap in 1979, and this flap was subsequently studied systematically. Although it can be used to repair and reconstruct the face and neck very well, it has the disadvantage of the donor site being on the shoulder, which is used for carrying burdens and is often exposed. The chest region is an ideal donor site, and has an abundant vessel network with an extensive blood supply, such as the cutaneous branch of the cervical segment of the transverse artery, the intercostal branch of the internal thoracic artery, the thoracoacromial artery, and the lateral thoracic artery.[20] In our experience, the TCAP flap is the first choice for face and neck reconstruction, because the pedicle is the nearest to the recipient site compared with other vessels; there is less wastage of the flap; and the area of the flap is adequate, especially after expansion.

Although the TCAP flap has a reliable and stable blood supply pedicled by the transverse cervical artery perforator, Doppler ultrasonography examination is needed preoperatively. In order to include the perforator and vessel network in the flap, the skin expander should be embedded beneath the deep fascia. The pre-expanded area

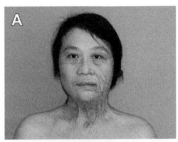
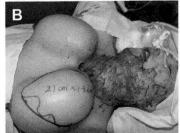
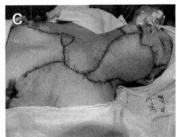
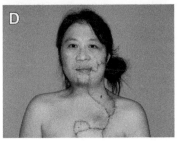

Fig. 3. A 38-year-old woman with severe scar and contracture (A). A 400-mL expander was positioned on each side, 1200 mL were injected on each side, and the scar contracture was excised and released (B). The flaps were elevated to reconstruct the wound (C). However, an extra scar was left on the breast skin. She was content with the facial and neck appearance and accepted the bilateral scar on the breast 15 days after the operation (D).

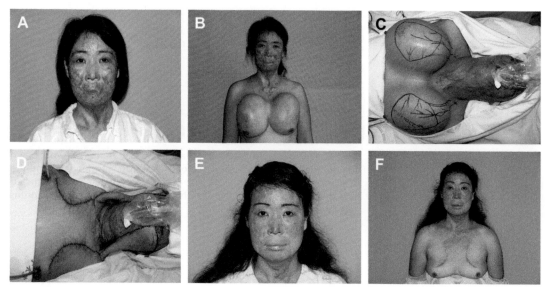

Fig. 4. A 44-year-old woman with bilateral burn scar (*A*). Two rectangular expanders were placed, which involved the upper breast skin (*B*). Intraoperative plan of the flap design (*C*). Bilateral flaps were raised to cover the lower and middle face wound (*D*). A satisfactory outcome (*E*). A symmetric scar was left on the breast, but the patient was satisfied with the result (*F*).

or the expander pocket should be defined precisely before the first operation, with the upper border below the clavicle, medial border near the thoracic median line, lateral border close to the anterior axillary line, and inferior border near the nipple level. After an adequate expansion period, usually lasting 4 to 6 months, the pre-expanded TCAP flap is formed and transferred to the recipient site. It is not necessary to make a complete dissection of the perforator, and some periperforator tissues should be kept for as a safeguard in case of trauma during the flap transplant.

The thickness of the pre-expanded TCAP flap is appropriate for face and neck reconstruction, but is not thin enough in some cases. It can be decreased by capsulectomy and immediate flap debulking without damage to the blood vessel network. Secondary liposuction is also available to improve the contour.

The pre-expanded TCAP flap is an ideal method for face and neck reconstruction, but the process of expansion should receive most attention to prevent complications. An sufficiently long expansion period is needed for the skin, soft tissue, and vessel network abundance. Adequate drainage and dressing with no pressure are the key points to prevent complications (especially no pressure on the marginal mandible).

In some cases, there is scar contracture of the incision. The multiple Z-plasty can be used to release it and achieve a better configuration and appearance at 6 months after the operation.

SUMMARY

The pre-expanded TCAP is one of the best options for cervicofacial reconstruction, with unique advantages of color and texture match, minimal flap complications, ease of operation, and only an inconspicuous linear scar on the donor site after being sutured directly. However, the selection of the flap for women involves the possibility of an extra scar on the chest or the deformity of the breast.

REFERENCES

1. Gillies HD. The tubed pedicle in plastic surgery. J Laryngol Otol 1923;38:503.
2. Kazanjian VH, Converse J. The surgical treatment of facial injuries. Baltimore (MD): Williams & Wilkins; 1949.
3. Lamberty BG. The supra-clavicular axial patterned flap. Br J Plast Surg 1979;32(3):207–12.
4. Lamberty BG, Cormack GC. Misconceptions regarding the cervico-humeral flap. Br J Plast Surg 1983;36(1):60–3.
5. Pallua N, Machens HG, Rennekampff O, et al. The fasciocutaneous supraclavicular artery island flap for releasing postburn mentosternal contractures. Plast Reconstr Surg 1997;99(7):1878–84.
6. Pallua N, Magnus Noah E. The tunneled supraclavicular island flap: an optimized technique for head and neck reconstruction. Plast Reconstr Surg 2000;105(3):842–51.

7. Pallua N, von Heimburg D. Pre-expanded ultra-thin supraclavicular flaps for (full-) face reconstruction with reduced donor-site morbidity and without the need for microsurgery. Plast Reconstr Surg 2005; 115(7):1837–44.

8. Hartman EH, Van Damme PA, Suominen SH. The use of the pedicled supraclavicular flap in noma reconstructive surgery. Plast Reconstr Surg 2006; 118(1):270–1.

9. Laredo Ortiz C, Valverde Carrasco A, Novo Torres A, et al. Supraclavicular bilobed fasciocutaneous flap for postburn cervical contractures. Burns 2007; 33(6):770–5.

10. Vinh VQ, Ogawa R, Van Anh T, et al. Reconstruction of neck scar contractures using supraclavicular flaps: retrospective study of 30 cases. Plast Reconstr Surg 2007;119(1):130–5.

11. Di Benedetto G, Aquinati A, Balercia P, et al. Supraclavicular island fascial flap in the treatment of progressive hemifacial atrophy. Plast Reconstr Surg 2008;121(5):247–50.

12. Chiu ES, Liu PH, Friedlander PL. Supraclavicular artery island flap for head and neck oncologic reconstruction: indications, complications, and outcomes. Plast Reconstr Surg 2009;124(1):115–23.

13. Ma X, Zheng Y, Xia W, et al. An anatomical study with clinical application of one branch of the supraclavicular artery. Clin Anat 2009;22(2):215–20.

14. Vinh VQ, Van Anh T, Ogawa R, et al. Anatomical and clinical studies of the supraclavicular flap: analysis of 103 flaps used to reconstruct neck scar contractures. Plast Reconstr Surg 2009;123(5):1471–80.

15. Kim RJ, Izzard ME, Patel RS. Supraclavicular artery island flap for reconstructing defects in the head and neck region. Curr Opin Otolaryngol Head Neck Surg 2011;19(4):248–50.

16. Epps MT, Cannon CL, Wright MJ, et al. Aesthetic restoration of parotidectomy contour deformity using the supraclavicular artery island flap. Plast Reconstr Surg 2011;127(5):1925–31.

17. Levy JM, Eko FN, Hilaire HS, et al. Posterolateral skull base reconstruction using the supraclavicular artery island flap. J Craniofac Surg 2011;22(5): 1751–4.

18. Khouri RK, Ozbek MR, Hruza GJ, et al. Facial reconstruction with prefabricated induced expanded (PIE) supraclavicular skin flaps. Plast Reconstr Surg 1995;95(6):1007–15.

19. Teot L, Cherenfant E, Otman S, et al. Prefabricated vascularised supraclavicular flaps for face resurfacing after postburns scarring. Lancet 2000; 355(9216):1695–6.

20. Song HF, Chai JK, Liu CM, et al. Application of thoracic skin flap with multiple blood supply in repair of tissue defects and deformities in jaw and neck. Chin J Burns 2009;25(1):15–7.

Pre-expanded Supraclavicular Artery Perforator Flap

Norbert Pallua, MD, PhD*, Bong-Sung Kim, MD

KEYWORDS

- Supraclavicular flap • Perforator flap • Head and neck reconstruction • Pre-expansion
- Maxillofacial reconstruction

KEY POINTS

- The pedicled anterior supraclavicular artery perforator (a-SAP) flap is a versatile flap in head and neck reconstruction.
- The a-SAP flap uses the anterior branch of the transverse cervical artery.
- The skin of the deltopectoral fossa is thinner, more pliable, and shows a better color match compared with the original supraclavicular artery perforator (SAP) flap.
- Pre-expansion allows the reconstruction of extended cervical and facial defects.

INTRODUCTION

Since its first description in 1997, the supraclavicular island flap (SIF) has emerged as a respected technique for the reconstruction of defects mainly located in the head and neck area, which remain a challenge to plastic and reconstructive surgeons.[1] The advantages of the SIF are manifold and include its minor donor site morbidity, its safety and reliability, and most importantly its favorable match in color and texture to tissue of the head and neck area. Over the years, the SIF underwent several decisive modifications. Although a more difficult procedure, tunneling of the SIF markedly reduces scars at the donor site.[2] In the same vein, the authors proposed a pre-expansion of the donor site, which permits an increase flap size and a considerable thinning of the flap with enhanced microcirculation.[3]

The most recent refinement of the SIF resulted in the renaming of the SIF to the SAP flap (because the supraclavicular artery pierces the platysma and is, therefore, considered a perforator in agreement with the Gent consensus on perforator flap terminology[4]), and the development of a new flap named the a-SAP flap.[5] The supraclavicular artery, which is the pedicle of the SAP flap, is a branch of the transverse cervical artery.[6] In the a-SAP flap, however, an anterior supraclavicular pedicle that originates separately from the transverse cervical artery serves as the main supplying artery. The anterior supraclavicular artery is as reliable as the supraclavicular artery but allows the harvest of a more anteriorly located flap. In the authors' department, the a-SAP flap is almost exclusively used due to its undeniable benefits over the SAP flap. This article reviews the surgical technique, complications, and postoperative outcomes of the pre-expanded a-SAP flap based on the current literature and many years of experience in the authors' department.

Disclosure: All authors declare no conflict of interest.
Department of Plastic and Reconstructive Surgery, Hand Surgery - Burn Center, University Hospital of the RWTH Aachen, Pauwelsstrasse 30, Aachen 52074, Germany
* Corresponding author.
E-mail address: npallua@ukaachen.de

Clin Plastic Surg 44 (2017) 49–63
http://dx.doi.org/10.1016/j.cps.2016.08.005

TREATMENT GOALS AND PLANNED OUTCOMES

As discussed previously, defects that are primarily reconstructed by the a-SAP flap are located in the head and neck area. The a-SAP flap is used to restore and improve defects that are congenital or related to infection, disease, tumors, and trauma, including burn injuries. The a-SAP flap unfolds its full benefits especially in large defects that cannot be satisfactorily covered by primary closure or other local solutions. Pre-expansion of the harvest area markedly increases flap size and allows the reconstruction of extensive facial and cervical defects. In some cases, the SAP and a-SAP flap also can be used as a free flap.

PREOPERATIVE PLANNING, PREPARATION, AND PATIENT POSITIONING

Defects of substantial size can be covered with a-SAP flaps without prior pre-expansion and primary closure of the donor site. To cover more extended defects, the authors routinely pre-expand the a-SAP flap. The donor site must be free of infection and patients and/or relatives must be well educated about the procedure and care, including pain that is par for the course, to reach high compliance during the arduous pre-expansion process. A sample of the defect may help to approximately estimate the position of the a-SAP flap and the size of the needed expander. Coverage by ipsilateral, contralateral, and even bilateral a-SAP flaps are commonly performed in the authors' department. The first surgery involves the implantation of a tissue expander above the muscle fascia in the deltopectoral fossa through a small axillary incision. The general concept of the pre-expanded a-SAP flap is shown in **Fig. 1**. Both operations, the implantation of the expander and the later defect coverage by the pre-expanded a-SAP flap, are performed in supine position with sufficient padding of the patient. When the defect is directly adjacent to the tissue flap, caution is warranted to prevent expansion of the defect tissue rather than the a-SAP flap. The port is usually placed in the medial part of the upper arm.

PROCEDURAL APPROACH

The operative procedure of a standard pre-expanded a-SAP flap is illustrated in **Figs. 2–4** in a 5-year-old male patient with extended burn scars in the head and neck area. The authors covered the left buccal area by a pre-expanded ipsilateral a-SAP flap. In **Figs. 2** and **3**, the inflated expander and the surgical transposition of the flap are shown. **Fig. 4** depicts the transaction procedure of the pedicle.

Once the donor site is sufficiently expanded to cover the recipient site, the second operation can be planned (see **Fig. 2**A, B). The a-SAP is a reliable vessel that allows the tissue harvest from a more anterior region than the SAP flap in the deltopectoral fossa (see **Fig. 2**C). It pierces the platysma between the origin of the 2 sternocleidomastoid muscle parts, crosses the clavicle in its junction between medial and central third, and runs down to the deltopectoral fossa (dashed line in **Fig. 2**C). The artery is preoperatively located by a Doppler probe and marked on the skin. A

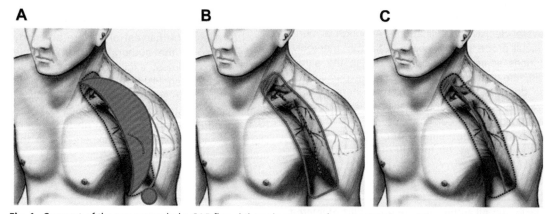

Fig. 1. Concept of the pre-expanded a-SAP flap. (*A*) Implantation of a crossaint-shaped tissue expander through a small incision roughly in the anterior axillary line. The port is positioned in the upper arm where it remains easily injectable. (*B*) Design of the a-SAP flap. The flap is located in the deltopectoral fossa and is perfused by the a-SAP. (*C*) The donor site can be close primarily after translocation of the a-SAP flap. (*From* Pallua N, Wolter TP. Moving forwards: the anterior supraclavicular artery perforator [a-SAP] flap: a new pedicled or free perforator flap based on the anterior supraclavicular vessels. J Plast Reconstr Aesthet Surg 2013;66(4):492; with permission.)

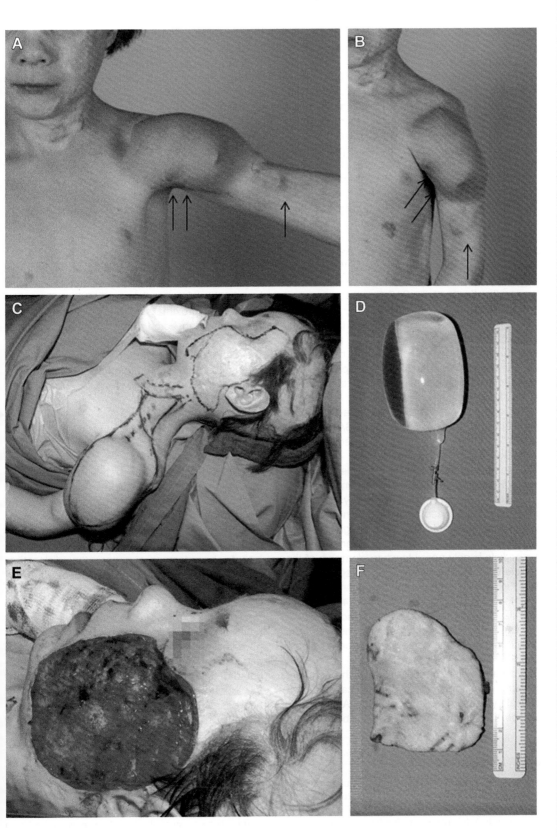

template is used to determine the exact location and size, and surplus length may be designed to avoid later dog ears.

First, the scar tissue of the recipient site is excised completely (see **Fig. 2**D, E). Next, the a-SAP flap is dissected. After skin incision, the expander and optionally its capsule are removed (see **Fig. 2**D). The flap is elevated above the muscle fascia from the lateral to the medial portion (see **Fig. 3**A), and the anterior branch is detected by intraoperative Doppler or diaphanoscopy (see **Fig. 3**B) when dissection reaches the clavicle. The anterior branch is traced to its origin where it takes off the transverse cervical artery. Two veins accompany the anterior branch, of which one drains into the transverse cervical vein and the other into the external jugular vein. When veins and artery are identified and dissected from the surrounding tissue, the a-SAP flap can be rotated into the recipient site (see **Fig. 3**C, D).

Final fixation of the flap is performed in a double-layered fashion with subcutaneous absorbable sutures and cutaneous sutures with nonabsorbable material. Wound drains are placed and removed in the early postoperative care; the donor site is closed primarily (see **Fig. 3**E).

The authors often perform the a-SAP in 2 surgical steps. In the first step, the a-SAP is transposed to its recipient site and the pedicle is not completely sutured. Instead, the pedicle is covered by a skin substitute (eg, Mepilex AG; Mölnycke Health Care, Düsseldorf, Germany) and transected after approximately 14 days when the a-SAP flap is perfused by the surrounding tissue of the recipient site. In **Fig. 4**, the surgical step of pedicle transection is illustrated. Transection of the pedicle is only possible when clamping of the pedicle does not significantly alter flap perfusion (see **Fig. 4**A). The flap is then disconnected and the blood vessels ligated (see **Fig. 4**B). The a-SAP flap is now perfused by its adjacent tissue. The flap is trimmed and superfluous tissue of the pedicle can be used to cover additional defects (see **Fig. 4**C, D).

In cases of distant localization of the recipient site from the donor site with significant amount of healthy tissue in between, the a-SAP flap also can be tunneled, which reduces visible scars in the neck area.[2] After complete incision of the flap, the pedicle with its surrounding fatty tissue is first dissected on the epifascial level and then in the subdermal layer. Finally, the a-SAP flap is gently pulled through a subcutaneous tunnel to its recipient site.

Under special circumstances, the a-SAP flap can be used as an osteocutaneous flap. When the incision reaches the periosteum, a bone chip is harvested from the lateral end of the clavicle or the acromion. The size of the bone chip may vary and should be adapted to the defect (eg, the cartilaginous defect of the trachea after decannulation). The a-SAP flap is then transposed to the tracheal defect and the bone chip is secured with slowly absorbable sutures.

The a-SAP flap also can be transferred as a free flap.[5] Flap dissection does not differ from the usual preparation of the pedicled a-SAP flap. The artery is followed proximally to the transverse cervical artery and transected when artery diameter reaches approximately 1.5 mm. After transection of the vein that drains into the external jugular vein, the flap can be anastomosed at the recipient site either end-do-end or end-to-side.

POTENTIAL COMPLICATIONS AND MANAGEMENT

Complications of the pre-expanded a-SAP flap can be divided into those related to the pre-expansion procedure and those that are caused by the explicit a-SAP flap transposition.

First, careful patient selection is the most important measure to avoid unfavorable results or complications during the tissue expansion. Those include hematomas, seromas, the dislocation, deflation, or exposure of the expander/port, infection, and necrosis. Minor hematomas and seromas may be aspirated preferably under ultrasound control to avoid damage to the expander and mostly resolve without surgical intervention. In other cases, however, a surgical evacuation of the hematoma and seroma, repositioning or replacement of dislocated/deflated expanders/ports, or even removal of the expander to manage infections and necrosis is necessary. To prevent infection and hematoma, meticulous intraoperative hemostasis and strict

Fig. 2. A 5-year-old boy with extended burn scars in the face, scalp, and neck area. Pictures after implantation of the expander for reconstruction by ipsilateral a-SAP flap. (*A, B*) Pre-expansion of the a-SAP flap, the port is placed in the medial part of the upper arm ([*single arrows*] port; [*double arrows*] scar of the incision for implantation of the expander). (*C*) Intraoperative view of the planned a-SAP flap. The course of the blood vessel is marked by a dashed line. (*D*) Explantation of the expander. (*E*) Excision of the scar tissue on the left buccal area. (*F*) Excised scar tissue.

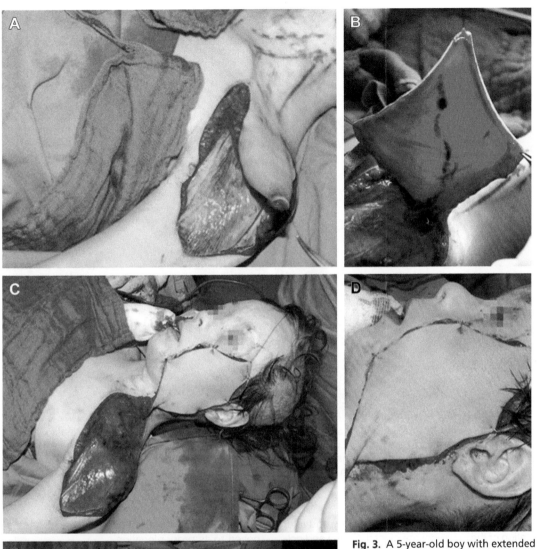

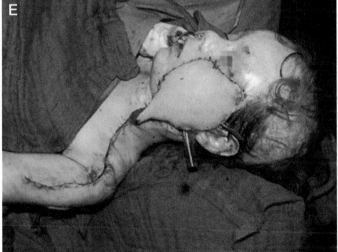

Fig. 3. A 5-year-old boy with extended burn scars in the face, scalp, and neck area. Reconstruction by pre-expanded ipsilateral a-SAP flap. (*A*) Dissection of a pedicled a-SAP flap after removal of the expander. (*B*) Elevated a-SAP flap with pedicle marked. (*C*) Transposition of the a-SAP flap to the recipient site with pedicle marked. (*D*) Transposed a-SAP flap with good vascularization. (*E*) Primary closure of the donor site and complete suturing of the a-SAP flap.

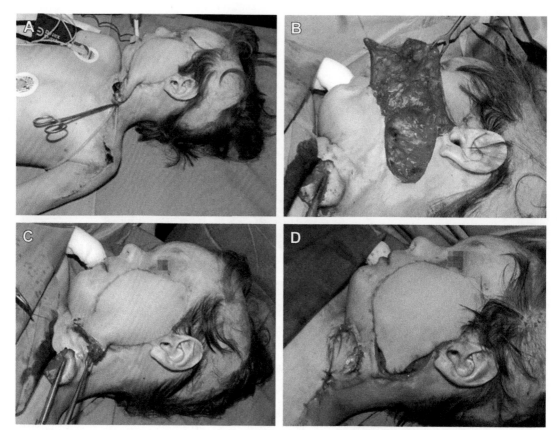

Fig. 4. A 5-year-old boy after closure of a buccal scar by pedicled pre-expanded ipsilateral a-SAP flap. Pictures show surgical transection of the pedicle 2 weeks after transposition of the a-SAP flap. (*A*) The pedicle is clamped, the flap shows good perfusion. (*B*) Transection of the pedicle. (*C*) Partial elevation of the flap in the dorsal portion to cover additional scar tissue in the infraauricular region. (*D*) Trimming and suturing of the pedicle and flap to the defect.

antiseptic precautions during the surgery and later inflation of the expander are pivotal. Cunha and colleagues[7] evaluated 315 tissue expanders in a total of 164 patients and found an average 22.2% of complications. The highest complication rates were found in the face and neck area and the scalp whereas the trunk showed the lowest. This report is in line with the authors' experience, rarely observing major complications of the tissue expansion in the deltopectoral fossa.

Although the vascularization of the a-SAP flap is reliable with a consistent artery and 2 veins, perfusion depending on the flap size is the most critical aspect. In cases of extended size of the flap or the iatrogenic damage of the pedicle during flap dissection, a delay procedure appears to be a potential remedy. Although the a-SAP is the main blood supplier of the flap, the flap also is party perfused via the surrounding tissue.[8] During the delay procedure, the a-SAP flap is incised at its borders enabling the pedicle to assume its role as the main circulation source. In a second

delayed procedure, the flap is raised and transposed to its proper location.

Other general complications may be considered, particularly in early postprocedural care, including hematomas, infections, wound healing disorders, donor site morbidity, and so forth, that may be managed with appropriate standardized measures. In larger studies involving more than 20 cases, a major complication rate of less than 5% and minor complication rate of approximately 10% for the SAP flap was reported.[2,9–14] Herr and colleagues[15] investigated the impact of the supraclavicular artery island flaps on shoulder function in 10 patients and found some limitation in the range of motion whereas the strength and function were not restricted.

POSTPROCEDURAL CARE, REHABILITATION, AND RECOVERY

The implantation of the tissue expander can be done as an outpatient operation. After 2 to 3 weeks

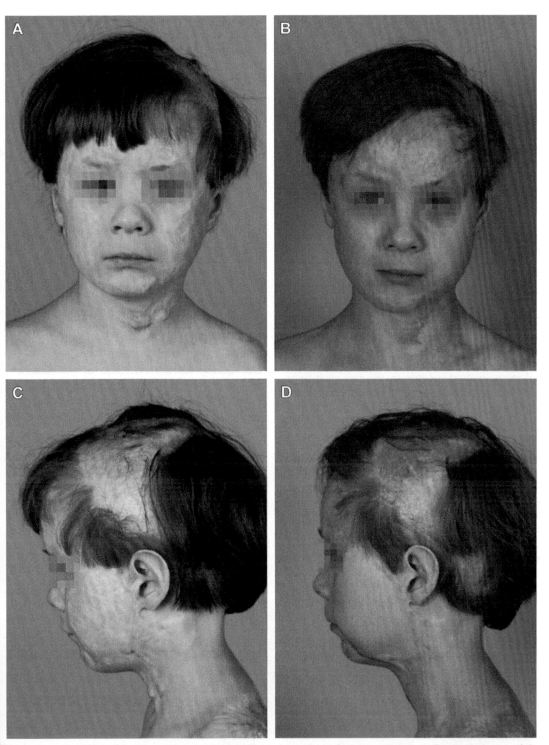

Fig. 5. Preoperative and postoperative views of a 5-year-old patient after reconstruction of extended scars of the left cheek by an ipsilateral pre-expanded a-SAP flap. The scars on the scalp were not reconstructed yet due to the soft skull bone. Reconstruction is planned after completion of growth. (*A*) Preoperative frontal view. (*B*) Postoperative frontal view 4 years after surgery. (*C*) Preoperative side view. (*D*) Postoperative side view 4 years after surgery.

of uneventful primary wound healing, the expander is perpetually filled through the port, which is normally placed at the medial upper arm where it is easily palpable. The inflation process is routinely performed as an office procedure on a weekly basis until the necessary expansion volume is reached. After a period of approximately 2 weeks after the final inflation, the surgical flap transposition is carried out, usually as an inpatient surgery. The postprocedural care does not vary markedly from other local flap surgeries. In the first days after surgery, disturbances of flap perfusion by mechanical stress should be avoided by adequate positioning of the arm and limited bed rest.

OUTCOMES
Case 1

Fig. 5 shows the preoperative and postoperative pictures of the 5-year-old patient with disfiguring facial burn scars who was treated by a ipsilateral pre-expanded a-SAP flap. The postoperative pictures taken 4 years after surgery show the good color match and the excellent reconstruction of the facial contour. The scars on the scalp were not reconstructed yet due to the soft skull bone and reconstruction is planned after completion of growth.

Case 2

Figs. 6 and **7** show the preoperative and postoperative pictures of a 30-year-old male patient who presented with extensive keloid formation on the ventral portion of the neck. To adequately address the keloid tissue, which not only entailed cosmetic issues but also led to functional impairment when reclining the head, a pre-expanded a-SAP flap was elevated from the left side, rotated 180°, and

sutured to the recipient site after meticulous keloid resection. Postsurgical pictures show the early outcome after 3 months.

Case 3

Fig. 8 shows preoperative, intraoperative, and postoperative pictures of a 47-year-old male patient with a preauricular defect measuring approximately 4 cm × 5 cm. The defect occurred from a radical excision of a basal cell carcinoma with numerous recurrences. Due to several surgical procedures in the past, a closure via local flap was not possible. Hence, a nonexpanded a-SAP flap was raised from the ipsilateral site and transferred in the first step with primary closure of the donor site. The pedicle was transected after 2 weeks and the flap healed without complications as seen in the pictures taken 8 months after surgery.

DISCUSSION

In agreement with the Gillies concept, stating that skin match increases with the proximity of donor and recipient site, the a-SAP flap offers optimal skin quality for the coverage of the face and neck. Furthermore, the donor sites of the SAP and a-SAP flap usually show little hair growth contributing to its cosmetic use in face and neck surgery especially in female patients.

In contrast to the classic SAP flap, the pedicle of the a-SAP flap is the anterior branch of the supraclavicular artery that originates separately from the transverse cervical artery. The so-called a-SAP supplies a tissue island that is located more anteriorly than the SAP flap. The great advantage of the a-SAP flap over the SAP flap is its tissue of the deltopectoral fossa which is even thinner and more flexible compared with the harvest tissue of the

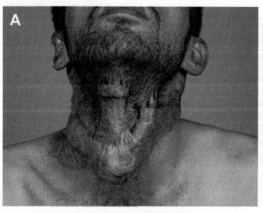
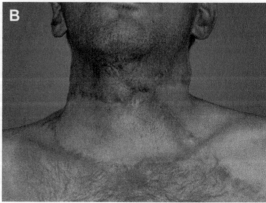

Fig. 6. Preoperative and postoperative views of a 30-year-old patient with keloid on the ventral part of the neck who was treated by a pre-expanded a-SAP flap from the left shoulder area. (*A*) Preoperative view of the reclined head. (*B*) Postoperative view of the reclined head 3 months after surgery.

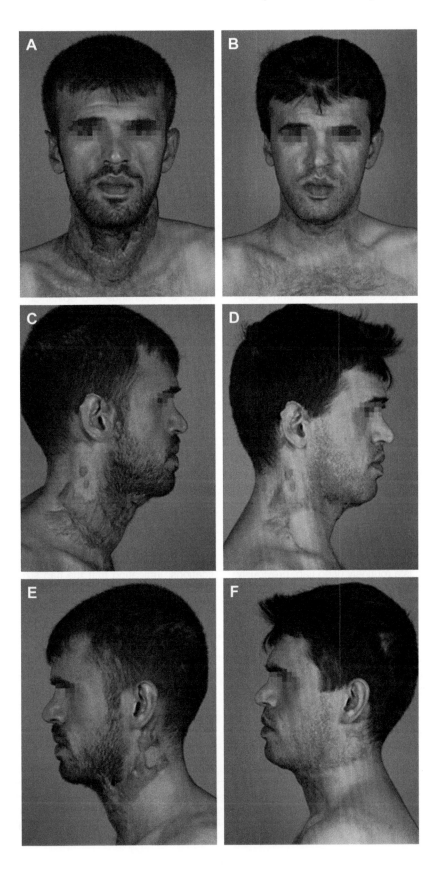

original SAP flap. Moreover, it shows superior color match to the SAP flap leading to a cosmetically more pleasing result. Especially the reconstruction of the face, where thin tissue with perfect color match is decisive, is improved by the a-SAP flap.

In the authors' experience, the pre-expansion of the SAP flap increased its size to flap dimensions (width of up to 15 cm and length of 35 cm) and a reduced thickness of only 2 mm to 3 mm. Internal tissue expansion was first described by Neumann,[16] who reconstructed the external ear after tissue expansion by a latex balloon. The routine use of tissue expanders with wide clinical applicability was further pioneered by Radovan[17] and Austad and Rose.[18] Pre-expansion not only increases size and reduces thickness but also enhances the microvascularization, which contributes to wound healing.[19,20] Another beneficial aspect of the pre-expanded SAP and a-SAP flap is that the expansion of the flaps is performed in a region that shows low complication rates unlike the expansion of tissue in the face and neck or scalp area.[7] Finally, pre-expansion leads to an atrophy of subcutaneous adipose tissue, which is favorable in the functional and cosmetic result in facial and cervical reconstruction.[21] Experimental studies have shown that expanders thinned tissue between the expander and skin but did not affect epidermal thickness.[22] Yang and colleagues[23] propose the incorporation of the capsule of the expander adds to the blood supply and constitutes a smooth interface between the recipient site and the SAP flap. The authors, however, in small to medium-sized flaps, commonly excise the capsule to reduce the risk of seroma formation. At last, pre-expansion allows primary closure of the donor site in all cases.

The SAP flap is a routinely used flap, previously suggested by Pallua and Wolter in 2013.[5] To avoid duplication of cases, the authors reviewed the literature published between 2013 and 2015 on PubMed with summarized data illustrated in **Table 1**. Supraclavicular flaps steadily gain interest as seen in the increase of relevant data found in PubMed (compare with the article of 2013[5]) with 6 relevant entries found in 2013, 10 in 2014, and 11 in 2015.

The versatility of the SAP flap and a-SAP in reconstructive surgery is impressive as investigators perpetually develop new areas of application. The authors reported the use of the SAP flap for the outer and inner lining of the SAP flap in combination with skin or mucosa grafts in stomatitis gangrenosa (also known as noma) patients requiring complex reconstruction.[24] In the literature, many more investigators documented the use of supraclavicular flaps for the reconstruction of defects of the oral cavity, oropharynx, laryngopharynx, esophagus, and trachea.[25] Tongue reconstruction was performed by different groups.[26–28] Zhang and colleagues[27] reported excellent speech and swallowing function of tongues in patients after hemiglossectomy and saw no marked difference to the free radial forearm flap (FRFF). Other investigators have successfully treated skull base and scalp defects.[29,30] Case reports further describe the utilization of the SAP flap in the reconstruction of the proximal esophagus and spinal defects.[31,32] The authors use the SAP and a-SAP flap to treat patients with tracheocutaneous fistulas by cotransferring a bone chip from the clavicle.[33] Although most scars heal without complication after decannulation and simple occlusive dressings, long-time ventilation, in particular, can lead do serious cartilaginous damage that requires reconstruction of the anterior tracheal wall.[34] Nicoli and colleagues[32] used an osteocutaneous supraclavicular flap for a composite nasal defect with damage to the skin, cartilage, and the nasal bone. Despite that the size of the vascularized clavicle fragment is limited, the pedicled osteocutaneous SAP and a-SAP flap may assume a more important role in the treatment of composite defects in the craniofacial area once plastic surgeons gain more experience and confidence with this technique.

Pre-expansion was reported in only 4 of 27 publications, indicating that the flap size is sufficient for most purposes even without pre-expansion.[23,35–37] But it also suggests that the benefits of pre-expansion, which were delineated earlier, and its advanced possibilities are not yet exhaustively utilized.

Although the SAP flap has been a workhorse in head and neck reconstruction since the early 1990s, the a-SAP flap was defined only 3 years ago.[5] Owing to the short history of this flap, the only other report of this particular modification was documented by Yoo and Belzile,[38] who

Fig. 7. Preoperative and postoperative views of a 30-year-old patient with keloid on the ventral part of the neck who was treated by a pre-expanded a-SAP flap from the left shoulder area. (*A*) Preoperative frontal view. (*B*) Postoperative frontal view 3 months after surgery. (*C*) Preoperative side view (*right*). (*D*) Postoperative side view 3 months after surgery (*right*). (*E*) Preoperative side view (*left*). (*F*) Postoperative side view 3 months after surgery (*left*).

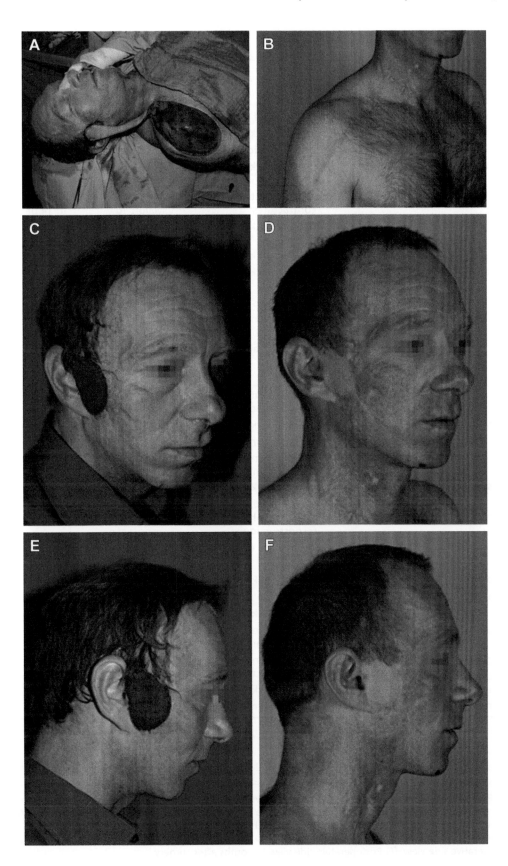

Table 1
Supraclavicular flaps in the literature between 2013 and 2015

Author, Year	Number of Cases	Indication	Complications (%)	Expansion
Dolan et al,[41] 2013	1	Perforation of piriform fossa	0	No
Granzow et al,[42] 2013	18	Head and neck reconstruction	39	No
Sever et al,[35] 2013	10	Postburn cervical contractures	0	Yes
Kokot et al,[25] 2013	45	Head and neck reconstruction	Minor: 5 Major: 24	No
Loghmani et al,[36] 2013	41	Postburn mentosternal contractures	Minor: 5 Major: 10	Pre-expansion in 14 patients
Shenoy et al,[43] 2013	11	Head and neck reconstruction	Minor: 18 Major: 9	No
Herr et al,[44] 2014	24	Head and neck reconstruction	Minor: 42	No
Kokot et al,[45] 2014	22	Head and neck reconstruction	Minor: 23 Major: 5	
Chen et al,[26] 2014	42	Tongue reconstruction	n/a	No
Emerick et al,[46] 2014	15	Reconstruction after laryngectomy	Minor: 40 Major: 7	No
Teymoortash et al,[47] 2014	4	Oropharyngeal defects	0	No
Yang et al,[23] 2014	18	Postburn contractures of the neck	0	Yes
Emerick et al,[29] 2014	10	Parotid and lateral skull base reconstruction	Minor: 60	No
Giordano et al,[28] 2014	3	Head and neck reconstruction	0	No
Hunt & Buchmann,[30] 2014	3	Lateral skull and scalp defects	Minor: 33	No
Sethi et al,[48] 2014	14	Reconstruction after laryngectomy	0	No
Yoo & Belzile,[38] 2015	7	Head and neck reconstruction	No major complications	No
Granzow et al,[49] 2015	1	Proximal esophageal reconstruction	100	No
Razdan et al,[31] 2015	1	Cervical spine defect	0	No
Nicoli et al,[32] 2015	1	Nasal defect	0	No
Razdan et al,[50] 2015	22	Head and neck reconstruction	Minor: 23	No
Chu et al,[51] 2015	5	Tracheostoma reconstruction	0	No
Yang et al,[37] 2015	16	Head and neck reconstruction	Minor: 6	Yes
Pabiszczak et al,[52] 2015	6	Reconstruction of cutaneopharyngeal fistulas	Minor: 17 Major: 17	No
Zhang et al,[27] 2015	12	Reconstruction after hemiglossectomy	Minor: 75	No
Kozin et al,[53] 2016	45	Head and neck reconstruction	13–29	No
Kucur et al,[54] 2015	1	Laryngopharyngeal defect	0	No

Fig. 8. Preoperative, intraoperative, and postoperative views of a 47-year old patient with a 4 cm × 5 cm large defect on the right preauricular area after resection of a basal cell carcinoma who was treated by an a-SAP flap from the left ipsilateral side. (*A*) Intraoperative view of the transferred flap. (*B*) Postoperative view of the donor site 8 months after surgery. (*C*) Preoperative oblique view. (*D*) Postoperative oblique view 8 months after surgery. (*E*) Preoperative side view. (*F*) Postoperative side view 8 months after surgery.

transferred an "infraclavicular" flap based on the anterior branch of the transverse cervical artery in 7 patients. The mean dimensions were 13.3 cm × 6.3 cm and the flap showed outcomes similar to other fasciocutaneous free flaps. The a-SAP supplies a tissue island in the supraclavicular and infraclavicular island but according to the international nomenclature the supplying vessels are decisive for the name of the angiosome. In the authors' department, the free a-SAP is considered an auspicious option for the coverage of defects on the foot and hand due to the thin and pliable tissue of the deltopectoral fossa.[5]

Ever since its first performance in 2005,[39] the facial allotransplantation gained popularity as a surgical option to restore severely disfigured facial defects in more than 30 cases to date. This non–life-saving procedure, however, entails lifelong immunosuppression with life-threatening side effects as well as ethical issues. Although long-term results are not available yet, Kueckelhaus and colleagues[40] reported significant volumetric and morphometric changes already in the first 36 months after transplantation. The increase of flap size by pre-expansion of the a-SAP flap enables the reconstruction of large superficial parts of the face without the need of complex tissue transfer and, therefore, may be regarded as a serious alternative to facial allotransplantation.

SUMMARY

The SAP flap has become a well-established flap in plastic and reconstructive surgery. Continued optimization and modifications in the last few years contributed to the versatility of the SAP and a-SAP flap, which may be regarded a key flap in the armamentarium of plastic surgeons. Unlike the classic SAP flap, the new a-SAP flap uses a skin flap that is located in the deltopectoral fossa and is supplied by an anterior branch of the transverse cervical artery. The improved color match and the thinner as well as more pliable tissue of this area lead to a more pleasing cosmetic and functional result compared with the SAP flap. Pre-expansion of the donor site allows even larger flap sizes that potentially may be used to cover extended defects in the face and neck area.

REFERENCES

1. Pallua N, Machens HG, Rennekampff O, et al. The fasciocutaneous supraclavicular artery island flap for releasing postburn mentosternal contractures. Plast Reconstr Surg 1997;99(7):1878–84 [discussion: 1885–6].

2. Pallua N, Magnus Noah E. The tunneled supraclavicular island flap: an optimized technique for head and neck reconstruction. Plast Reconstr Surg 2000;105(3):842–51 [discussion: 852–4].

3. Pallua N, von Heimburg D. Pre-expanded ultra-thin supraclavicular flaps for (full-) face reconstruction with reduced donor-site morbidity and without the need for microsurgery. Plast Reconstr Surg 2005; 115(7):1837–44 [discussion: 1845–7].

4. Blondeel PN, Van Landuyt KH, Monstrey SJ, et al. The "Gent" consensus on perforator flap terminology: preliminary definitions. Plast Reconstr Surg 2003;112(5):1378–83 [quiz: 1383, 1516; discussion: 1384–7].

5. Pallua N, Wolter TP. Moving forwards: the anterior supraclavicular artery perforator (a-SAP) flap: a new pedicled or free perforator flap based on the anterior supraclavicular vessels. J Plast Reconstr Aesthet Surg 2013;66(4):489–96.

6. Lamberty BG. The supra-clavicular axial patterned flap. Br J Plast Surg 1979;32(3):207–12.

7. Cunha MS, Nakamoto HA, Herson MR, et al. Tissue expander complications in plastic surgery: a 10-year experience. Rev Hosp Clin Fac Med Sao Paulo 2002;57(3):93–7.

8. Farber N, Haik J, Weissman O, et al. Delay techniques for local flaps in dermatologic surgery. J Drugs Dermatol 2012;11(9):1108–10.

9. Di Benedetto G, Aquinati A, Pierangeli M, et al. From the "charretera" to the supraclavicular fascial island flap: revisitation and further evolution of a controversial flap. Plast Reconstr Surg 2005; 115(1):70–6.

10. Rashid M, Zia-Ul-Islam M, Sarwar SU, et al. The 'expansile' supraclavicular artery flap for release of post-burn neck contractures. J Plast Reconstr Aesthet Surg 2006;59(10):1094–101.

11. Vinh VQ, Ogawa R, Van Anh T, et al. Reconstruction of neck scar contractures using supraclavicular flaps: retrospective study of 30 cases. Plast Reconstr Surg 2007;119(1):130–5.

12. Ma X, Zheng Y, Xia W, et al. An anatomical study with clinical application of one branch of the supraclavicular artery. Clin Anat 2009;22(2):215–20.

13. Vinh VQ, Van Anh T, Ogawa R, et al. Anatomical and clinical studies of the supraclavicular flap: analysis of 103 flaps used to reconstruct neck scar contractures. Plast Reconstr Surg 2009;123(5):1471–80.

14. Chen WL, Zhang DM, Yang ZH, et al. Extended supraclavicular fasciocutaneous island flap based on the transverse cervical artery for head and neck reconstruction after cancer ablation. J Oral Maxillofac Surg 2010;68(10):2422–30.

15. Herr MW, Bonanno A, Montalbano LA, et al. Shoulder function following reconstruction with the supraclavicular artery island flap. Laryngoscope 2014; 124(11):2478–83.

16. Neumann CG. The expansion of an area of skin by progressive distention of a subcutaneous balloon; use of the method for securing skin for subtotal reconstruction of the ear. Plast Reconstr Surg (1946) 1957;19(2):124–30.

17. Radovan C. Breast reconstruction after mastectomy using the temporary expander. Plast Reconstr Surg 1982;69(2):195–208.

18. Austad ED, Rose GL. A self-inflating tissue expander. Plast Reconstr Surg 1982;70(5):588–94.

19. Kaner D, Zhao H, Terheyden H, et al. Improvement of microcirculation and wound healing in vertical ridge augmentation after pre-treatment with self-inflating soft tissue expanders - a randomized study in dogs. Clin Oral Implants Res 2015;26(6): 720–4.

20. Maitz PK, Pribaz JJ, Hergrueter CA. Impact of tissue expansion on flap prefabrication: an experimental study in rabbits. Microsurgery 1996;17(1):35–40.

21. Margulis A, Agam K, Icekson M, et al. The expanded supraclavicular flap, prefabricated with thoracoacromial vessels, for reconstruction of post-burn anterior cervical contractures. Plast Reconstr Surg 2007;119(7):2072–7 [discussion: 2078–9].

22. Cherry GW, Austad E, Pasyk K, et al. Increased survival and vascularity of random-pattern skin flaps elevated in controlled, expanded skin. Plast Reconstr Surg 1983;72(5):680–7.

23. Yang Z, Hu C, Li Y, et al. Pre-expanded cervico-acromial fasciocutaneous flap based on the supraclavicular artery for resurfacing post-burn neck scar contractures. Ann Plast Surg 2014;73(Suppl 1):S92–8.

24. Heitland AS, Pallua N. The single and double-folded supraclavicular island flap as a new therapy option in the treatment of large facial defects in noma patients. Plast Reconstr Surg 2005;115(6): 1591–6.

25. Kokot N, Mazhar K, Reder LS, et al. The supraclavicular artery island flap in head and neck reconstruction: applications and limitations. JAMA Otolaryngol Head Neck Surg 2013;139(11):1247–55.

26. Chen WL, Zhang DM, Yang ZH, et al. Functional hemitongue reconstruction using innervated supraclavicular fasciocutaneous island flaps with the cervical plexus and reinnervated supraclavicular fasciocutaneous island flaps with neurorrhaphy of the cervical plexus and lingual nerve. Head Neck 2014;36(1):66–70.

27. Zhang S, Chen W, Cao G, et al. Pedicled supraclavicular artery island flap versus free radial forearm flap for tongue reconstruction following hemiglossectomy. J Craniofac Surg 2015;26(6):e527–30.

28. Giordano L, Bondi S, Toma S, et al. Versatility of the supraclavicular pedicle flap in head and neck reconstruction. Acta Otorhinolaryngol Ital 2014; 34(6):394–8.

29. Emerick KS, Herr MW, Lin DT, et al. Supraclavicular artery island flap for reconstruction of complex parotidectomy, lateral skull base, and total auriculectomy defects. JAMA Otolaryngol Head Neck Surg 2014; 140(9):861–6.

30. Hunt JP, Buchmann LO. The supraclavicular artery flap for lateral skull and scalp defects: effective and efficient alternative to free tissue transfer. J Neurol Surg Rep 2014;75(1):e5–10.

31. Razdan SN, Ro T, Albornoz CR, et al. Case report of a supraclavicular artery island flap for reconstruction of a nonhealing cervical spine wound. J Reconstr Microsurg 2015;31(3):236–8.

32. Nicoli F, Orfaniotis G, Gesakis K, et al. Supraclavicular osteocutaneous free flap: clinical application and surgical details for the reconstruction of composite defects of the nose. Microsurgery 2015; 35(4):328–32.

33. Pallua N, Wolter TP. Defect classification and reconstruction algorithm for patients with tracheostomy using the tunneled supraclavicular artery island flap. Langenbecks Arch Surg 2010;395(8): 1115–9.

34. Cacciaguerra S, Bianchi A. Tracheal ring-graft reinforcement in lieu of tracheostomy for tracheomalacia. Pediatr Surg Int 1998;13(8):556–9.

35. Sever C, Kulahci Y, Eren F, et al. Reconstruction of postburn cervical contractures using expanded supraclavicular artery flap. J burn Care Res 2013; 34(4):e221–7.

36. Loghmani S, Eidy M, Mohammadzadeh M, et al. The supraclavicular flap for reconstruction of post-burn mentosternal contractures. Iran Red Crescent Med J 2013;15(4):292–7.

37. Yang Y, Ren J, Pang X, et al. Reconstruction of facial and cervical scar with the expanded supraclavicular island flaps. Zhonghua Zheng Xing Wai Ke Za Zhi 2015;31(1):11–3 [in Chinese].

38. Yoo J, Belzile M. Infraclavicular free flap for head and neck reconstruction: surgical description and early outcomes in 7 consecutive patients. Head Neck 2015;37(3):309–16.

39. Devauchelle B, Badet L, Lengele B, et al. First human face allograft: early report. Lancet 2006; 368(9531):203–9.

40. Kueckelhaus M, Turk M, Kumamaru KK, et al. Transformation of face transplants: volumetric and morphologic graft changes resemble aging after facial allotransplantation. Am J Transplant 2016; 16(3):968–78.

41. Dolan RT, O'Duffy F, Seoighe DM, et al. Novel use of a supraclavicular transverse cervical artery customised perforator flap: a paediatric emergency. J Plast Reconstr Aesthet Surg 2013;66(8): 1138–41.

42. Granzow JW, Suliman A, Roostaeian J, et al. Supraclavicular artery island flap (SCAIF) vs free

fasciocutaneous flaps for head and neck reconstruction. Otolaryngol Head Neck Surg 2013; 148(6):941–8.

43. Shenoy A, Patil VS, Prithvi BS, et al. Supraclavicular artery flap for head and neck oncologic reconstruction: an emerging alternative. Int J Surg Oncol 2013; 2013:658989.

44. Herr MW, Emerick KS, Deschler DG. The supraclavicular artery flap for head and neck reconstruction. JAMA Facial Plast Surg 2014;16(2):127–32.

45. Kokot N, Mazhar K, Reder LS, et al. Use of the supraclavicular artery island flap for reconstruction of cervicofacial defects. Otolaryngol Head Neck Surg 2014;150(2):222–8.

46. Emerick KS, Herr MA, Deschler DG. Supraclavicular flap reconstruction following total laryngectomy. Laryngoscope 2014;124(8):1777–82.

47. Teymoortash A, Mandapathil M, Hoch S. Indications for reconstruction of mucosal defects in oropharyngeal cancer using a supraclavicular island flap. Int J Oral Maxillofac Surg 2014;43(9):1054–8.

48. Sethi RK, Kozin ED, Lam AC, et al. Primary tracheoesophageal puncture with supraclavicular artery island flap after total laryngectomy or laryngopharyngectomy. Otolaryngol Head Neck Surg 2014;151(3):421–3.

49. Granzow JW, Li AI, Boyd JB, et al. Use of dual, tubularized supraclavicular artery island flaps in series to restore gastrointestinal continuity after a failed ileocolic esophageal reconstruction. Ann Plast Surg 2015;75(3):306–8.

50. Razdan SN, Albornoz CR, Ro T, et al. Safety of the supraclavicular artery island flap in the setting of neck dissection and radiation therapy. J Reconstr Microsurg 2015;31(5):378–83.

51. Chu MW, Levy JM, Friedlander PL, et al. Tracheostoma reconstruction with the supraclavicular artery island flap. Ann Plast Surg 2015;74(6): 677–9.

52. Pabiszczak M, Banaszewski J, Pastusiak T, et al. Supraclavicular artery pedicled flap in reconstruction of pharyngocutaneous fitulas after total laryngectomy. Otolaryngol Pol 2015;69(2):9–13.

53. Kozin ED, Sethi RK, Herr M, et al. Comparison of perioperative outcomes between the supraclavicular artery island flap and fasciocutaneous free flap. Otolaryngol Head Neck Surg 2016;154(1): 66–72.

54. Kucur C, Durmus K, Ozer E. Supraclavicular artery island flap reconstruction of a contralateral partial laryngopharyngeal defect. Acta Otorhinolaryngol Ital 2015;35(2):121–4.

Pre-expanded Internal Mammary Artery Perforator Flap

Stacy Wong, MD, James D. Goggin, MD,
Nicholas D. Webster, MD, Michel H. Saint-Cyr, MD*

KEYWORDS

- Internal mammary artery perforator flap • IMAP • Pre-expansion • Tissue expansion

KEY POINTS

- Advantages of the pre-expanded internal mammary artery perforator (IMAP) flap include increased vascularity from delay phenomenon, primary closure of donor site, decreased donor site morbidity, local tissue use, and no need for microsurgery.
- Disadvantages include staged reconstruction, protracted timeline for serial expansion, and risks/complications associated with tissue expansion.
- During pre-expansion, make the incision according to final flap design, fixate the tissue expander in the subcutaneous plane, and wait a minimum of 4 weeks between final expansion and flap harvest.
- A pinch test should be performed to ensure that direct primary closure can be obtained for the donor site.
- Confirm internal mammary perforator integrity, and adequate flow (visible pulse, loud audible venous, and arterial signals) before making a complete circumferential incision of the flap.

INTRODUCTION

Historically a mainstay of head and neck reconstruction, the deltopectoral flap[1–3] is perfused by multiple perforators of the internal mammary artery (IMA). Potential pitfalls of this flap, however, included high rate of flap necrosis, donor site skin grafting, and inability to island the flap leading to dog-earing.[4–6] Refinement of the original deltopectoral flap, based on the same perforator vessels, resulted in the IMAP flap, which was first described by Yu and colleagues.[7] Initially described for tracheostomy reconstruction, the IMAP flap is applicable toward various defects of the head, neck, and chest. Perforator flaps throughout the body have become essential tools for plastic surgery reconstruction. Recent advances in the vascular anatomy knowledge and dominant perforator location have increased flap selection options.

Perforator mapping and anatomic studies have elucidated the perforasome theory, which was outlined by Saint-Cyr and colleagues.[8] The perforasome describes the arterial vascular territory of a single perforator. Its characteristics and relationship to neighboring vascular territories were studied, revealing general principles pertaining to surgical vasculature.[8] Clinical application of this knowledge allows for more predictable and dependable results in perforator flap surgery (**Fig. 1**).

Tissue expansion has been used throughout the body to increase skin and cutaneous tissue. It has the added benefit of improving vascularity and allowing for primary donor site closure. Tissue expansion is commonly performed with traditional

Disclosure Statement. Pacira consultant (Dr M.H. Saint-Cyr).
Division of Plastic Surgery, Baylor Scott & White Health, 2401 South 31st Street, Temple, TX 76508, USA
* Corresponding author.
E-mail address: Michel.SaintCyr@BSWHealth.org

Clin Plastic Surg 44 (2017) 65–72
http://dx.doi.org/10.1016/j.cps.2016.09.001

plasticsurgery.theclinics.com

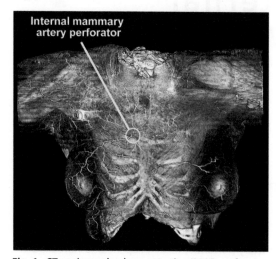

Fig. 1. CT angiography demonstrating IMAP perforator.

flaps, and it has only more recently been applied to perforator flaps. Pre-expansion of the pedicled IMAP flap is an excellent choice for reconstruction in select cases that require a large flap for the head, neck, or chest region—often in patients who have limited other options.

ANATOMY OF INTERNAL MAMMARY ARTERY PERFORATORS

The IMA runs 1 cm to 2 cm lateral to the edge of the sternum and divides into the deep superior epigastric artery and musculophrenic artery between the sixth costal cartilage and intercostal space. There are 2 venae comitantes distally, which merge between the third and fourth intercostal spaces to form 1 internal mammary

vein.[9–11] The internal mammary vessels tend to be larger on the right side.

The perforating branches of the IMA pass through the intercostal muscles and medial pectoralis major. These cutaneous perforating branches are given off by the IMA in the first 5 to 6 intercostal spaces. The second perforator is generally the largest (usually >0.8 mm).[11,12] In an anatomic study conducted by Wong and colleagues,[13] the mean perforator diameter among IMA perforators was 1.50 mm in the first intercostal space, 1.83 mm in the second intercostal space, and 1.47 mm in the third intercostal space. The IMAPs have been demonstrated to vary in size and dominance between patients and chest side.[14–16] The IMAP flap is based on a single or double perforator of the IMA, and it can generally extend from the midline of the chest to the anterior axillary line.

The arterial territory, the perforasome, of the IMA perforators explains the characteristics of the IMAP flap. The foundation of the perforasome theory[8] consists of the following 4 principles:

1. Direct and indirect linking vessels (**Fig. 2**). Direct linking vessels are large vessels that communicate directly from one perforator to the next, and indirect linking vessels maintain perfusion between perforators through recurrent flow from the subdermal plexus.
2. Flap design and skin paddle orientation are dependent on linking vessel direction. Orientation of the linking vessels demonstrates direction of maximal blood flow. For the IMAP flap, this is perpendicular to the midline. The IMAP flap has a fairly large perforasome, which allows for greater customization for flap planning, including horizontal, vertical, and oblique designs.[11]

INDIRECT FLOW THROUGH THE SUBDERMAL PLEXUS

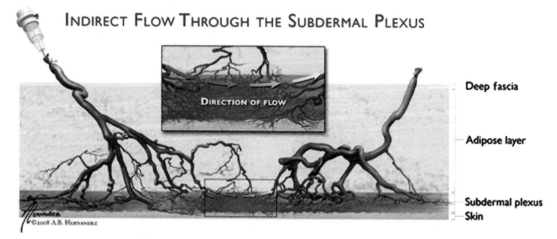

Fig. 2. Indirect linking vessels. (Printed with permission from A.B. Hernandez of Gory Details Illustration, Grapevine, TX.)

3. Preferential filling of perforasomes. Perforators of the same source artery are preferentially filled first, followed by perforators of other adjacent source arteries.
4. Perfusion is directed away from points of articulation. Perforators for the IMAP flap have multidirectional blood flow.

The IMAP flap can be sensate through the preservation of the anterior cutaneous branch of the intercostal nerve, and large areas can be covered with raising bilateral flaps. The IMA perforators may occasionally, but not always, communicate with the lateral thoracic arteries through linking vessels in the subdermis or between the dermis and pectoral fascia,[13] allowing for greater flap size. Occasionally, an even larger area is required, in which tissue expansion may be applied to have primary closure of the donor site.

TREATMENT GOALS AND PLANNED OUTCOMES

Soft tissue defects of the head, neck, and anterior chest wall often call for thin pliable tissue. Deltopectoral flaps, latissimus dorsi flaps, and other muscle flaps often do not provide adequate skin islands and may sacrifice muscles important for function in some patients. Other patients have already undergone failed reconstructions or have had recurrences with need for a new reconstruction. The expanded IMAP provides another option for these difficult reconstructions and provides thin pliable tissue with skin. Tissue expansion in particular provides a delay phenomenon, decreases the arc of rotation and allows for larger flaps with less donor site morbidity and avoidance of skin grafting.

Due to the delay of weeks to months required for tissue expansion, this technique is not applicable for reconstructions that must be performed urgently.

PREOPERATIVE PLANNING AND PREPARATION

All candidates for reconstruction should undergo a complete history and thorough physical examination. Patients undergoing major head and neck surgical procedures frequently have significant comorbidities that increase their risk for perioperative complications. History of tobacco/alcohol abuse, previous radiation, cardiac or pulmonary disease, and nutritional status should be investigated. A precise surgical history should be obtained. Preoperative perforator mapping is essential to surgical success. Use of CT angiogram to identify critical vascular territories helps guide intervention (see **Fig. 1**). Flap design should be based on the axial anatomy of the IMA perforator's linking vessels, which course horizontally and obliquely across the chest wall (**Fig. 3**). Preoperative mapping of the perforators can be performed using pencil Doppler to identify the perforators seen on CT angiography. Maximal flap length is gained by designing the flap in an inferior oblique direction (**Fig. 4**). It is critical to balance the choice of flap orientation for length, the arc of rotation, and choice of a vigorous perforator to ensure a viable reconstruction.

PATIENT POSITIONING

Placement of the tissue expander requires the patient to be placed in supine position to provide access to the anterior chest wall. Due to the arc of rotation of all flap designs, pedicled reconstructions are limited to head, neck, and anterior chest. For flap elevation and insetting after expansion, the patient may be in supine position. To provide better access to the neck, it may be helpful to place a patient's head on a horseshoe headrest. Consider whether a nasal right angle endotracheal tube allows better access to the lower two-thirds of the face and neck.

PROCEDURAL APPROACH
Expander Placement and Expansion Process

Using a lateral approach, the dominant perforator is found approximately 10 mm to 23 mm lateral to the sternal border using pencil Doppler and preoperative CT angiography imaging. A pre-chosen tissue expander is placed lateral to the second intercostal IMA perforator. The incision should be designed to be part of the design of the final flap. The expander should be placed subcutaneously and care must be taken not to disrupt the IMA perforators while dissecting the pocket for the expander or during the expansions process. Drains are placed at the

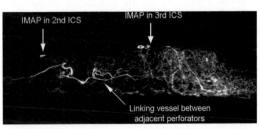

Fig. 3. CT angiography showing linking vessels between second and third intercostal IMA perforators. ICS, intercostal space.

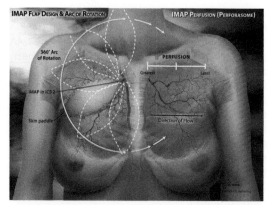

Fig. 4. IMAP perfusion and flap design. ICS, intercostal space. (Printed with permission from A.B. Hernandez of Gory Details Illustration, Grapevine, TX.)

time of tissue expander placement and kept in place for 5 to 7 days to help prevent seroma. During the period when the drains are in place, prophylactic antibiotics should be provided. The expansion process typically takes several weeks and requires multiple outpatient visits. Serial expansion is performed every 2 to 3 weeks until desired tissue gain is achieved.

Flap Harvest/Inset

After tissue expansion is complete and desired flap size is achieved, the IMAP flap is harvested at a second stage. Flap harvest usually occurs 4 to 6 weeks after final expansion is complete. Skin paddle design may be varied. Z-plasty/zigzag-type incisions have been used to avoid scar contracture of the neck. The IMAP flap is harvested in a suprafascial plane above the pectoral fascia without skeletonizing the pedicle. During dissection frequent examination of the flap for evidence of venous congestion and arterial inflow with pencil Doppler is helpful. The use of muscle relaxants in anesthesia can help to facilitate this dissection. Pre-expansion of the adjacent tissue allows for greater arc of rotation, whereas morbidity of the pectoralis major and costal cartilage is avoided. The flap can also be harvested as a sensory flap by incorporating the anterior cutaneous branch of the intercostal nerve accompanying the perforator. The distal third of the flap is generally poorly perfused and should be discarded. The flap is transposed into the defect and inset in such a way to minimize the arc of rotation. Any twisting or kinking of the internal mammary perforator should be avoided and Doppler signal for venous and arterial flow should be confirmed after flap inset. Further pedicle

dissection can be performed to minimize any risk of kinking. The corresponding costal cartilage cephalad to the perforator can be removed and the caudal internal mammary vessels ligated in order to increase the arc of rotation and reach of the flap. Generally, flap rotation occurs at 90° and proceeds in clockwise direction for right-sided flaps and counterclockwise for left-sided flaps. Supercharging venous outflow should be strongly considered if there is any concern for venous congestion. Drains are placed to prevent seroma.

POTENTIAL COMPLICATIONS AND MANAGEMENT

Complications of tissue expansion include seroma, hematoma, extrusion, infection, and wound dehiscence. Cases of hematoma and extrusion are managed with return to the operating room. Seroma may be drained percutaneously with ultrasound guidance. Infected tissue expanders require prompt removal and often result in significant delays in reconstruction.

The most common acute flap complication is venous congestion. This can be caused by hematoma, flap design, or tight inset that causes compression of the vein. It is important to identify venous congestion early with swift return to the operating room for reinsetting, evacuation of hematoma, or supercharging to help prevent flap loss. Flaps in the head and neck are at risk for compromise from compression from tracheostomy ties and pressure from items used for head positioning postoperatively. Writing on the flap and communicating directly with the nursing staff, family, and patient about avoiding pressure is helpful. Drains remain in place for 2 to 3 weeks.

POSTPROCEDURAL CARE

Like other pedicled perforator flaps, the expanded IMAP requires postoperative monitoring similar to free flaps. Complications that can benefit from rapid operative intervention are most likely to occur in the first 24 hours after surgery; therefore, patients remain in the hospital at least 1 day. Patients with head and neck defects often have other complicating factors that require prolonged treatment and observation and may require longer hospital stays. Avoidance of hypotension and medications that cause peripheral vasoconstriction is critical in the immediate postoperative period.

Flap monitoring is generally performed using pencil Doppler and clinical examination. It is imperative that the nursing staff is trained to monitor the flap using temperature, capillary refill, color Doppler, or any other adjunct. Hand-offs between staff should have both parties present so there is no confusion about the status of the flap. It is sometimes helpful to provide an immediate postoperative color photo as a point of comparison at bedside. There is limited evidence about pedicled perforator flap monitoring but hourly checks for the first 24 hours and then every 4 hours while hospitalized are prudent.

REHABILITATION/RECOVERY

Drains remain in place for 5 to 7 days after tissue expander placement and 2 to 3 weeks after flap inset. To assist with postoperative pain, intercostal nerve blocks can be placed at the conclusion of the case.

OUTCOMES

The pre-expanded IMAP flap was used by the senior author (M.H. Saint-Cyr) for reconstruction of severe neck contracture secondary to burn injury in a young woman. Due to large size, the deformity

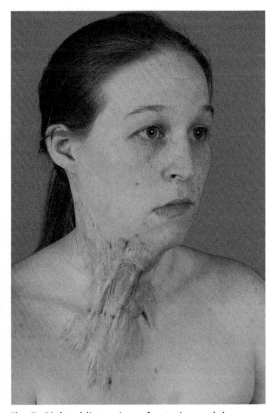

Fig. 5. Right oblique view of anterior neck burn scar contracture.

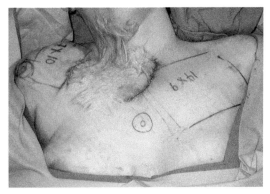

Fig. 6. Status post–tissue expander placement.

could not be entirely covered using a single pre-expanded thoracodorsal artery perforator or parascapular flap alone (**Fig. 5**). A 500-cm^3 rectangular tissue expander was placed lateral to the second intercostal IMAP (**Figs. 6–8**), serial expansion was performed, and a pedicled perforator flap of 12 cm × 8 cm was obtained. The flap was harvested in a suprafascial plane, and the donor site was closed primarily[17] (**Figs. 9** and **10**).

DISCUSSION

Zan and colleagues[18] Present an extensive series of pre-expanded flaps of the anterior chest wall. In particular, they present a series of 11 pedicled IMAP flaps. These flaps were generally performed for burn scars of the neck and neck and lower cheek. These flaps average 18 cm × 10 cm in size. They also have a series of 8 free IMAP flaps, which averaged 18 cm × 9 cm and were transferred to the cheek, forehead, nose, and perioral areas without any episodes of flap loss. Hocaoğlu and colleagues[19] and Cherry and colleagues[20] present 2 cases of pre-expanded IMAP flaps in a

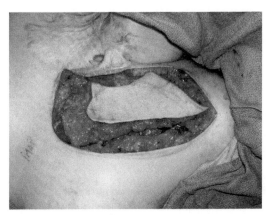

Fig. 7. Incised IMAP flap.

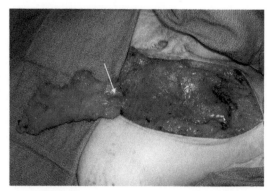

Fig. 8. IMAP flap and pedicle (*arrow* demonstrates internal mammary artery pedicle).

series of pre-expanded perforator flaps evaluating postexpansion perforator diameter to pre-expansion size. One case was a large burn contracture of the anterior neck treated with bilateral pre-expanded IMAP pedicled flaps (19 cm × 6 cm and 19 cm × 7 cm) without any complication. The other was an esophagocutaneous fistula with flap size of 36 cm × 9 cm without complication (**Table 1**).

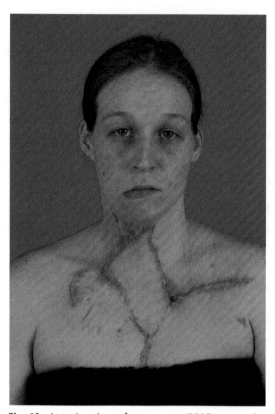

Fig. 10. Anterior view of status post-IMAP to anterior neck.

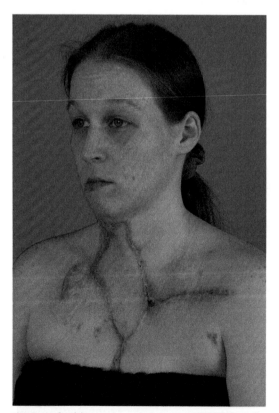

Fig. 9. Left oblique view of status post-IMAP to anterior neck.

Perforator flaps are the product of better understanding of perforators and elucidation of the perforasome theory. Pedicled flaps decrease operative time by obviating microsurgery. IMAP flaps are a lifeboat for patients who have undergone multiple failed reconstructions and require large amounts of soft tissue and lack other donor sites.

IMA-based pedicled perforator flaps can be used to reconstruct defects of the neck and anterior chest wall. Pre-expanding IMAP flaps causes a delay phenomenon improving flap survival as well as decreases donor site morbidity and increases the area that can be covered. Pre-expansions can also allow for perforator flaps that require a shorter arc of rotation. Pre-expansion requires more procedures, has risk of extrusion and infection, causes temporary contour deformity during the expansion process, and requires a longer course. Patient selection is especially important in the use of tissue expansion.

It is important to adequately free up the perforator to prevent kinking. The flap must be monitored in a similar manner to a free flap. Supercharging can decrease the risk of venous congestion. All members of the team caring for a patient postoperatively should be familiar with

Table 1
Literature reports of the pre-expanded internal mammary artery perforator flap for reconstruction; including location of defect, size of defect/flap, and pertinent points

Author	Location of Defect	Size of Defect/Flap	Notes
Zan et al,[18] 2013	Neck 9, neck and lower cheek 2	Average size 18 cm × 10 cm	Pedicled flaps, no tip necrosis or total necrosis
Zan et al,[18] 2013	Cheek 3, forehead 3, nose and perioral 2	Average size 18 cm × 9 cm	Free flaps, no necrosis
Hocaoğlu et al,[19] 2014	Anterior neck and lower face, anterosuperior neck	19 cm × 6 cm, 19 cm × 7 cm, 36 cm × 9 cm	Pedicled flaps, for burn scar contractures, 2 cases with 1 case of bilateral expanded flaps, no necrosis
Saint-Cyr et al,[17] 2009	Anterior neck	12 cm × 8 cm	Pedicled flaps, anterior neck burn scar contracture case report, no flap necrosis

flap monitoring techniques to allow for rapid return to the operating room for any necessary salvage procedures.

SUMMARY

Pre-expanded IMAP flaps can be a useful for patients who have few other options in covering vital structures of the neck and dealing with complex defects of the chest wall with good reconstructive outcome but minimal donor site complications.

REFERENCES

1. Bakamjian VY. A two-stage method for pharyngoesophageal reconstruction with a primary pectoral skin flap. Plast Reconstr Surg 1965;36:173–84.
2. Krizek TJ, Robson MC. The deltopectoral flap for reconstruction of irradiated cancer of the head and neck. Surg Gynecol Obstet 1972;135:787–9.
3. Sherlock EC, Maddox WA. The versatile deltopectoral skin flap in reconstruction about the head and neck. Am J Surg 1969;118:744–51.
4. Bakamjian VY, Long M, Rigg B. Experience with the medially based deltopectoral flap in reconstructive surgery of the head and neck. Br J Plast Surg 1971;24:174–83.
5. Gilas T, Sako K, Razack MS, et al. Major head and neck reconstruction using the deltopectoral flap: a 20 year experience. Am J Surg 1986;152:430–4.
6. Krizek TJ, Robson MC. Potential pitfalls in the use of the deltopectoral flap. Plast Reconstr Surg 1972;50:326–31.
7. Yu P, Roblin P, Chevray P. Internal mammary artery perforator (IMAP) flap for tracheostoma reconstruction. Head Neck 2006;28:723–9.
8. Saint-Cyr M, Wong C, Schaverien M, et al. The perforasome theory: vascular anatomy and clinical implications. Plast Reconstr Surg 2009;124(5):1529–44.
9. Arnez ZM, Valdatta L, Tyler MP, et al. Anatomy of the internal mammary veins and their use in free TRAM flap breast reconstruction. Br J Plast Surg 1995;48:540–5.
10. Ninkovic M, Anderl H, Hefel L, et al. Internal mammary vessels: a reliable recipient system for free flaps in breast reconstruction. Plast Reconstr Surg 1995;48:533–9.
11. Vesely MJ, Murray DJ, Novak CB, et al. The internal mammary artery perforator flap: an anatomical study and a case report. Ann Plast Surg 2007;58:156–61.
12. Cormack GC, Lamberty BGH. The arterial anatomy of skin flaps. Edinburgh (United Kingdom): Churchill Livingstone; 1986.
13. Wong C, Saint-Cyr M, Rasko Y, et al. Three- and four-dimensional arterial and venous perforasomes of the internal mammary artery perforator flap. Plast Reconstr Surg 2009;124:1759–69.
14. Taylor GI, Palmer JH. The vascular territories (angiosomes) of the body: experimental study and clinical applications. Br J Plast Surg 1987;40:113–41.
15. Yu BT, Hsieh CH, Feng GM, et al. Clinical application of the internal mammary artery perforator flap in head and neck reconstruction. Plast Reconstr Surg 2013;131:520e–6e.
16. Takeuchi M, Sakurai H. Internal mammary artery perforator flap for reconstruction of the chest wall. J Plast Surg Hand Surg 2013;47:328–30.
17. Saint-Cyr M, Schaverien M, Rohrich RJ. Preexpanded second intercostal space internal mammary

artery pedicle perforator flap: case report and anatomical study. Plast Reconstr Surg 2009;123: 1659–64.

18. Zan T, Li H, Du Z, et al. Reconstruction of the face and neck with different types of pre-expanded anterior chest flaps: a comprehensive strategy for multiple techniques. J Plast Reconstr Aesthet Surg 2013; 66(8):1074–81.

19. Hocaoğlu E, Emeklı U, Çızmecı O, et al. Suprafascial pre-expansion of perforator flaps and the effect of pre-expansion on perforator artery diameter. Microsurgery 2014;34:188–96.

20. Cherry GW, Austad E, Pasyk K, et al. Increased survival and vascularity of random-pattern skin flaps elevated in controlled, expanded skin. Plast Reconstr Surg 1983;72:680–7.

Pre-expanded Intercostal Perforator Super-Thin Skin Flap

Yunjun Liao, MD[a], Yong Luo, MD[a], Feng Lu, MD[a],
Hiko Hyakusoku, MD[b], Jianhua Gao, MD[a],*,
Ping Jiang, MD[a],*

KEYWORDS

- Intercostal perforator • Skin flap • Super-thin • Expanded

KEY POINTS

- When the intercostal perforator flap is thinned after expansion, it is slightly thicker than a full thickness skin graft and can be used to repair face and neck defects, thereby simultaneously restoring function and cosmetic appearance.
- Its benefits include a surgical delay after expansion, which allows the flap to be trimmed into a thinner flap while avoiding necrosis and reducing the risk of long- and short-term skin contracture.
- Pre-expanded intercostal perforators enhance the blood flow of the flap and yields a flap with an above-average length-to-width ratio. However, it is a time-consuming three-stage procedure that is difficult for elderly patients and patients with cervical problems.

 Video content accompanies this article at http://www.plasticsurgery.theclinics.com.

INTRODUCTION

The pre-expanded super-thin perforator flap was developed by combining the super-thin flap with a perforator and expansion. Alternatively, it is seen as a perforator flap that has been processed by super-thinning and pre-expansion. The super-thin flap, or the subdermal vascular network flap, was first reported by Situ[1] in 1986. Thereafter, it gained wide attention in P.R. China, thus resulting in the late 1980s and early 1990s in the publication of many experimental and clinical studies in Chinese journals.[2–5]

Surgeons have sought to develop thin flaps for many decades. In 1966, Colson and Janvier[6] trimmed the distal end of a flap, thus forming a flap-graft. In 1980, Thomas[7] also reported a thin flap. However, this thin flap was still a conventional flap because it required a delay of 3 weeks to achieve flap transposition and another 3 weeks before the pedicle could be divided after flap transposition. Unlike the conventional thin flap, the super-thin flap reported here is revolutionary in that a delay in flap transposition is not required and the pedicle division occurs about 1 week postoperatively. Later, the free thin flap and the narrow pedicled super-thin flap without an axial vessel were also developed.[8,9] In 1992, Gao and coworkers[10,11] (one of the authors of this article) introduced a super-thin (intercostal) perforator flap with a perforator from subcutaneous vessels. It was later improved as the perforator-supercharged flap with

Disclosures: The authors have nothing to disclose.
[a] Department of Plastic and Aesthetic Surgery, Nanfang Hospital, Southern Medical University, 1838 North Guangzhou Avenue, Guangzhou 510515, P.R. China; [b] Department of Plastic and Aesthetic Surgery, Nippon Medical School, Sendagi 1-1-5, Benkyoku 113-8602, Tokyo, Japan
* Corresponding author.
E-mail addresses: gaopsnf@163.com; jp9585@126.com

Clin Plastic Surg 44 (2017) 73–89
http://dx.doi.org/10.1016/j.cps.2016.09.005

vessel anastomosis at its distal end[12-15] and, as reported here, the pre-expanded super-thin (intercostal) perforator flap.[16] These developments in perforator flap design enlarged and stabilized the dimension of flaps.

The perforator flap was initially introduced by Kroll and Rosenfield[17] in 1988, whereas the expansion technique started in 1957.[18] Perforators increase the blood supply to the super-thin flap, whereas expansion enhances the tolerance of the flap to ischemia and hypoxia, thus augmenting the subdermal vascular plexus and reducing the risk of flap failure. The pre-expanded super-thin perforator flap is thinner than the regular flap and has a larger survival area: the length-to-width ratio is 1.5 to 2:1. Thus, it improves the viability of the distal flap. Other advantages of the procedure are that the donor site requires only primary suture and that there is no secondary thinning of the flap. However, this flap also has several disadvantages, including its time intensiveness, the need for staged procedures, and that the patients must adopt an uncomfortable position during healing.

Theoretically, any donor site with a known perforator can be used to generate a pre-expanded super-thin perforator flap, especially those sites with large and stable perforators. The chest and abdomen are often used to generate super-thin perforator flap designs because they are conventional donor sites and are usually covered by clothes. In clinical practice, perforators from the first to third intercostal spaces are frequently used to reconstruct defects on the face and neck,[16] whereas perforators from the fourth to the twelfth intercostal spaces are used to reconstruct the hands.[19,20] The chest and abdomen have abundant skin that is suitable for transposition, and the donor sites can be easily closed primarily. For this reason, pre-expansion is rarely required when the perforators are from the fourth to the twelfth intercostal spaces. Therefore, this article mainly discusses the pre-expanded super-thin perforator flap whose perforator comes from the first to third intercostal spaces.

TREATMENT GOALS AND PLANNED OUTCOMES

The pre-expanded super-thin flap with an intercostal perforator from the first to the third intercostal spaces is suitable for the following: (1) reconstruction of a large defect or scar on the face and neck, (2) compulsory transposition of a local flap or a pre-expanded local flap, and (3) patients who have zero tolerance to a scar caused by an additional local incision (Fig. 1). This flap is preferable to other conventional flaps for reconstructing face and neck defects for the following reasons. First, the color of the flap is similar to that of the face and neck: the color differences between the donor and recipient sites are small. Second, this flap does not require secondary thinning and is not bulky. Third, this procedure is less invasive than others because the perforator can supply blood to a large flap and the donor site is closed primarily. Most importantly, the flap is pliable and does not readily contract. Given its promising long-term outcomes, it is now the flap of choice for reconstruction of large defects on the face and neck in our institution.

PREOPERATIVE PLANNING AND PREPARATION
Clinical Anatomy

The intercostal perforators derive from the internal mammary artery. This artery arises from the first part of the subclavian artery, travels along the medial scalenus anterior muscle, and crosses the clavicle to enter the thorax. It then descends 1 to 1.5 cm laterally off the lateral sternum with intercostal perforating branches running in parallel to the intercostal plane. The perforators end at the inner margin of the thoracoacromial artery. They are subcutaneous arteries and many anastomose with the thoracoacromial artery and with subcutaneous branches of the cervical part of the transverse cervical artery. These anastomoses constitute wide blood supply sources. The intercostal perforators from the second intercostal spaces are the most commonly used perforators because they have a relatively large diameter of 1.2 mm and their perforating points in the deep fascia are relatively fixed. In this case, the second intercostal perforator serves as the axial vessel of the flap, whereas the accompanying perforating vein, in which the blood flows back to the internal thoracic vein, serves as the vein of the flap (Fig. 2).

Surgical Planning

Three-stage procedure
Stage 1 is insertion of an expander subcutaneously in the chest and shoulder region. After the patient is discharged, the expander is inflated with saline solution for 3 months in the outpatient department. Stage 2 is flap transposition. Stage 3 is pedicle division about 10 days after flap transposition.

Flap dimensions
The upper margin of the flap reaches the lower clavicle. The inner margin is 2 cm off the lateral sternum. The outer margin touches the deltoid. The lower margin is at the fifth rib level. The

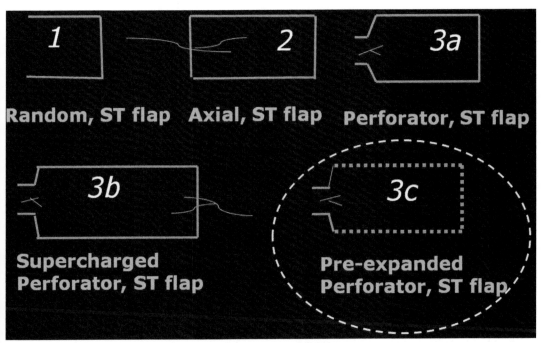

Random, ST flap   Axial, ST flap   Perforator, ST flap

Supercharged
Perforator, ST flap

Pre-expanded
Perforator, ST flap

Fig. 1. The pre-expanded super-thin perforator flap (3c). ST, super-thin.

rotation point is at the intercostal space between the first and second ribs, 2 cm off the lateral sternum. The expander should be placed in the area described previously (10 cm × 12 cm). The width

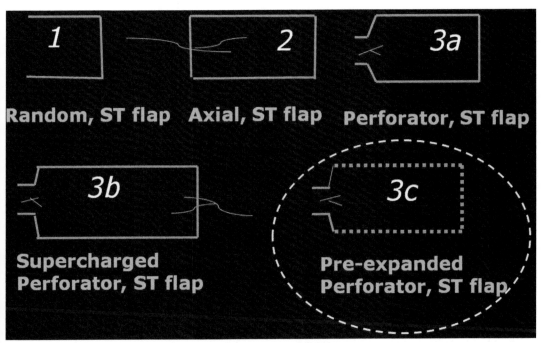

Fig. 2. Anatomy of the perforators from the second intercostal space. (a) Perforators from the second intercostal artery of the internal thoracic artery. (b) Perforators from the transverse cervical artery of the thyrocervical trunk. (c) Perforators from the thoracoacromial artery. (*From* Dang R, Zhang C. Object atlas of human regional anatomy[M]. Shanghai: Second Military Medical University Press, 2011:183; with permission.)

of the flap doubles after expansion, which is sufficient for reconstructing defects on the face. Primary closure at the donor site is also feasible.

Expander selection
Cylindrical and crescent-shaped expanders (range, 350–600 mL) are commonly used in clinical practice, but the crescent-shaped expander (usually 400 mL) is the most frequently used expander because it matches the curve of the lower clavicle and the anatomic shape of the chest and shoulder. The volume of the crescent-shaped expander depends on the cervical length of the patient and the coverage required.

Other considerations
Measure the coverage and arc of flap rotation required, determine the appropriate inflation of the expander, and decide whether the flap should have one or two perforators.

PATIENT POSITIONING

The patient takes a supine position. In stage 2, when the flap is transposed to the face and neck, a pillow should be given to elevate the patient's head and neck and the patient should tilt his or her head toward the involved side to relieve tension on the pedicled flap. After pedicle division, the patient must again adopt the supine position with a pillow under the shoulder and the head falling backward to relax the contracted neck.

PROCEDURAL APPROACH
Stage 1: Expander Placement

Flap design
Mark the surface projection of the perforators in the first and second intercostal spaces with methylene blue. The incision should be parallel to the axillary folds on the medial wall of the axilla and approximately 7 cm in length. After sterilization and draping, leakage of the 400-mL crescent-shaped expander should be checked by filling it with air. Then empty the expander, flatten it, and place it on the operating field with its base plate downward and the injection port pointing toward the axilla. Mark the expander with methylene blue (**Fig. 3**).

Tissue separation and expander placement
Make an incision to the muscle fascia and separate the tissue by blunt dissection to avoid impairing the perforators, especially those from the second intercostal space and the transverse cervical artery. After meticulous hemostasis and irrigation, place the expander flat into the cavity with its base plate downward and the injection port at one side of the incision near the anterior axillary line. Routinely install a negative pressure drain and then inject air into the expander to check the folding of the fill tube and the roll-over of the expander. Finally, evacuate all air from the expander.

Postoperative inflation
Place pressure on the expander area with a sandbag and maintain the negative pressure drain after the operation. When the drain fluid is dark red or yellow serum-like in color, and the drainage is

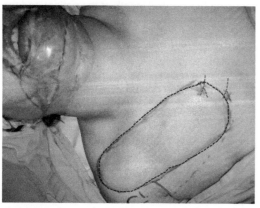

Fig. 3. Designing the incision and separation areas. Solid red line, the incision; dashed red line, the perforators; dashed blue line, the separation area.

less than 5 mL, remove the drain tube. Remove the incision suture on Day 7 and start to slightly inflate the expander with saline solution. The expander should be inflated once every 3 days in the early stage and will be filled in a month. Maintain the inflated expander by injecting saline solution once every 7 days for 2 more months. Thus, the inflation takes about 3 months in total and the total volume that is injected is 800 to 1000 mL. When the skin in the center of the expander area is expanded and thin enough that small blood vessels that stretch parallel to the longitudinal axial of the flap are visible, it is time to perform the second operation.

Precautions
Do not overinflate at each injection because it can cause excessive tension and/or pain and result in dermis tearing and "stretch marks," or even ulceration and exposure of the expander. The inflation process should be aseptic to prevent infection. In the late stage of expansion, the expander reaches a certain volume and is likely to slip downward because of gravity. In this case, an elastic bandage should be placed underneath the expander to fix it in place and preparations for the stage 2 operation should be started.

Stage 2: Expander Removal and Flap Transposition

Flap design
Identify the candidate pedicled vein using the transillumination test and mark the artery branches in the flap in red and blue using Doppler flowmetry (**Fig. 4**). Based on the preferred candidate pedicle vessels and the coverage required, decide on the number of perforators, direction of flap, and dimensions of the flap to be transposed in the stage 2 operation. Generally, the intercostal perforator from the second intercostal space serves as the pedicle. Perforators from the transverse cervical artery can also be included if necessary. The flap should be more than large enough to cover the defect with a redundant rim of about 1 cm. Stimulate flap rotation with a cloth, then decide the arc of rotation.

Flap elevation
Elevate the flap from the middle and distal periphery to elevate half or two-thirds of the total flap. The incision should be made to the capsule of the expander. Then open the capsule with scissors and remove the expander. Maintain the intactness of the flap vascular plexus as much as possible. During surgery, if part of the flap periphery cannot be transposed because of excessive tension,

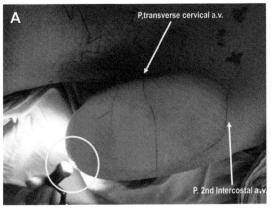
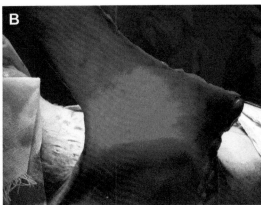

Fig. 4. Transillumination test (*circle* indicates the light source direction) before (*A*) and during (*B*) surgery.

consider cutting through the epidermis only but leaving the subcutaneous vascular plexus as it is.

Flap thinning

Flip the flap over and remove the expander capsule with blunt straight scissors to expose the subcutaneous adipose tissue of the flap, where the adipose globules among the fibrous septa bulge if gently pressed with scissors. Prick the globule capsules and remove the entire adipose globules. This thinning strategy guarantees maximal adipose removal while protecting the vascular plexus in the fibrous septa. After trimming off the deep subcutaneous adipose tissue, the subdermal vascular plexus becomes visible. It is important to maintain the intactness of the subdermal vascular plexus because this ensures favorable flap blood supply. Use low-energy electrocoagulation or multiple clamping to achieve hemostasis after thinning. Thereafter, pack the flap with wet gauze (**Fig. 5**). Slightly cut through the epidermis along the markings in the pedicle area using the back of the scalpel and stain the incision with gentian violet. It marks the incision that is to be used in pedicle division (**Fig. 6**).

Recipient site preparation

Make an incision along the edge of the scar contracture to the superficial adipose layer and elevate the scar flap. The elevated scar flap should have the same dimensions as the elevated super-thin flap. Completely stop bleeding by electrocoagulation. Rotate the scar flap downward and anastomose it to the super-thin flap. As much as possible, prevent the pedicles folding into tubes; this prevents compression caused by postoperative swelling (see **Fig. 6**; **Fig. 7**).

Inset of the flaps

Using a pillow, orient the patient so that the head tilts toward the involved side. Pull the scar flap down until it is tight and align it with the donor site margin under tension. The tension should be

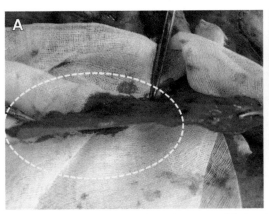
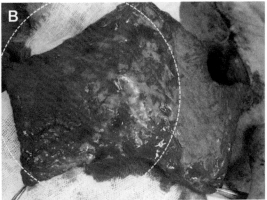

Fig. 5. Photographs showing the side view and front view of thinned flaps (*A, B*) and a video showing the flap-thinning method (Video 1). (*Dotted circle* indicates the thickness of thinned flaps.)

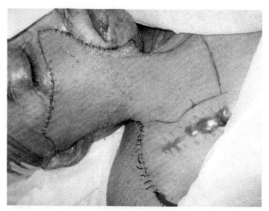

Fig. 6. Marking the incision to be used in pedicle division, transposing the flap at the recipient site. The anastomosis of the transposed flap and the scar flap forms the pedicle.

borne by the scar flap only: the pedicle of the super-thin flap should not bear any tension. Fix the joining points of the super-thin flap and the faciocervial wound with 4–0 Vicryl sutures and close the epidermis with 6–0 nylon sutures. If a vacuum develops under the pedicles of the two flaps, suture the subcutaneous tissue to the base. Place a negative pressure drain under the flaps (see **Figs. 6** and **7**).

Donor site management
The defect in the donor site is sutured primarily. In rare cases, the defect may have to be repaired by local flap transplantation. A negative pressure drain should also be placed in the donor site.

Postoperative fixation
Make sure to place an elastic net over the thinned distal flap and pack it with compression bandages for 3 days if necessary. However, no pressure should be placed on the pedicles. Fix the hand

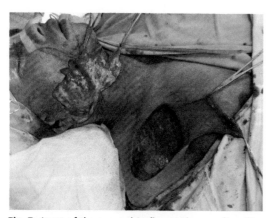

Fig. 7. Inset of the super-thin flap to the scar flap. The scar flap was rotated downward to anastomose to the super-thin flap.

and the upper arm with a bandage with the head tilting toward the pedicle. Wrap a piece of cloth around the upper arm to inhibit upper body mobility so that the patient cannot move during anesthesia recovery or when dreaming. When the drain fluid is dark red or yellow serum-like in color and the drainage is less than 5 mL, remove the drain tube.

Stage 3: Pedicle Division

Timing of pedicle division
Pedicle division is generally performed 10 days after flap transposition. Although the authors initially performed pedicle division on Day 7 after super-thin flap transposition,[20] and early animal experiments indicate that the pedicle will survive if the division is performed on postoperative Day 5,[3] the authors, who have many years of clinical experience, currently believe that the pedicle of pre-expanded super-thin flaps should be divided a bit later, namely, on postoperative Day 8 to 12 because of the flap size and patient position. The decision when to divide the pedicle depends on clinical observations. If the flap completely interweaves with the wound, pedicle division can be performed on Day 8. However, if the flap interweaves with only half of the wound, pedicle division should be performed on Day 11, whereas flap interweave with two-thirds of the wound means pedicle division can be performed on Day 10. If there is severe skin contraction at the donor site after Day 14, it is likely that it will be difficult to close the donor site defect. In general, there is no need to perform a division test before pedicle division.

Dividing the pedicle
The patient takes a supine position with the head on a pillow. Make an incision along the marks made in the last operation to expose the former expander cavity. Divide the pedicle completely. Remove the pillow immediately after pedicle division and place the head at a level position. If the surgery aims to repair a cervical scar contracture, a pillow should be placed under the shoulder so that the head falls backward. Remove scar tissue at the anastomosis site and irrigate thoroughly.

Flap thinning
Thin the flap as described previously. Align and suture the flap to the wound margin. Set up a negative pressure drain subcutaneously. Place an elastic net over the flap for compression.

POTENTIAL COMPLICATIONS AND THEIR MANAGEMENT
Circulatory Problems

Ischemia in the distal flap and venous congestion are the most common complications of the pre-expanded super-thin intercostal perforator flap. In most cases, the flap is pale cyan or pale blue after surgery and the capillary refill time takes 2 to 3 seconds. The color generally normalizes within 3 days. However, if the skin is extremely pale, exhibits cyanosis, and/or becomes blackened, this indicates that there are circulatory problems.

Ischemia of the distal flap

Symptoms of ischemia are paleness, low cutaneous temperature, long ($\geq$4 second) capillary refill time or no capillary refill in the early stage, and grayish purple skin, piebaldness, and no capillary refill in the late stage. It should be managed by correcting the patient's position, reducing flap tension, releasing the twisted flap, and/or adjusting the compression generated by the dressing (**Fig. 8**). If the ischemia cannot be alleviated by these methods, implement vascular dilation, spasm alleviation, local thermal therapy, hyperbaric oxygen therapy, or other therapies and perform secondary surgery if necessary. This surgery involves trimming and thinning the disordered area and then packing the flap with pressure dressings and applying a full thickness skin graft.

Venous congestion

Symptoms of venous congestion consist of reddish purple skin, high cutaneous temperature, and a short (<2 second) capillary refill time. In 2 to 4 hours, the flap becomes dark purple, even blackish purple, with localized swelling and no capillary refill. Venous congestion is managed by releasing the tension on the pedicle, removing stitches in the distal flap at intervals, exsanguinating the congestion with acupuncture, and wet dressing the wound with heparin (**Fig. 9**). The congestion should be evacuated from the distal end to the rim. Increase the pressure from the elastic net when the skin color turns red. Implement hyperbaric oxygen treatment when necessary.

Hematoma

Subcutaneous swelling, abnormal bulging of the flap, and large-volume and scarlet drain fluid usually indicate hematoma. Blood clots are visible when squeezing the incision margin. The hematoma should be managed by removing some of the stitches, squeezing out the blood clots, increasing pressure over the bleeding area, and administering a hemostatic systematically. Perform exploratory surgery to stop the bleeding if necessary.

Infection

Infection occurs rarely after flap transposition and pedicle division. However, it can develop after expander placement in stage 1 because of inadequate sterilization, the presence of foreign matter in the cavity, or expander exposure caused by overthinning of the flap and ulceration. It is managed by standard antibiotics treatment, asepsis, and timely dressing changes.

Complications in Expansion

The expansion may be complicated by hematoma, expander exposure, ulceration caused by an overthinned flap, infection, and other complications. For details, please refer to the article on expanders elsewhere in this issue.

POSTPROCEDURAL CARE
Postural Care

The procedure demands stringent maintenance of specific patient positions, especially after flap transposition. It is vitally important that the patient maintains a fixed posture. Two pillows should be given to support the head in a tilting forward position. The patient should lean toward the flap pedicle to keep the pedicle skin loose. Twisting is prohibited. The patient has a painful neck for the first day or 2; thereafter, the patient becomes

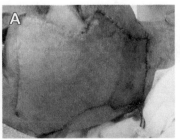 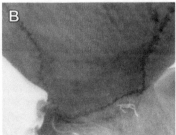 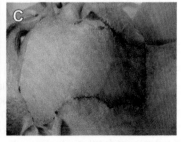

Fig. 8. Hemodynamic disorder caused by elastic net compression that was relieved by timely decompression. (*A*) The flap was compressed for about 12 hours after surgery. (*B*) Two days after decompression. (*C*) One week after the operation.

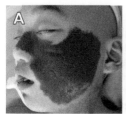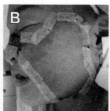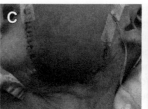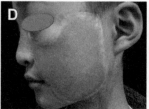

Fig. 9. Venous congestion of the super-thin perforator flap. (*A*) Patient with a melanocytic nevus on the left cheek, 3 months after expander placement. (*B*) The pedicle was divided 10 days after removing the melanocytic nevus and transposing a second intercostal perforator super-thin flap. (*C*) Venous congestion developed the day after pedicle division. It was relieved by increasing the pressure of the dressing and by hyperbaric oxygen treatment. (*D*) One year after the super-thin intercostal perforator flap procedure.

accustomed to the position. An analgesia pump and massage help to relieve the discomfort.

Incision Care

The patient may vomit during recovery from the anesthesia. The vomit should be quickly cleaned off the operative site, and the dressing should be changed. There could be considerable exudate in the early stage after the operation. Moreover, the invisible area between the pedicle and the neck usually contains exudate residue. Thus, it is necessary to clean the wound regularly and sterilize the surgical site to prevent infection.

Dietary Care

Patients take a liquid diet during the first 3 days after surgery, after which they change to a semi-liquid diet. The patient can commence a regular diet 5 days after the operation.

REHABILITATION AND RECOVERY

The patient should keep wearing the elastic net after surgery to ensure compression on the wound, because this can inhibit scar development, accelerate swelling relief, and help shape the wound. Patients should place skin closures, scar creams, or other methods of scar prevention on the incision uninterruptedly for 6 months to prevent scar formation. After reconstruction of a cervical scar, the patient should exercise by tilting their head backward for 6 months.

OUTCOMES

Since 2003, the authors have used pre-expanded super-thin intercostal perforator flaps to reconstruct defects on the face and neck in 279 cases. The largest flap was 25 cm × 10 cm, whereas the smallest was 16 cm × 5 cm. All of the flaps survived except for three that developed a hemodynamic disorder at the 2-cm margin of the distal end. These three flaps were processed into full

thickness skin grafts within 24 hours. All patients were followed up for between 3 months and 4 years. To date, all have a favorable prognosis. The flaps have a texture, color, and thickness that is almost identical to that of the normal skin in the periphery. There were no cases of skin contracture after the procedure, and there was no need for secondary flap thinning in the procedure. Thus, the pre-expanded super-thin intercostal perforator flap has become the option of choice for large defect reconstruction.

CLINICAL CASE DEMONSTRATIONS
Case 1

A 19-year-old male patient had facial disfigurement caused by burns 10 years ago. The contracted scars around corners of the mouth resulted in microstomia. Three months after the expansion, the flaps were transferred on the face for reconstruction.

Capillary refilling was tested after the scar removal and flap transposition on the left cheek. Results were normal (Video 2).

Thinned flap on the right. The flap was slightly darker than normal skin but capillary refilling was normal (Video 3).

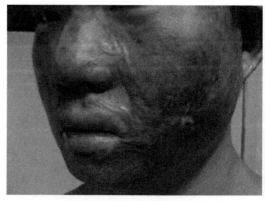

Before surgery, side view.

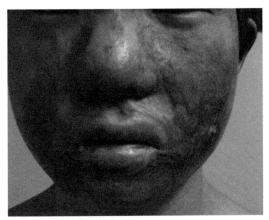

Before surgery, front view.

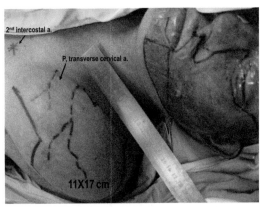

Scars on the left cheek were removed first. The flap design was marked before removal of the left expander and flap transposition.

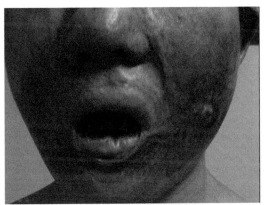

Scars contracted around corners of the mouth, resulting in microstomia.

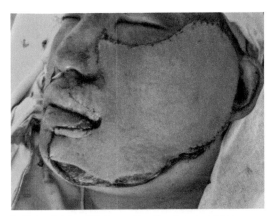

Pedicle division 10 days after flap transposition.

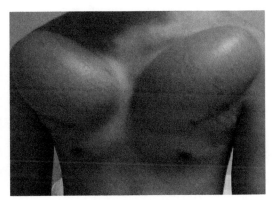

Three months after expander placement on both sides.

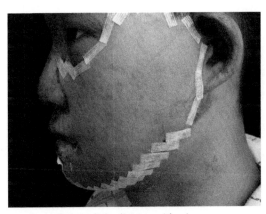

Ten days after pedicle division, side view.

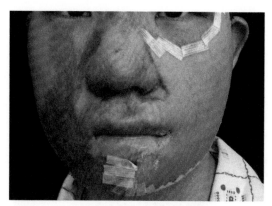

Ten days after pedicle division, front view.

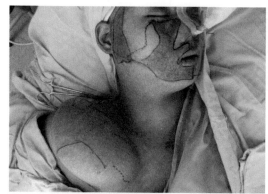

Scars were removed on the right cheek. Flap design was marked before removal of the right expander and flap transposition.

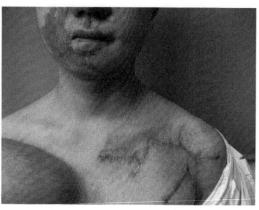

Recovery at donor and recipient sites 1.5 months after pedicle division.

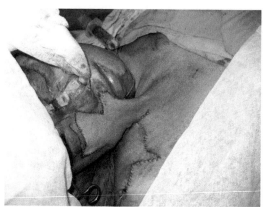

Flap transposition on the right, during surgery.

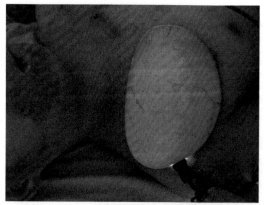

One and a half months after pedicle division on the left, before flap transposition on the right.

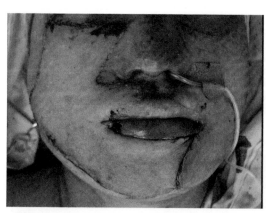

Pedicle on the right was divided 9 days after flap transposition.

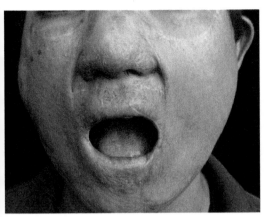

One year after the procedure.

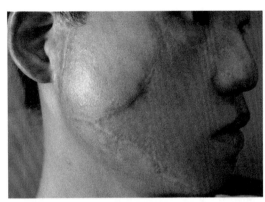

Four years after the procedure.

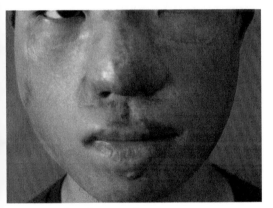

Four years after the procedure.

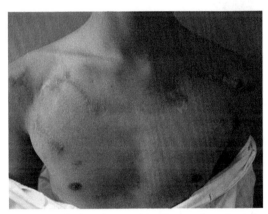

Recovery of the donor site 15 months after the procedure.

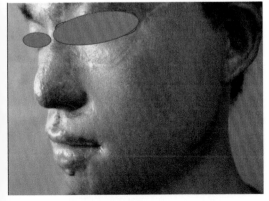

Four years after the procedure.

Case 2

A 34-year-old female patient had full facial disfigurement caused by burns 32 years ago. We removed scars on her left cheek and performed intercostal perforator super-thin flap transposition in the first, then reconstructed her oral clefts. Finally we reconstructed her right cheek in the operation.

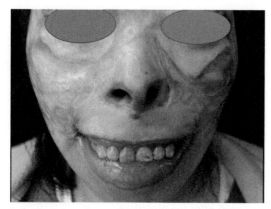

Before surgery, front view.

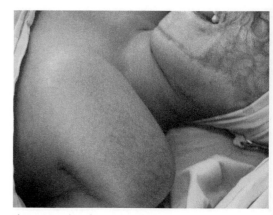

Three months after expander placement.

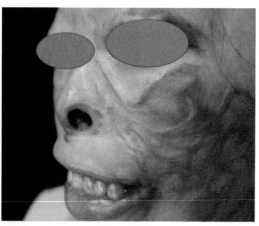

Before surgery, left side view.

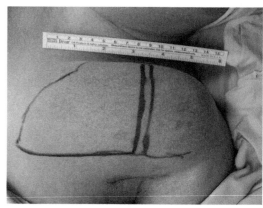

Flap design was marked before expander removal and flap transposition.

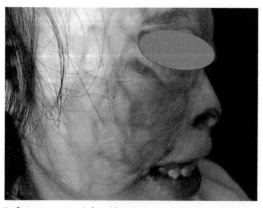

Before surgery, right side view.

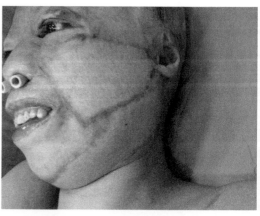

Four months after the flap transposition on the left.

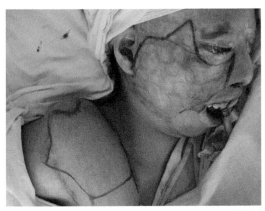

Scars on the right cheek were to be removed and flap transposition was to be performed.

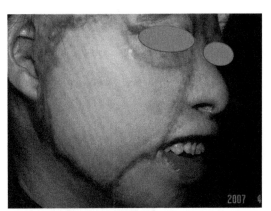

Two and a half months after the procedure on the right.

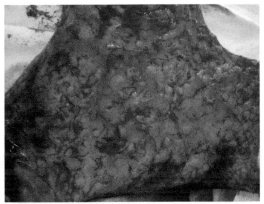

Subcutaneous vessel plexus were visible after flap thinning.

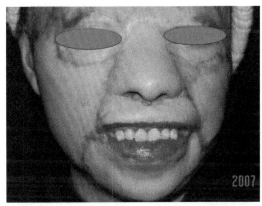

Two and a half months after the procedure on the right.

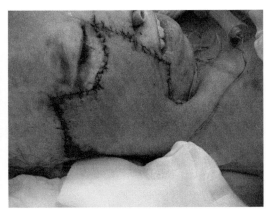

Three days after the procedure on the right.

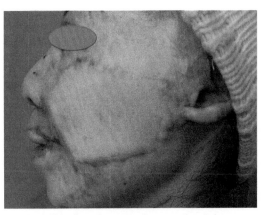

Four months after the procedure on the right.

Case 3

A 32-year-old female patient had disfigurement on the left cheek caused by burns 29 years ago. The patient also had oral clefts and incomplete closure of the mouth. Using this flap, we reconstructed her facial appearance.

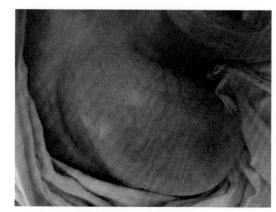

Before scar removal on the left cheek and super-thin intercostal perforator flap procedure.

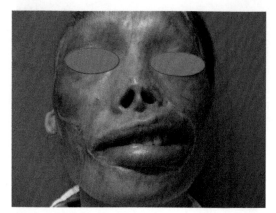

Before surgery, front view.

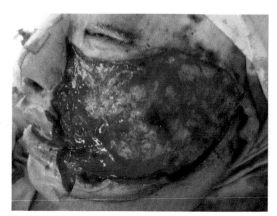

Scars at the recipient site were removed. The lower end of the scar flap was reserved for anastomosis to the pedicle.

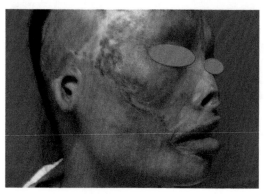

Before surgery, side view.

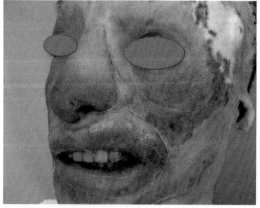

Before surgery, side view.

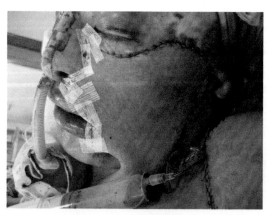

The transposed flap was pale blue.

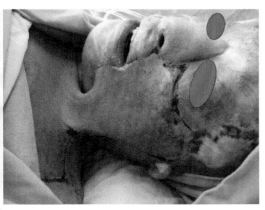

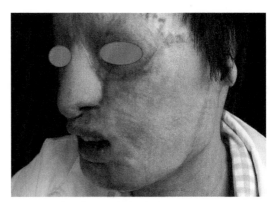

The flap resumed normal color 3 days after transposition, 10 days before pedicle division.

Four months after pedicle division.

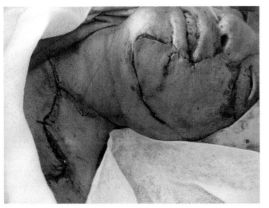

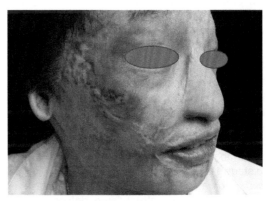

After pedicle division.

Four months after pedicle division.

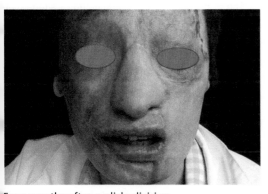

Four months after pedicle division.

DISCUSSION

Theoretically, a pre-expanded super-thin perforator flap can be generated at any donor site with a known intercostal perforator. However, intercostal perforator flaps generated from the chest and abdomen require no pre-expansion and the donor site can be closed primarily. Moreover, these flaps are too far away from the face and neck to reconstruct defects. Therefore, the pre-expanded super-thin perforator flap is usually generated from the first and second intercostal spaces.

The pre-expanded super-thin perforator flap is currently the second largest flap used to reconstruct face and neck defects following free flaps. Its perfect thickness exempts a secondary thinning procedure and the donor site can be closed primarily. Thus, it becomes the flap of choice for reconstruction of large defects on the face and neck. However, compulsory position is the most undesirable disadvantage for this procedure, which is not suitable for elderly patients.

What is important in the procedure is to protect the perforator, meaning the tissue separation should go deep enough for perforator substitution in case the planned perforator is damaged or too thin. The substitute could be either from the transverse cervical artery or the thoracoacromial artery. What is difficult in the procedure is to keep the subdermal vascular plexus intact when supperthinning the flap. The key for postoperative management is to adjust the pressure on the flap. This is different from the management of a traditional flap, which requires no pressure. It is also different from the management of a skin graft, which should be packed with pressure dressing for 7 to 10 days. The super-thin perforator flap prefers a pressure in between. It should be managed with single-layer elastic net for 3 days or so, and the pressure should respond to the flap color. Release the pressure a bit if the flap is pale and increase the pressure if it is purple.

SUMMARY

The pre-expanded super-thin intercostal perforator flap mostly takes perforators from the first or second intercostal space as the pedicle and carries with it large areas of soft tissue from between the lower clavicle and the fifth rib in the chest and shoulder region. The flap is expanded in stage 1 and then thinned and elevated with the perforator as the pedicle. The elevated flap is transposed to reconstruct large defects, scars, or disease-related impairments on the face and neck. The flap has a similar texture and thickness as the original skin but does not contract or swell. The donor site is closed primarily. Because this flap can provide function and cosmetic reconstruction simultaneously, it is recommended for the reconstruction of large defects on the face and neck.

SUPPLEMENTARY DATA

Supplementary data related to this article can be found online at http://dx.doi.org/10.1016/j.cps.2016.09.005.

REFERENCES

1. Situ P. Pedicled flap with subdermal vascular network. Academic J First Medical College of PLA 1986;6:60–1 [in Chinese].
2. Chen B, Xu D, Situ P. Anatomic basis of subdermal vescular networkskin flap in cervico-shoulder-humeral region. Chinese Journal of Clinical Anatomy 1993;11(4):245 [in Chinese].
3. Yuan XB, Chen WP, Yang Y, et al. Experimental study of island super thin flap. Chinese J Microsurgery 1993;16:188–90 [in Chinese].
4. Gao JH, Hyakusoku H, Sato M, et al. Analysis of transcutaneous gas and blood flow in narrow pedicled flap with subdermal vascular network. Chinese J Microsurgery 1994;17:248–50 [in Chinese].
5. Chen B, Situ P, Wu S, et al. Free radical production in the subdermal vascular network thin skin flap. Chinese Journal of Plastic Surgery 1995;11(2):87 [in Chinese].
6. Colson P, Janvier H. Le degraissage primaire et total des lambeaux d'autoplastic a distance. Ann Chir Plast 1966;11:11–20.
7. Thomas CV. Thin flaps. Plast Reconstr Surg 1980;65:747–52.
8. Koshima I, Fukuda H, Utunomiya R, et al. The anterolateral thigh flap; variations in its vascular pedicle. Br J Plast Surg 1989;42:260–2.
9. Yang ZY, Chen BB, Huong YM, et al. The use of the pedicled over-thin flap of the acromiopectoral region in repair of face and neck. J Rep Reconstr Surg 1991;5:141–2 [in Chinese].
10. Gao JH, Hyakusoku H, Akimoto M, et al. Experiences in using the super-thin flap. Jpn J Plast Reconstr Surg 1992;35:1097–103 [in Japanese].
11. Gao JH, Hyakusoku H, Luo JH, et al. El colgajo occipito-cervico-hombro (OCH) con pediculo estrecho, para la reconstruccion de cara y Cuello. Cirugía plástica ibero-latinoamericana 1995;21:127–41.
12. Hyakusoku H, Pennington DG, Gao JH. Microvascular augmentation of the super-thin occipitocervico-dorsal flap. Br J Plast Surg 1994;47:465.
13. Hyakusoku H, Gao JH. The super thin flap. Br J Plast Surg 1994;47:457–64.
14. Gao JH, Hyakusoku H, Luo JH, et al. The clinical application of subdermal vascular network flaps and their supercharged versions. Jpn J Plast Reconstr Surg 1995;38:1067–77 [in Japanese].
15. Hyakusoku H, Gao JH, Pennington DG, et al. The microvascular augmented subdermal vascular network (ma-SVN) flap. Br J Plast Surg 2002;55(5):402.
16. Lu F, Gao JH, Ogawa R, et al. Preexpanded distant "super-thin" intercostals perforator flaps for facial reconstruction without the need for microsurgery. J Plast Reconstr Aesthet Surg 2006;59:1203–8.
17. Kroll SS, Rosenfield L. Perforator-based flaps for low posterior midline defects. Plast Reconstr Surg 1988;81(4):561–6.
18. Neumann CG. The expansion of an area of skin by progressive distention of a subcutaneous balloon; use of the method for securing skin for subtotal

reconstruction of the ear. Plast Reconstr Surg 1957; 19(2):124–30.

19. Gao JH, Hyakusoku H. Stage transposition of the intercostal cutaneous perforator (ICP) flap as a subdermal vascular network flap for coverage of the land. Cirugía plástica ibero-latinoamericana

1996;12(1):69. Plast Reconstr Surg 1999;3:1104 (Summary).

20. Gao JH, Hyakusoku H, Inoue S, et al. Usefulness of narrow pedicled intercostal cutaneous perforator flap for coverage of the burned hand. Burns 1994; 20(1):65.

Pre-expanded Thoracodorsal Artery Perforator Flap

Yalcin Kulahci, MD[a],[*], Cihan Sahin, MD[b],
Huseyin Karagoz, MD, PhD[b], Fatih Zor, MD[c]

KEYWORDS

- Expanded • Pre-expanded • Thoracodorsal • Perforator • Flap

KEY POINTS

- Mark the perforator arteries and anterior border of the latissimus dorsi muscle before surgery with the patient in the lateral decubitus position.
- Perform subfascial dissection to find the perforator.
- Place the tissue expander precisely according to the pedicle and its vascular territory to avoid complications.
- Perform the dissection meticulously in the second operation based on the high risk of injuring the pedicle in scar tissue.
- Do not skeletonize the pedicle in both stages and dissect the pedicle with a small amount of fibrotic and soft tissue around in case of necessity.

INTRODUCTION

The thoracodorsal artery perforator (TDAP) flap was first described in 1995 as "latissimus dorsi musculo-cutaneous flap without muscle," and is based on perforators from the thoracodorsal artery.[1] Therefore, its proper name is the thoracodorsal artery perforator flap.[2] It has been used for reconstruction of head and neck, extremities, axillary region, chest wall, and the back.[3–7] However, the disadvantages of the flap are perforator anatomy variations, difficulties in preoperative localization of a reliable perforator, and intramuscular dissection. Furthermore, if the TDAP flap is large, necrosis at the distal site of the flap is possible. Pre-expansion of the flap provides a delay phenomenon and probably increases the flap survival area.

The use of the TDAP flap has increased recently because of its advantages.[3,8–10] The factors that affect the widespread use of the flap are summarized as follows: basic and reliable anatomy, the ability to be thinned without compromising blood supply, the possibility of obtaining a long pedicle, the pliability of the flap, and the lack of significant donor site morbidity. However, in a number of situations, the size of the flap or pedicle can be found to be inadequate. To provide a solution in these cases, pre-expansion of the TDAP flap may be used to increase the size of the flap.

A pre-expanded TDAP flap can be especially useful in releasing axillary burn contractures that require large amounts of skin flap. Another

Disclosure: None of the authors has a financial interest in any of the products, devices, or drugs mentioned in this article.
[a] Department of Hand and Upper Extremity Surgery, Gulhane Military Medical Academy, General Dr Tevfik Saglam Cad, Etlik 06010, Ankara, Turkey; [b] Department of Plastic and Reconstructive Surgery, Haydarpasa Training Hospital, Gulhane Military Medical Academy, Tibbiye Caddesi, Üsküdar 34668, Istanbul, Turkey; [c] Department of Plastic, Reconstructive, and Aesthetic Surgery, Gulhane Military Medical Academy, General Dr Tevfik Saglam Cad, Etlik 06010, Ankara, Turkey
* Corresponding author.
E-mail address: yakulahci@yahoo.com

Clin Plastic Surg 44 (2017) 91–97
http://dx.doi.org/10.1016/j.cps.2016.08.010

important advantage of the technique is that it allows primary closure of the donor site.[11]

PREOPERATIVE PLANNING AND PREPARATION

Before surgery, the perforator arteries are marked using a handheld Doppler ultrasound apparatus (Huntleigh dopplex, Cardiff, United Kingdom) with the patient in the lateral decubitus position. If the surgeon adheres to the previously defined surgical determinants, success is very likely while planning and harvesting the flap. A line indicating the anterior border of the latissimus dorsi (LD) muscle is drawn. The first perforator usually emerges from a point 8 to 10 cm inferior to the posterior axillary fold and 1 to 2 cm posterior to the anterior border of the LD muscle.[4,12] Another landmark is 4 cm (range, 3–6 cm) below the tip of the scapula and 2.5 cm posterior to the anterior border of the LD muscle (**Fig. 1**). The thoracodorsal artery bifurcates at that point to medial (or horizontal) branch and lateral (or descending) branch. Both branches of the thoracodorsal artery are

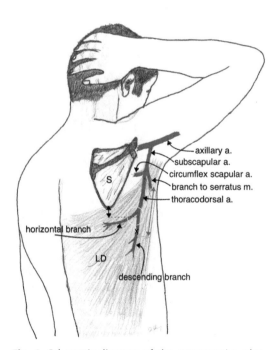

Fig. 1. Schematic diagram of the preoperative planning. a, artery; LD, latissimus dorsi muscle; m, muscle; S, scapula; X, first thoracodorsal artery perforator. Blue double arrow is approximately 8 to 10 cm inferior to the posterior axillary fold, green double arrow is approximately 1 to 2 cm and shows the distance posterior to the anterior border of the LD muscle, black double arrow is 4 cm (range, 3–6 cm) diameter below the tip of scapula, and yellow circle shows the possible bifurcation location of thoracodorsal artery.

under the surface of the LD muscle throughout the course.[2,13,14]

PATIENT POSITIONING AND SURGICAL TECHNIQUE

Once anesthesia is used, the patient should be placed in the lateral decubitus position with the arm abducted 90° over. In this position, an incision is made in the area corresponding to the anterior border of the LD muscle. After revealing the anterior border of the LD muscle, a subfascial dissection is performed to find the perforator and create a pocket for the tissue expander (**Fig. 2**A). Exposing the pedicle completely at this stage of surgery should be avoided. However, many perform suprafascial dissection.[15] Both surgical plans can be executed; it is up to the surgeon's preference. Afterward, a tissue expander is placed (**Fig. 2**B) and 2 weeks after surgery, serial expansions start.

A second operation is carried out a minimum of 4 weeks after completion of the expansion. In the second stage, dissection should begin at the anterior side of the flap using the previous incision. Subfascial dissection is performed to find the perforator initially. At this stage, one needs to be very careful because the perforator can be injured easily based on the scar tissue. It is suggested to not skeletonize the perforator as it should be dissected with a little bulk around it. Next, intramuscular dissection toward the descending branch and the thoracodorsal artery is performed.

The pre-expanded TDAP flap is harvested with the capsule following pedicle dissection. The dissection should be performed precisely because of the adherence of the expander capsule to the perforator (**Fig. 3**). The TDAP flap donor site can be sutured primarily.

Placing the tissue expander meticulously according to the pedicle and its vascular territory increases the reliability of the flap and avoids complications. At the time of placement, partial filling of the expander ensures that the implant is positioned properly.

MANAGEMENT OF THE POTENTIAL COMPLICATIONS

The main complication of the pre-expanded TDAP flap is the potential for perforator injury, especially during the second stage. As well, this is indicated as one of the main disadvantages of TDAP flaps in the literature.[8] Therefore, perforator marking before surgery should be performed carefully for both stages of the surgery. It is crucial during the first stage not to place the tissue expander close

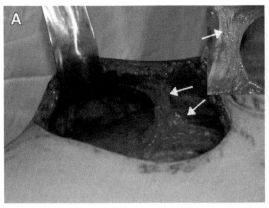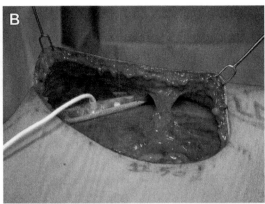

Fig. 2. (*A*) Intraoperative view of the prepared pocket for the tissue expander and the pedicle. White arrows show the pedicle (the inset at the *right top* shows the zoom-in view of the pedicle). (*B*) After the tissue expander was placed in the pocket.

to the vessels because during expansion, the pedicle can be injured, especially if the expander is inflated too much and too quickly. Correct positioning of the tissue expander is very important in the first operation because if the tissue expander is placed near the vessels, this can ultimately cause vessel obstruction and thrombosis. In the second operation, scar tissue can be the cause of pedicle injury as it is hard to dissect the vessels in scar tissue. In the first operation, marking the vessels with a suture can be helpful for the second operation. In addition, using a handheld Doppler apparatus is helpful while looking for the pedicle. The authors suggest not skeletonizing the pedicle and dissecting it with small amounts of fibrotic and soft tissue in the vicinity. These precautions are beneficial in avoiding injury to the vessels. Moreover, a small amount of muscle tissue around the

pedicle can be included if the perforators are too small.[8–11]

Another disadvantage of using the pre-expanded flap is the need to perform the procedure in 2 stages. Usually, 2 weeks after surgery, serial expansions begin and this sometimes may be uncomfortable for the patient.

Risk of infection, implant exposure, and flap ischemia are also existing disadvantages related to tissue expanders.

POSTPROCEDURAL CARE

A drain is implanted near the expander, and taken out when drainage is lower than 30 mL a day. Two weeks after the operation, serial expansion started twice weekly. Expansion is terminated when the size exceeds approximately 25% more of the expander volume. A second operation is carried out a month after completion of the expansion. Mild venous congestion could be seen in the early postoperative period, but usually recovers spontaneously in a few days.

REHABILITATION AND RECOVERY

Physical therapy is started after the incision lines have healed for the patients who had axillary or antecubital contractures. We recommend the use of elastic bandages to the patients, where their use is possible for such extremities. This application accelerates recovery and decreases the edema faster.

OUTCOMES

All of the flap donor sites were closed primarily. Both the aesthetic and the functional results were satisfactory to the patients and the physicians (**Figs. 4**D, **5**D, and **6**D).

Fig. 3. Intraoperative view of the elevated flap. White arrows show the pedicle.

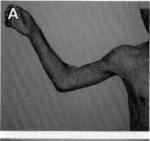
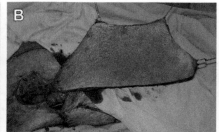
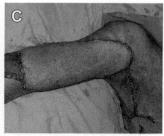
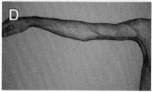

Fig. 4. (*A*) Preoperative appearance of the patient with right axillary contracture. (*B*) Intraoperative view of the patient after pre-expanded pedicled TDAP flap was harvested. (*C*) Intraoperative view of the patient after the flap was transferred to the recipient area. (*D*) Appearance of the patient 3 months postoperatively displaying rather favorable results.

Case 1

Fig. 4 portrays a patient who had been injured by a flame burn 12 years earlier. Planning for a pre-expanded TDAP flap began for reconstruction of the antecubital and axillary contractures. First, a rectangular tissue expander was placed under the flap and expanded to reach the desired size. In the second operation, the pre-expanded TDAP flap was harvested and transferred to the defect.

Case 2

A 21-year-old man had sustained burns to the right cubital region 15 years earlier due to flame burn (**Fig. 5**A). The pre-expanded pedicled TDAP flap

was planned for reconstruction (**Fig. 5**B). In the first stage, a 950-mL rectangular tissue expander was inserted. After 12 weeks, a total of 1250 mL saline was injected to reach the maximum expansion volume (**Fig. 5**C). In the second stage, the contracted scar tissue was completely excised and reconstructed with the pre-expanded TDAP flap (**Fig. 5**D).

Case 3

A 20-year-old man presented with congenital melanocytic nevi on his left ankle (**Fig. 6**A). A pre-expanded TDAP flap was planned to close the defect site. After 10 weeks of serial saline injection, a maximum expansion volume of 800 mL was

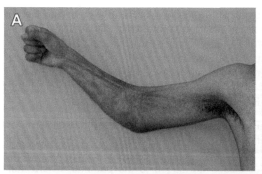
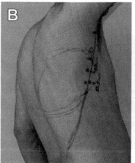
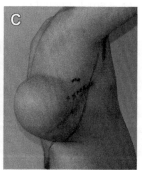
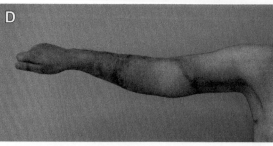

Fig. 5. (*A*) Preoperative appearance of the patient with right cubital contracture. (*B*) Preoperative view of the planning. (*C*) Preoperative appearance of the expanded flap. (*D*) Appearance of the patient 3.5 months postoperatively.

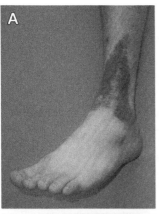
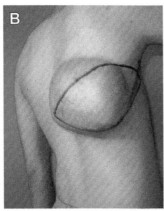
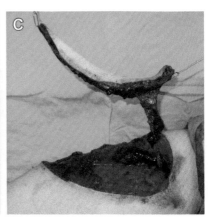
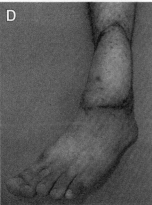

Fig. 6. (*A*) Preoperative appearance of the patient with melanocytic nevi on his left ankle. (*B*) Preoperative appearance of the expanded flap. (*C*) Intraoperative view of the harvested TDAP flap. (*D*) Appearance of the patient 1.5 months postoperatively.

reached (**Fig. 6**B). In the second stage, melanocytic nevi were excised and the flap was transferred to the defect (**Fig. 6**C, D).

DISCUSSION

TDAP flaps have been used progressively in reconstructive surgery as pedicled flaps or free flaps. The wide preference for the TDAP flap is attributable to its following characteristics: the basic and reliable anatomy, the ability to be thinned, obtaining a long pedicle, lack of significant donor site morbidity, and the pliability of the flap.[3,8] However, the requirement of a large flap will increase the donor site problems. If the width of the flap is less than 8 cm, the donor area can be closed directly without skin grafting. If it exceeds 8 cm, the donor site must be skin grafted. Pre-expanding the TDAP flap provides closure to the donor site primarily. Besides this, pre-expansion provides the flap that also has good vascularity and more dependable perforators.

Careful surgical planning by preoperative perforator mapping is necessary because it is possible to damage the perforators during dissection.[3]

Therefore, careful surgical planning by preoperative perforator mapping is needed. In the first operation, accurate positioning of perforators of flaps is essential for insertion of the tissue expander. The tissue expander should be inserted precisely over the central portions of the skin paddle supplied by perforators. This is also important for the accurate positioning of the expander. There are also some difficulties during the second stage. Identification of the perforator intraoperatively in the second stage of the operation may be difficult

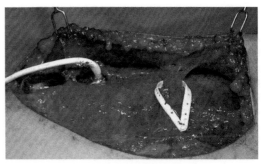

Fig. 7. Intraoperative view of the application of the silicone band around the vascular pedicle.

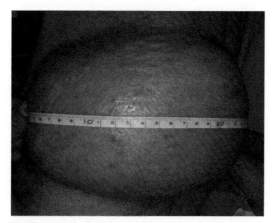

Fig. 8. A total of 1050 mL saline was injected to reach the desired size.

due to fibrotic tissue around the pedicle. Thus, it is useful to place a silicone band around the pedicle at the first surgical stage (**Fig. 7**). This facilitates the pedicle dissection in the second stage. Furthermore, it is better and safer to include a small amount of muscle and fibrotic tissue around the pedicle. The TDAP flap can be elevated up to 10 × 25 cm in size[8]; however, a pre-expanded TDAP flap can be elevated to 18 × 28 cm in size and the flap donor site can be closed primarily without difficulty. One perforator usually supplies enough blood to the flap that is indeed as large as 18 × 28 cm (**Fig. 8**). According to the authors' experiences, expanders of 650 to 950 mL can provide tissues of adequate size.

Kim and colleagues used a thinned TDAP flap for axillary burn scar contracture, and they obtained aesthetically desirable results.[16] In this study, we did not perform flap thinning. It is known that the dermal, fatty, and muscular components are thinned after expansion.[17] We observed that pre-expanded TDAP flaps were thinned in these series when we compared our previous experiences with the TDAP flap.[18,19]

SUMMARY

Although flap dissection is challenging in the second operation because of the scar tissue, pre-expansion of the TDAP flap provides the opportunity to use a large-sized flap with a reliable anatomy. This flap can be used in a wide variety of areas, including the axillary, antecubital, hand, and foot.[3,4,8,11,20] Besides this, a pre-expanded flap also has the advantage of primary closure at the donor site and also possibly being preferred in the following situations: need for extensive tissue, no desire for use of a muscle flap, wanting to hide the scar, intention to close the donor site primarily, requirement for using hairless tissue, and necessitating a long pedicle or a thin flap.

REFERENCES

1. Angrigiani C, Grilli D, Siebert JW. Latissimus dorsi musculocutaneous flap without muscle. Plast Reconstr Surg 1995;96:1608–14.
2. Heitmann C, Guerra A, Metzinger SW, et al. The thoracodorsal artery perforator flap: anatomic basis and clinical application. Ann Plast Surg 2003;51(1):23–9.
3. Er E, Uçar C. Reconstruction of axillary contractures with thoracodorsal perforator island flap. Burns 2005;31:726–30.
4. Ayhan S, Tuncer S, Demir Y, et al. Thoracodorsal artery perforator flap: a versatile alternative for various soft tissue defects. J Reconstr Microsurg 2008;24: 285–93.
5. Hamdi M, Van Landuyt K, Monstrey S, et al. A clinical experience with perforator flaps in the coverage of extensive defects of the upper extremity. Plast Reconstr Surg 2004;113:1175–83.
6. Jeon B, Lim SY, Pyon JK, et al. Secondary extremity reconstruction with free perforator flaps for aesthetic purposes. J Plast Reconstr Aesthet Surg 2011;64: 1483–9.
7. Mun GH, Lim SY, Hyun WS, et al. Correction of temporo-masseteric contour deformity using the dual paddle thoracodorsal artery perforator adiposal flap. J Reconstr Microsurg 2006;22:335–42.
8. Ortiz CL, Mendoza MM, Sempere LN, et al. Versatility of the pedicled thoracodorsal artery perforator (TDAP) flap in soft tissue reconstruction. Ann Plast Surg 2007;58:315–20.
9. Scaglioni MF, Chen YC, Yanko-Arzi R, et al. Upper extremity sarcoma reconstruction with a pedicle thoracodorsal artery perforator flap. J Reconstr Microsurg 2015;31(8):617–20.
10. Gunnarsson GL, Børsen-Koch M, Nielsen HT, et al. Bilateral breast reconstruction with extended thoracodorsal artery perforator propeller flaps and implants. Plast Reconstr Surg Glob Open 2015;3(6):e435.
11. Kulahci Y, Sever C, Uygur F, et al. Pre-expanded pedicled thoracodorsal artery perforator flap for postburn axillary contracture reconstruction. Microsurgery 2011;31:26–31.
12. Sever C, Bayram Y, Sahin C. Thoracodorsal artery perforator flap: basic surgical determinants. Arch Clin Exp Surg 2012;1(4):270–1.
13. Mun GH, Lee SJ, Jeon BJ. Perforator topography of the thoracodorsal artery perforator flap. Plast Reconstr Surg 2008;121(2):497–504.
14. Guerra AB, Metzinger SE, Lund KM, et al. The thoracodorsal artery perforator flap: clinical experience and anatomic study with emphasis on harvest

techniques. Plast Reconstr Surg 2004;114(1):32–41 [discussion: 42–3].

15. Hocaoğlu E, Emeklı U, Çızmecı O, et al. Suprafascial pre-expansion of perforator flaps and the effect of pre-expansion on perforator artery diameter. Microsurgery 2014;34(3):188–96.

16. Kim DY, Jeong EC, Kim KS, et al. Thinning of the thoracodorsal perforator-based cutaneous flap for axillary burn scar contracture. Plast Reconstr Surg 2002;109:1372–7.

17. Slavin SA. Improving the latissimus dorsi myocutaneous flap with tissue expansion. Plast Reconstr Surg 1994;93:811–24.

18. Uygur F, Kulahci Y, Sever C, et al. Reconstruction of postburn thenar contractures using the free thoracodorsal artery perforator flap. Plast Reconstr Surg 2009;124:217–21.

19. Uygur F, Sever C, Tuncer S, et al. Reconstruction of postburn antebrachial contractures using pedicled thoracodorsal artery perforator flaps. Plast Reconstr Surg 2009;123:1544–52.

20. Hocaoğlu E, Arıncı A, Berköz Ö, et al. Free pre-expanded lateral circumflex femoral artery perforator flap for extensive resurfacing and reconstruction of the hand. J Plast Reconstr Aesthet Surg 2013; 66(12):1788–91.

Pre-expanded Paraumbilical Perforator Flap

Yuanbo Liu, MD*, Mengqing Zang, MD, Shan Zhu, MD,
Bo Chen, MD, Qiang Ding, MD

KEYWORDS

- Perforator flap • Pre-expansion • Paraumbilical perforators • Upper extremity reconstruction

KEY POINTS

- Paraumbilical perforator flap is based on deep inferior epigastric artery perforators, with a supero-lateral extension of skin paddle to the lateral chest wall.
- Many of the disadvantages of pedicled paraumbilical perforator flaps are offset by pretransfer expansion.
- With proper planning and precise definition of the pre-expansion area, the expander placement is quick and safe.
- Because there is no need to dissect the perforators through the muscle, expanded pedicled para-umbilical perforator flaps are reliable and easy to elevate.
- Capsulectomy and primary thinning of the flap are safely performed.

INTRODUCTION

The paraumbilical perforator flap is a paraumbilical flap based on the perforators derived from the deep inferior epigastric artery (DIEA). According to the "Gent" consensus on perforator flap terminology,[1] it should be called DIEA perforator flap. The paraumbilical perforator flap was first described by Koshima and coworkers in 1991.[2] He later described this flap as a superthin DIEA perforator flap[3] or paraumbilical perforator flaps without DIEA[4] that required supermicrosurgery for vascular anastomosis. Nowadays, most authors use the name "paraumbilical perforator flap" to address a flap design that is different from the DIEA perforator flap with the transverse skin paddle for breast reconstruction.[4,5]

The early anatomic study of Taylor and colleagues[6] showed that the perforators from DIEA extended radially like the spokes of a wheel.[7] The perforators connect with other artery systems in anterior trunk via choke vessel, including deep superior epigastric artery, intercostal artery, and superficial inferior epigastric artery. The flap can be elevated in many directions along the axes that radiated from the umbilicus. However, because of the dominant connections with intercostal artery perforators, the best flap design seems to be the one planned along the axis between the umbilicus and the inferior angle of the scapula.[6,7]

The flap based on DIEA perforators with supero-lateral extension of skin paddle was called the oblique paraumbilical perforator flap by some and the extended DIEA perforator flap by others.[5,8] Compared with the transversely designed DIEA perforator flap, this obliquely extended flap has longer pedicle and larger arc of rotation, and its

Disclosures: The authors have nothing to disclose.
Department of Plastic and Reconstructive Surgery, Plastic Surgery Hospital, Peking Union Medical College and Chinese Academy of Medical Sciences, Ba-Da-Chu Road 33#, Beijing 100144, P.R. China
* Corresponding author.
E-mail address: ybpumc@sina.com

Clin Plastic Surg 44 (2017) 99–108
http://dx.doi.org/10.1016/j.cps.2016.08.003

distal portion from the chest wall was relatively thin, thus it was suggested as a good distant pedicled flap option for upper extremity reconstruction.[6] The flap was found to offer reliable coverage for the hand, wrist, and forearm.[9–14]

However, the usage of this flap in upper extremity reconstruction is limited by several factors. The donor tissue can be insufficient when dealing with massive wounds. The relative thick abdominal portion of the flap, especially in obese patients, appears bulky and unnatural in the upper extremity. In addition, the pedicled flap, owing to the limited pedicle length, can hardly reach defects beyond the proximal forearm. To overcome those limitations, we combined the flap transfer with pretransfer expansion. In this article, we demonstrate the value of pre-expanded perforator-based paraumbilical flaps in upper extremity reconstruction and summarize our experiences of using this technique in patients with extensive upper extremity soft tissue defects.

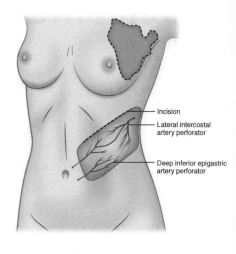

Fig. 1. Graphic scheme of the design of the pre-expanded flap design.

TREATMENT GOALS AND PLANNED OUTCOMES

We applied the pre-expanded paraumbilical perforator flap mainly in patients with extensive scar and giant congenital melanocytic nevi in upper extremity, to achieve excellent functional and aesthetic outcomes. This technique provides a large, thin flap with similar color and texture for upper extremity reconstruction. Our experience with more than 90 flaps supports the claim that this technique is safe and successful in achieving superior aesthetic results. When properly planned and performed, these operations have a low complication rate and minimal donor site morbidity.

PREOPERATIVE PLANNING AND PREPARATION

Before implantation of the tissue expander, the dimension of the wound is evaluated (**Figs. 1** and **2**). In the cases of burn reconstruction, the defect size following scar contracture release is estimated by referring to the corresponding area in the unaffected side. Doppler ultrasound probe is used to identify at least two large perforators adjacent to the ipsilateral umbilicus.

The pre-expanded area is designed slightly larger than the estimated defect dimension in the anterior abdomen, and is oriented along the axis between the umbilicus and the inferior angle of the scapula. We plan the medial border of pre-expanded area just lateral to the points where we

detect the perforators. The pre-expanded area can be extended to the posterior axillary line, creating a sufficient space for placing a large expander in adult and pediatric patients. The pre-expansion area usually includes the lower ribs superiorly in the chest wall. Because the hard thoracic cage cannot absorb the expansion force of tissue expanders, the tissue expansion over the chest wall is effective. However, in the female patient, expansion of the area immediately below the inframammary fold should be avoided to prevent breast deformation.

PATIENT POSITIONING

For tissue expander placement and removal, the patient should be in the supine position with the affected upper extremity abducted. For the second stage-procedure, we usually plan the lateral border of the flap at the posterior axillary line. To give a better exposure of this area, cushions should be put under the patients' buttock and shoulder. This maneuver facilitates the flap elevation and closure of the donor site.

PROCEDURAL APPROACH
Pre-expansion of the Paraumbilical Perforator Flap

The superior edge of the designed area is selected as the incision for expander placement. The incision is made down to the deep fascia and a pocket is created superficially to the external oblique aponeurosis within the marked

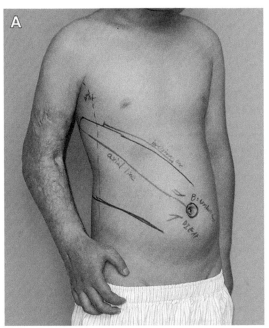
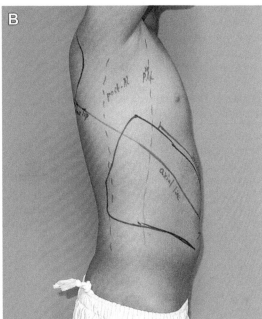

Fig. 2. (*A*) Two large perforators in the paraumbilical area were detected by using Doppler ultrasound probe. The pre-expanded area was oriented along the axis between the umbilicus and the inferior angle of the scapula. The superior border was selected as the incision for expander placement. (*B*) The pre-expanded area was extended laterally to the posterior axillary line.

pre-expansion area. The dissection is carried out quickly by using electrotome until the selected perforators are visualized. To avoid potential damage to the perforators, we do not expose the penetrating point from the anterior sheath of the perforator (**Fig. 3**A). Other perforators emerging during the dissection, especially from the intercostal artery system, are ligated using bipolar coagulator or clips (**Fig. 3**B). Then the rectangular expanders with proper size are placed into the pocket. In some adult patients, two large expanders might be implanted. The filler valves are routinely positioned over the lateral chest wall.

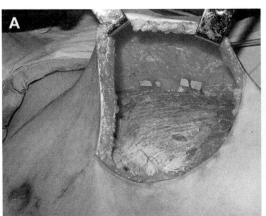
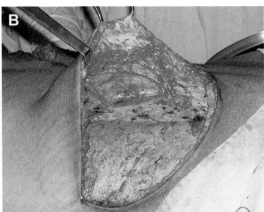

Fig. 3. (*A*) During the dissection, several perforators were observed penetrating the external oblique abdominal muscle. These perforators derived from intercostal artery and were ligated to initiate a delay effect. (*B*) The paraumbilical perforators previously detected were visualized and the dissection was terminated at this point to avoid incidental damage of the pedicle perforators.

Expansion is begun 14 days later with normal saline added on a weekly interval until adequate volume has been achieved. The flap is always overexpanded to obtain more donor tissue and to achieve direct closure of the donor site.

Transfer of Pre-expanded Paraumbilical Perforator Flap

The perforators are relocated using the Doppler probe. A pattern is made and placed over the expanded skin. The dimension of the flap is marked making the previous incision the flap superior border. A wide pedicle is designed to include the preoperatively identified perforators and to facilitate skin tube formation.

With consideration of minimal pedicle tension and most comfortable arm position following flap transfer, only half of the upper extremity lesion is resected. The flap is elevated following the expander removal (**Fig. 4**A). As a pedicle flap, dissection of the perforators during the flap elevation is unnecessary. Capsulectomy and immediate flap debulking are performed in some patients with relatively thick flaps. The capsule near the pedicle is preserved to protect the perforators and their branches (**Fig. 4**B, C). The flap is then transferred and inset to the upper extremity wound, with its proximal portion sutured as a skin tube. The donor site is directly closed after drainage placement. The patient's arm is immobilized to avoid pedicle avulsion with assistance of a circumferential bandage.

Division of Pre-expanded Paraumbilical Perforator Flap Pedicle

Three weeks after flap transfer, the pedicle is divided at its desired length. The perforators in the pedicle are ligated. The residual lesion in upper extremity is excised and reconstructed. Because the pedicle area is not efficiently expanded, flap debulking is usually performed. The extra tissue is reinserted back to the donor site.

POTENTIAL COMPLICATIONS AND MANAGEMENT
Complications Associated with the Expansion

Tissue expansion is associated with a high rate of complication with initial attempt. However, as more experiences accumulate, the incidence of complications decreases. The complications include, but are not limited to, hematoma, infection, implant failure, and exposure. In our cases, the rate of complication associated with the expansion was low. Hematoma occurred in one pediatric patient after the surgery and required surgical exploration. A new expander was placed following the hematoma debridement. The postoperative course was uneventful. Because of the extensive dissection, perfect hemostasis should constantly be sought in every case, especially for pediatric patients. Early mobilization is not encouraged in the first 48 hours after surgery.

Vascular Complications of the Flaps

There was no total flap loss in our series. Partial flap necrosis and venous congestion in the distal part of the flap were observed in our earlier cases. They happened when we tried to recruit more tissue beyond the posterior axillary line or when the pedicle was kinking, compressed, or stretched. Local debridement was performed if partial flap was lost. The wound was either healed secondarily, closed directly, or skin grafted, depending on the size of the resultant defects.

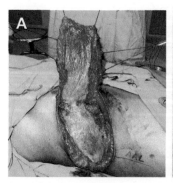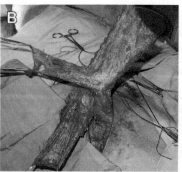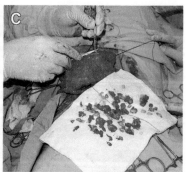

Fig. 4. (*A*) The perforators from DIEA could be observed through the thin capsule after the elevation of the pre-expanded flap. (*B*) The capsule and Scarpa fascia could be removed quickly by using electrotome or tissue scissors. (*C*) The large fat lobules in the deep layer of the Camper fascia were carefully removed using microsurgical dissection.

Complications of the Donor Site

Seroma formation developed in some flaps and the abdominal donor site after the second stage of surgery, which was treated with repeated aspiration and resolved. It is important to exert proper compression on the flap to prevent seroma formation under the flap. The seroma blocks vascular ingrowth into the flap from the wound bed. Flap division was delayed in such situations. Seroma in the donor site often causes wound-healing problems, so these areas should be drained with suction drains until all excess drainage stops. A compression garment can also be used postoperatively.

Infection occurred in the abdominal donor sites in some cases after the pedicle division. Infection was usually caused by the introduction of bacteria to the unhealed wound. We suggest antibiotics be given if there is an open wound in the donor site before the pedicle division.

POSTPROCEDURAL CARE

After the expander implantation, drainage and temperature of patients need to be carefully monitored. Drains are usually taken out on postoperative day 2 or 3 when drainage decreased to 30 mL per day. Expansion is begun 14 days after surgery with normal saline added on a weekly interval.

Flap monitoring is performed clinically after the expanded flap is transferred. If the distal portion of the flap shows sign of venous congestion, one should check if the pedicle tube is twisted or kinking. A circumferential bandage is used to immobilize the upper extremity to avoid avulsion of the pedicle. Patients are usually discharged on postoperative day 4 to 6.

Dress changing is performed every 3 days. The patients usually get used to the gesture 7 days later and the bandage can be loosened to allow limited movement of the shoulder and elbow. Vascular ingrowths of the flap are confirmed by clamping the pedicle, following 7-day pedicle clamping training.

Followed the pedicle division, flap monitoring is performed as mentioned previously. Flap debulking and scar revision are performed 3 months later if necessary.

REHABILITATION AND RECOVERY

Oral analgesics are routinely given for 2 days to alleviate pain caused by shoulder movement after long-time immobilization. Patients are asked to use silicone gel sheet to prevent scar proliferation in donor and recipient sites for 6 months.

OUTCOMES

The perforator-based paraumbilical flaps were expanded over 10 to 24 weeks. The expander ranged in size from 300 mL to 800 mL. Single expander was used in most cases. Some adult patients required double expanders. Expanded flaps were used to resurface wounds of the hand, forearm, elbow, and upper arm. For circumferential lesions of upper extremity, bilateral paraumbilical perforator flaps were expanded and used for reconstruction. The maximum size of the expanded flap was 30 cm × 14 cm. All abdominal donor sites were closed directly. Flap with the width up to 10 cm to 14 cm is harvested without displacing the nipple and umbilicus. Widening of the abdominal scar is expected as the children grow up. Scar revision might be required in upper extremity and abdomen. Repeated flap debulking was demanded by patients with extremely thick abdominal flaps.

CASE 1

A 9-year-old boy presented with congenital melanocytic nevi on his left dorsal hand. A 400-mL expander was placed and expansion was performed for 11 weeks. The defect following the nevi resection was reconstructed with an 8 cm × 7 cm pedicle paraumbilical perforator flap. Capsulectomy and flap debulking was performed at the same time. The patient's flap survived without complications (**Fig. 5**).

CASE 2

A 4-year-old girl had congenital giant melanocytic nevi on her right forearm. One 600-mL rectangular expander was placed through the superior incision. After expansion for 7 months, a 19 cm × 14 cm flap was elevated based on the paraumbilical perforators. The postoperative course was uneventful. The patient underwent flap debulking twice in the following 3 years. The final aesthetic results were satisfactory (**Fig. 6**).

CASE 3

A 12-year-old boy had a burn scar contracture of his right elbow. A 600-mL expander was placed and expanded for 22 weeks. A 20 cm × 8 cm pedicle paraumbilical flap was transferred to repair his elbow defect following the scar contracture release. The flap survived completely without complications (**Fig. 7**).

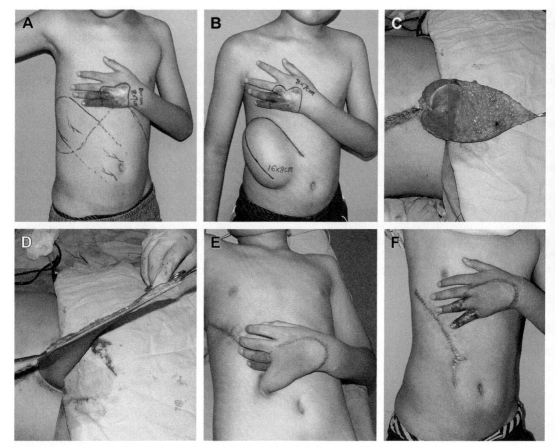

Fig. 5. (*A*) Preoperative flap design and the defect location. (*B*) The expander has been adequately expanded. (*C*) A pedicle paraumbilical perforator flap has been raised. (*D*) A thin flap was obtained by capsulectomy and flap debulking. (*E*) The distal portion of the flap was attached to the dorsum of the hand. (*F*) Postoperative view.

CASE 4

A 4-year-old girl had circumferential melanocytic nevi on her right forearm and wrist, extending to her dorsal hand. Bilateral paraumbilical perforator flaps were designed to resurface the resultant defect following the nevi resection. A 600-mL rectangular expander was placed in each side of her abdomen. After expansion for 4 months, the ipsilateral expanded paraumbilical perforator flap first resurfaced the extensor region of her forearm, wrist, and dorsal hand. After 3 weeks, at the same time of pedicle division, the expander at the left side was removed and the expanded flap was formed into a tube. The flexor region of the forearm and wrist was resurfaced by the contralateral paraumbilical perforator flap 3 weeks later. After the pedicle division, the residual expanded flap was used for skin grafting the dorsal area of the thumb and fingers. The patient was followed up for 2 and half years (**Fig. 8**).

DISCUSSION

The oblique skin paddle design of the abdominal flap was introduced by Taylor and colleagues[6] in 1983. Based on their delicate anatomic study of the DIEA system, the constant cluster of large paraumbilical perforators from DIEA could support a cutaneous flap extending from umbilicus for a considerable distance onto the chest wall.[6,7] The paraumbilical perforator flaps have several advantages for complex upper extremity wounds resurfacing, including largest cutaneous flap dimension, reliable blood supply, similar skin characteristics, and allowing relatively comfortable arm position.[15] Long-term arm immobilization and an additional surgery present great disadvantages of the pedicled paraumbilical perforator flap. However, we still prefer pedicle flap to free flaps. Free flap transfer is technically challenging in pediatric patients. In addition, the pedicle flap, although perforator-based, does not require

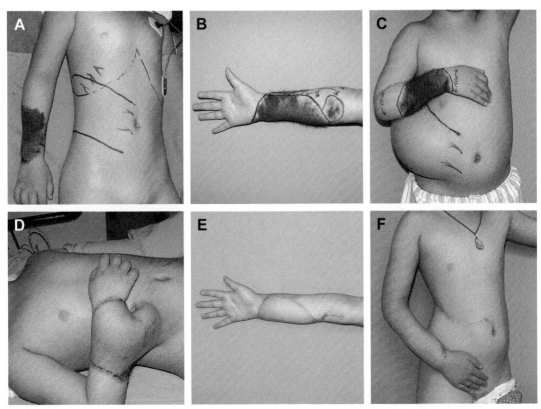

Fig. 6. (*A, B*) Preoperative views showing the flap design and location of the congenital melanocytic nevi. (*C*) The expander has been completely inflated. (*D*) The pre-expanded paraumbilical perforator flap was transferred to repair the dorsal defect of the forearm. (*E, F*) Postoperative views showing the appearance of both the donor and recipient sites.

dissecting out the perforators through the rectus abdominis muscle, reducing surgical time and complication risks. The wide pedicle of the flap usually included more than one perforator.

Pre-expansion made this flap a more effective tool for upper extremity reconstruction. Pre-expansion increased the flap length, allowing some range of motion of the shoulder and

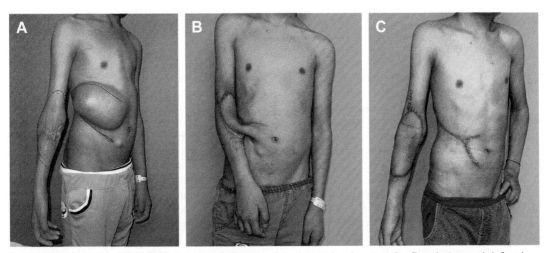

Fig. 7. (*A*) Preoperative view after complete inflation of the expander showing the flap design and defect location. (*B*) The distal portion of the right pre-expanded paraumbilical perforator flap was transferred to repair the elbow defect following partial removal of the scar. (*C*) Postoperative view showing the complete release of the scar contracture and also the appearance of the abdominal donor site.

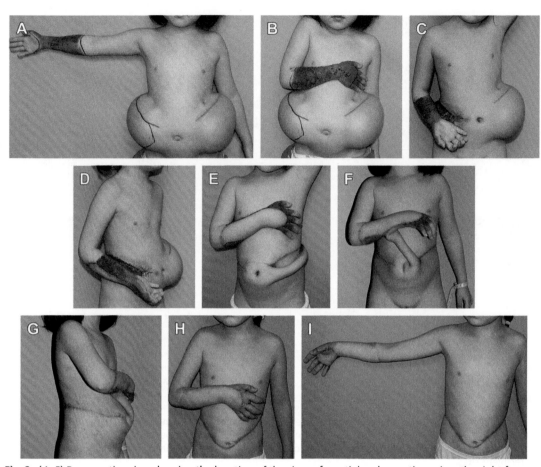

Fig. 8. (*A, B*) Preoperative view showing the location of the circumferential melanocytic nevi on the right forearm and wrist. Bilateral paraumbilical perforator flaps were adequately expanded. (*C, D*) The ipsilateral pre-expanded paraumbilical perforator flap was firstly used to resurface the extensor region of the forearm, wrist, and dorsal hand. (*E*) The right paraumbilical perforator flap was completely transferred to the right upper extremity. The expander at the left side was removed and the expanded paraumbilical perforator flap was formed into a tubed flap simultaneously. (*F, G*) The contralateral paraumbilical perforator flap was used to reconstruct the defect in the flexor region of the forearm and wrist. (*H, I*) Postoperative views showing the appearance of both the donor and recipient sites.

elbow during the immobilization period. The long pedicle also allowed the flap to reach the elbow and upper arm comfortably. Flap expansion produced thinning of the abdominal portion in all cases, improving the final contour of upper extremity. Donor site morbidity was decreased by pre-expansion, although the long scar in the abdominal region was unavoidable.[15]

Tissue expansion is a useful tool in prefabrication of flaps.[16] Our series demonstrated that the pretransfer expansion produced a more reliable and larger paraumbilical flap. The elongation of the flap was achieved not only by physical expansion but also by including additional component of distal skin. The anatomic study by injecting DIEA showed that skin staining was carried through the choke vessel onto the chest wall, reaching the anterior axillary line.[6,7] We demonstrated that it was safe to extend the flap to the posterior axillary line.[15] Both dissection of expander pocket and expansion can initiate delay effects, which allow the flap to catch more adjacent angiosomes.[17–19]

It was reported that perforator-based tissue expansion could be challenging, because of the possible damage of perforators.[20] However, with the precise preoperative design, pre-expansion is safely performed. Up to 100% of perforators are found within 5 cm of the umbilicus and the perforators are detected by using Doppler ultrasound probes.[21] The paraumbilical perforators run obliquely toward the chest wall in the fascial framework on the undersurface and within the subcutaneous fat.[6,7] In our series, the pre-expansion area was planned along the axis between the umbilicus and the inferior angle of scapula. The dissection was made above the deep fascia, which proved to be a safe surgical plane for flap elevation. To prevent incidental damage and capsule adherence to the musculocutaneous perforators during the expansion, dissection was stopped at visualization of the selected perforators. With precise definition of the pre-expansion area, we found the expander insertion and flap transfer was quick and straightforward.

Although the thickness of the flap was reduced by pre-expansion, the flap was sometimes still not thin enough to achieve a perfect contour of upper extremity. We tried to further decrease the flap thickness by capsulectomy and immediate flap debulking. Koshima and coworkers[2,3] first described the use of thin paraumbilical perforator-based flaps. He showed that it was possible to obtain a thin DIEA perforator flap by resecting most of the pannicular fat. Because vascular anastomoses are formed primarily in the subdermal vascular plexus, the subcutaneous fatty tissue in the distal portion of the flap can be extensively reduced without damaging the subdermal plexus.[2,3] However, other authors suggested that the thinning procedure was risky and should be performed at a later procedure.[22] Based on our experiences, we found that removal of the capsule, the Scarpa fascia, and the deep layer of the Camper fascia was safe in the primary procedure. We observed that there is always a small vessel in the cell of a large fat lobule. By preserving those vessels using microsurgical dissection, large fat lobules could be removed from the Camper fascia without compromising flap viability.

Despite several advantages, inherent disadvantages of pretransfer expansion, such as additional procedure, time investment of patients, and possible complications associated with the expansion, should be considered and communicated with patients. Although a relatively invisible site, the trade of the abdominal morbidities for upper extremity reconstruction should be carefully weighed.

SUMMARY

With the considerations of excellent functional and aesthetic outcomes, we think this pre-expanded paraumbilical flap is a good option for patients who have extensive, severe scarring in their upper extremities and high demand of aesthetic outcomes, with the premise that they are willing to invest more time in their treatment.

REFERENCES

1. Blondeel PN, Van Landuyt KH, Monstrey SJ, et al. The "Gent" consensus on perforator flap terminology: preliminary definitions. Plast Reconstr Surg 2003;112:1378–83.
2. Koshima I, Moriguchi T, Fukuda H, et al. Free, thinned, paraumbilical perforator-based flaps. J Reconstr Microsurg 1991;7:313–6.
3. Koshima I, Moriguchi T, Soeda S, et al. Free thin paraumbilical perforator-based flaps. Ann Plast Surg 1992;29:12–7.
4. Koshima I, Inagawa K, Urushibara K, et al. Paraumbilical perforator flap without deep inferior epigastric vessels. Plast Reconstr Surg 1998;102:1052–7.
5. Lassus P, De Leo A, Moussa IH, et al. Paraumbilical perforator flap for reconstruction of the external auditory meatus: a case report. Microsurgery 2015;35:573–5.
6. Taylor GI, Corlett R, Boyd JB. The extended deep inferior epigastric flap: a clinical technique. Plast Reconstr Surg 1983;72:751–65.
7. Boyd JB, Taylor GI, Corlett R. The vascular territories of the superior epigastric and the deep inferior epigastric systems. Plast Reconstr Surg 1984;73:1–16.
8. Masia J, Sommario M, Cervelli D, et al. Extended deep inferior epigastric artery perforator flap for head and neck reconstruction: a clinical experience with 100 patients. Head Neck 2011;33:1328–34.
9. Gutwein LG, Merrell GA, Knox KR. Paraumbilical perforator flap for soft tissue reconstruction of the forearm. J Hand Surg Am 2015;40:586–92.
10. Kamath BJ, Verghese T, Bhardwaj P. "Wing flaps": perforator-based pedicled paraumbilical flaps for skin defects in hand and forearm. Ann Plast Surg 2007;59:495–500.
11. O'Shaughnessy KD, Rawlani V, Hijjawi JB, et al. Oblique pedicled paraumbilical perforator-based flap for reconstruction of complex proximal and midforearm defects: a report of two cases. J Hand Surg Am 2010;35:1105–10.
12. Shukla L, Taylor GI, Shayan R. The pedicled inferior paraumbilical perforator (I-PUP) flap for a volar wrist defect: a reconstructive solution across the ages. J Plast Reconstr Aesthet Surg 2013;66:1613–5.
13. Yilmaz S, Saydam M, Seven E, et al. Paraumbilical perforator-based pedicled abdominal flap for extensive soft-tissue deficiencies of the forearm and hand. Ann Plast Surg 2005;54:365–8.
14. Hu XH, Qin FJ, Chen Z, et al. Combined rectus abdominis muscle/paraumbilical flap and lower abdominal flap for the treatment of type III circumferential electrical burns of the wrist. Burns 2013;39:1631–8.
15. Zang M, Zhu S, Song B, et al. Reconstruction of extensive upper extremity defects using pre-expanded oblique perforator-based paraumbilical flaps. Burns 2012;38:917–23.

16. Abbase EA, Shenaq SM, Spira M, et al. Prefabricated flaps: experimental and clinical review. Plast Reconstr Surg 1995;96:1218–25.

17. Leighton WD, Russell RC, Marcus DE, et al. Experimental pretransfer expansion of free-flap donor sites: I. Flap viability and expansion characteristics. Plast Reconstr Surg 1988;82:69–75.

18. Leighton WD, Russell RC, Feller AM, et al. Experimental pretransfer expansion of free-flap donor sites: II. Physiology, histology, and clinical correlation. Plast Reconstr Surg 1988;82:76–87.

19. Russell RC, Khouri RK, Upton J, et al. The expanded scapular flap. Plast Reconstr Surg 1995;96:884–95 [discussion: 896–7].

20. Tsai FC. A new method: perforator-based tissue expansion for a preexpanded free cutaneous perforator flap. Burns 2003;29:845–8.

21. Ireton JE, Lakhiani C, Saint-Cyr M. Vascular anatomy of the deep inferior epigastric artery perforator flap: a systematic review. Plast Reconstr Surg 2014;134:810e–21e.

22. Wei FC, Mardini S. Flaps and reconstructive surgery. Philadelphia: Elsevier Health Sciences; 2009.

Pre-expanded Deep Inferior Epigastric Perforator Flap

Sharon E. Monsivais, MD, Nicholas D. Webster, MD,
Stacy Wong, MD, Michel H. Saint-Cyr, MD*

KEYWORDS

- Deep inferior epigastric perforator flap • DIEP • Pre-expansion • Tissue expansion

KEY POINTS

- Advantages of the pre-expanded deep inferior epigastric perforator (DIEP) flap include increased vascularity, primary closure of donor site, decreased donor site morbidity, local tissue use, and no need for microsurgery.
- Disadvantages include staged reconstruction, protracted timeline for serial expansion, and risks/complications associated with tissue expansion.
- During pre-expansion, make the incision according to final flap design, fixate the tissue expander in the subcutaneous plane, and wait a minimum of 4 weeks between final expansion and flap harvest.
- During flap harvest and inset, discard the lateral one-third of the flap, implement intraoperative Doppler monitoring throughout, and perform a pinch test prior to circumferential incision.

INTRODUCTION

The perforator flap has become an essential tool in the plastic surgeon's reconstructive armamentarium since its introduction by Kroll and Rosenfield in 1988.[1] Although initially described for lower posterior midline defects, perforator flaps have since been designated for use throughout the body. Understanding the vascular anatomy and dominant perforator location has increased flap selection options and improved customization for patients.

Taylor and Palmer[2] mapped skin and cutaneous vascular anatomy in 1987, identifying an average of 374 major perforators per subject and introducing the concept of the "angiosome." Perforator mapping laid the foundation for the "perforasome" theory, outlined by Saint-Cyr and colleagues,[3] which encompasses the arterial vascular territory of a single perforator. Its characteristics and relationship to neighboring vascular territories were studied, and optimal surgical techniques were conjectured based on those principles. Clinical application of this knowledge allows for more predictable and dependable results in perforator flap surgery (**Fig. 1**).

This article aims to delineate the anatomy, treatment goals, preoperative planning, operative principles, postprocedure care, and clinical results of the pre-expanded DIEP flap.

ANATOMY OF DEEP INFERIOR EPIGASTRIC PERFORATOR FLAP

First characterized by Koshima and Soeda in 1989, the DIEP flap is a transverse lower abdominal flap perfused by perforators of the DIEA.[4] Nuances of DIEP flap anatomy are complex and variable; however, recent anatomic studies have elucidated major principles to optimize its use.

Disclosure Statement: Pacira consultant (M.H. Saint-Cyr).
Division of Plastic Surgery, Baylor Scott & White Health, 2401 South 31st Street, Temple, TX 76508, USA
* Corresponding author.
E-mail address: Michel.SaintCyr@BSWHealth.org

Clin Plastic Surg 44 (2017) 109–115
http://dx.doi.org/10.1016/j.cps.2016.09.002

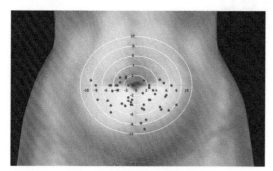

Fig. 1. Periumbilical DIEPs, external view.

The DIEA is the most significant artery supplying the skin of the anterior abdominal wall, and its pedicle ranges from 7.5 cm to 20.5 cm in length and 3.3 mm ± 0.4 mm in diameter, with 2 accompanying venae comitantes.[5] Although there are anatomic variations,[2] there are most commonly 2 main branches giving off medial and lateral row of perforators in the medial and lateral third of the rectus abdominis muscle, respectively.[6] The most robust perforators are typically in the periumbilical region (see **Fig. 1**; **Fig. 2**).

Schaverien and colleagues[7] used 3-D and 4-D CT angiography (CTA) and venography to study the arterial and venous anatomy of the DIEP flap. Their anatomic study determined that all perforators were located within 10 cm of the umbilicus. They found a mean of 5.3 perforators (range, 2 to 8) perforators greater than or equal to 0.5 mm in diameter per specimen. Perfusion occurred mostly through recurrent flow through the subdermal plexus, with horizontally oriented perforator complexes at the suprafascial level. Branches of the medial row perforators were seen to communicate with the medial row perforators across the midline at the level of the subdermal plexus as well as

perfusing lateral row perforators bilaterally, with extension to zone IV (of Hartrampf zones of perfusion [**Fig. 3**]). Lateral perforator vasculature, however, directed laterally with no visible perfusion of zone IV.[7]

Wong and colleagues[8] also expounded on the difference between medial and lateral row perforators in terms of DIEP flap vascular flow in their anatomic study. They determined that zone II perfusion was greater in medial perforators compared with lateral perforators, and zone III had greater perfusion from lateral perforators. Whereas medial perforators perfused zone II prior to zone III, the sequence of perfusion in lateral perforators was reversed.[8]

TREATMENT GOALS AND PLANNED OUTCOMES

Pre-expansion of the DIEP flap allows it to attain reconstructive goals, including coverage of large defects, primary closure of the donor site, and minimizing morbidity. Well known for its role in autologous breast reconstruction as a free flap, the DIEP flap also has been described in its pedicled form to repair defects of the proximal lower extremity,[9–11] abdominal wall,[12–14] perineum,[15,16] vulva,[17–20] and buttock.[21] Despite its versatility and reliability, local donor tissue availability may limit its utilization for large defects. Through use of tissue expansion, the pre-expanded DIEP flap can now cover large defects in those regions. Tissue expansion is a principle of reconstructive plastic surgery in which mechanical stress applied to skin provides additional cutaneous tissue with the added benefit of improved vascularity through mechanical and biologic creep. Pre-expansion has routinely been performed with traditional flaps and only more recently utilized in perforator flaps. Pre-expansion of the pedicled DIEP flap allows for reconstruction of a variety of defects in select cases, maximizing the benefits of tissue expansion and pedicled perforator flaps while minimizing patient morbidity.

PREOPERATIVE PLANNING AND PREPARATION

As with any major surgical procedure, it is imperative that surgeons optimize patients to the best of their ability and ensure that patients are able to withstand the rigors of surgery and the postoperative course. This includes preoperative work-up of patient comorbidities, especially those that might compromise healing or vasculature. Additionally, the use of CTA to assist in identification of perforators has become an integral step in preoperative

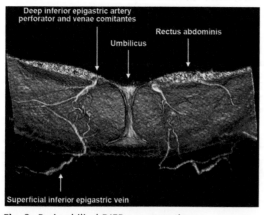

Deep inferior epigastric artery perforator and venae comitantes

Rectus abdominis

Umbilicus

Superficial inferior epigastric vein

Fig. 2. Periumbilical DIEPs, cross-section.

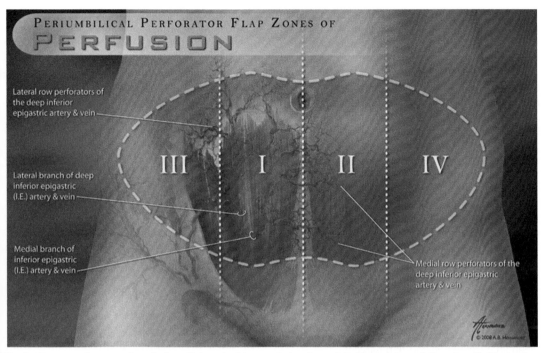

Fig. 3. Hartrampf zones of perfusion. (Printed with permission from A.B. Hernandez of Gory Details Illustration, Grapevine, TX.)

planning (**Fig. 4**). Imaging allows a surgeon to identify major perforators and thus the ability to reduce operating time. Keys and colleagues[22] note that although it can be extremely useful, clinical judgment is ultimately the deciding factor in determining which perforator to isolate and use; therefore, surgeons cannot solely rely on preoperative imaging for perforator selection.

PATIENT POSITIONING

Patient positioning for tissue expander placement can be successfully performed for the most part with supine positioning and sterile

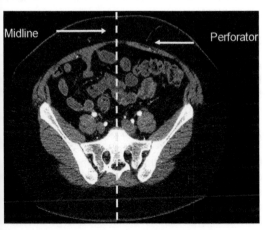

Fig. 4. CTA demonstrating a DIEA perforator.

preparation to the lateral flanks bilaterally. Positioning for the flap harvest and inset depends on the location of proposed reconstruction. Supine is sufficient for upper abdominal and anterior proximal lower extremity defects; however, lithotomy may be required for vulvar/perineal defects and frog leg position for the medial proximal lower extremity.

PROCEDURAL APPROACH
Expander Placement and Expansion Process

Tissue expander selection is dictated by anatomic site as well as amount of tissue needing to be expanded. Shapes include round, rectangular, and crescent as well as anatomic for breast pocket expansion. Expanders are also available to be customized with regard to final fill volume.

In designing the pre-expanded DIEP, ideally the incision line should be placed within the incision design of the flap and oriented along the long axis of the expander. A transverse skin paddle design accommodates this nicely. A subcutaneous plane is chosen because it has the advantages of precise pocket creation, has a lower risk of seroma, and allows for a faster expansion process postoperatively. It is important to have the expander placed over an area in the abdomen where it can be against a bony structure, such as ribs or the iliac crest. This not only provides more control of the projection of expansion but also decreases patient discomfort. The final position of the expander should be beneath perfusion zones I and II of the flap. Fixation of the expander is important to reduce the risk of migration or rotation of the expander. Ports can be integrated within the expander itself or be connected by customizable length tubing, which is outside of the body. Selection of the port is at the discretion of the surgeon; an incorporated port has the risk of expander compromise if the port is missed during filling, but an exteriorized port has the risk of introducing bacteria via the tubing.

Postoperatively, drains are placed to reduce the risk of seroma formation for the first 5 to 7 days, and prophylactic antibiotics are imperative as long as the drains remain in place. The expansion process does not move forward until the incision site is well healed, which can potentially be within 7 days as long as the skin flaps appear well perfused and healthy. Expansion can occur once per week every 2 to 3 weeks depending on local tissue laxity, patient comfort level, and anticipated final volume. There is a minimum of 4 weeks between final expansion and flap harvest.

Flap Harvest/Inset

Pedicle flaps offer the advantage of no microsurgery, which can theoretically decrease operative time. Surgeons must always remain cognizant of certain crucial details. Once the perforator has been identified and dissected, care must be taken to ensure it does not become twisted or kinked during the inset. Additional perforator length can be obtained to prevent kinking or twisting, with curvilinear pedicle inset. Doppler signal of the selected perforator should occur regularly through the dissection, prior to any mobilization, and after inset. Arterial and venous Doppler signal, capillary refill, and signs of venous congestion should be assessed. The superficial inferior epigastric vein may be harvested and anastomosed when additional venous outflow is needed. It is also imperative to perform a pinch test of the tissue prior to any final circumferential excisions, to ensure adequate tissue laxity for closure. Minimizing the degree of rotation decreases flap complications; flap rotation should ideally be 90° from its native position. Lastly, the lateral one-third of the flap has the highest risk for ischemia and, thus, should be discarded.

POTENTIAL COMPLICATIONS AND MANAGEMENT

The most common acute complication is venous congestion. This can be caused by tight inset that causes compression of the vein, hematoma,

and flap design. Progressive tension sutures can offset any tension when insetting the flap and should be used liberally. It is important to identify venous congestion early and return to the operating room for reinset, evacuation of hematoma, or supercharging to help prevent flap loss. Flaps that cross joints are at higher risk for mechanical compression with ambulation, and those on the perineum or buttock can be compressed with sitting and laying down. It is important to be aware of this and avoid pressure and compression postoperatively. Other potential complications include seroma, hematoma, extrusion, infection, and wound dehiscence. Cases of hematoma and extrusion are managed with return to the operating room. Seroma may be attempted to be drained percutaneously. Infected tissue expanders require removal.

POSTPROCEDURAL CARE

Like other pedicle perforator flaps, the expanded DIEP requires postoperative monitoring similar to free flaps. Complications that can benefit from rapid operative intervention are most likely to occur in the first 24 hours after surgery, so patients remain in the hospital 1 day on average. Avoidance of hypotension and medications that cause peripheral vasoconstriction are critical.

Flap monitoring is generally performed using pencil Doppler and clinical examination. It is imperative that the nursing staff is trained to monitor the flap using temperature, capillary refill, color, Doppler, or any other adjunct. Hand-offs between staff should have both parties present so there is no confusion about the status of the flap. It is sometimes helpful to provide an immediate postoperative color photo as a point of comparison at bedside. There is limited evidence about pedicled perforator flap monitoring but hourly checks for the first 24 hours or while hospitalized are prudent.

REHABILITATION/RECOVERY

After inset of the flap, drains remain in place for 2 to 3 weeks. A locoregional block can be performed to assist with postoperative pain, along with other enhanced recovery after surgery protocols.

OUTCOMES

In the experience of the senior author (M.H. Saint-Cyr), the pre-expanded pedicled DIEP flap was applied in conjunction with a pre-expanded contralateral superficial inferior epigastric artery flap for staged reconstruction of a large anterior abdominal scar and soft tissue defect status

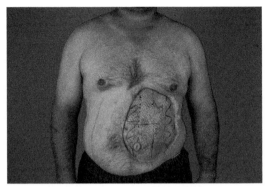

Fig. 5. Preoperative anteroposterior view of large burn defect, nipple asymmetry, and healed skin grafts. The surrounding tissue laxity was insufficient for complete primary closure.

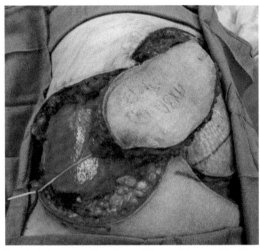

Fig. 7. Intraoperative view of the right propeller DIEP flap rotated into the defect. The prior skin graft is now completely excised and the left expander has been removed to permit advancement of the left abdominal skin flap using progressive tension sutures. The flap is completely inset with several drains and primary closure of the donor site.

post–burn injury. The patient experienced improved abdominal contour with primary closure of the donor sites and minimal donor site morbidity (**Figs. 5–8**).[23]

DISCUSSION

The pre-expanded pedicled DIEP flap is indicated for use in the anatomic distribution of the pedicled DIEP flap, including the proximal lower extremity, abdominal wall, perineum, vulva, and buttock, but provides a larger donor surface area with

potentially enhanced circulation. By pre-expanding the DIEP flap, the flap benefits from a delay phenomenon with enhanced vascularity. It has been firmly established that the number and caliber of vessels in an expanded flap are superior to its nonexpanded counterpart.[24] Shang and colleagues[25] described their series of 18 patients who suffered burn contracture of the hand, wrist, and/or forearm. The investigators performed buried pre-expanded DIEP flaps with good functional

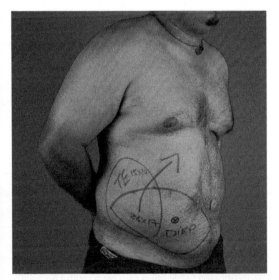

Fig. 6. Oblique view of the planned pre-expanded DIEP flap from the right abdomen based on a lateral row DIEP (*blue*) identified using pencil Doppler; CTA imaging is shown with TE (*green*) indicating the expander position and the skin island is marked (*purple*).

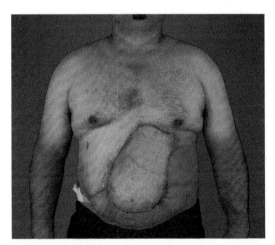

Fig. 8. Postoperative anteroposterior view demonstrating improvement in the abdominal soft tissue contour, minimal donor site distortion, and improved nipple position symmetry.

Table 1
Clinical results of the pre-expanded deep inferior epigastric perforator flap

Author	Location of Defect	Size of Defect/Flap	Notes
Cheng & Saint-Cyr,[23] 2013	Anterior abdomen	30 cm × 24 cm	Used in conjunction with pre-expanded contralateral superficial inferior epigastric artery flap
Shang et al,[25] 2011	Upper extremity	14 cm × 8 cm to 25 cm × 12 cm	Survival of 16 of 18 flaps; anatomic studies demonstrated 32.5% increase in mean diameter of perforator after expansion.
Song et al,[26] 2013	Forearm	22 cm × 9 cm	Anticipated abdominoplasty flap prefabricated and expanded, then used as a free flap for burn contracture of forearm
Margulis et al,[27] 2010	Posterior neck and upper back	21 cm × 15 cm	For giant congenital melanocytic nevus in a 4-year-old boy; six months later, successful in situ re-expansion for further excision of nevus
Grinsell et al,[28] 2012	Lower extremity	26 cm × 19 cm	Bipedicled pre-expanded DIEP flap

result and high patient satisfaction in the 16 flaps that survived. They also used CTA before and after expansion. They noted an increase in perforator diameter by an average of 32.5%.[25]

The pre-expanded DIEP flap has also been used as a free flap. Song and colleagues[26] reported their use of the flap for a forearm burn scar deformity. The deep inferior epigastric vessels were anastomosed to the radial artery and vein. Anastomosis of the deep inferior epigastric vessels was performed with the facial vessels in an account by Margulis and colleagues[27] for a child with giant congenital melanocytic nevus of the posterior neck and upper back. Grinsell and colleagues[28] used the pre-expanded pedicled DIEP flap for reconstruction of a large lower extremity wound (26 cm × 19 cm) in a pediatric patient after removal of a neurofibroma (**Table 1**).

The pre-expanded DIEP flap is an excellent reconstructive option with appropriate patient selection. Because the flap requires staged operations and multiple outpatient appointments for progressive tissue expansion, patients need to be amenable to a protracted timeline. It is better used in patients with posttraumatic or burn deformities and less suitable for cancer patients who may require more immediate reconstruction.

Perforator flaps are the product of better understanding of perforator anatomy and elucidation of the perforasome theory. Pedicled flaps decrease operative time by obviating microsurgery.

DIEP-based pedicled perforator flaps can be used to cover defects of the proximal lower extremity, abdominal wall, perineum, vulva, and buttock. Free flaps can be designed using this perforator as well.

Pre-expanding DIEP flaps causes a possible delay phenomenon improving flap survival, decreases donor site morbidity, and increases the area that can be covered. Pre-expansion requires more procedures, has risk of extrusion and infection, has temporary contour deformity during the expansion process, and requires a longer course. Patient selection is especially important in the use of tissue expansion.

It is important to adequately free up the perforator to prevent kinking. The flap must be monitored in a similar manner to a free flap. Supercharging can decrease the risk of venous congestion. All members of the team caring for patients postoperatively should be familiar with flap monitoring techniques to allow for rapid return to the operating room for any necessary salvage procedures.

SUMMARY

Pre-expanded DIEP flaps can be a useful flap with proper patient selection and planning for reconstructing various large adjacent or distant defects, especially for abdominal wall defect with good reconstructive outcome but minimal donor site morbidity.

REFERENCES

1. Kroll SS, Rosenfield L. Perforator-based flaps for low posterior midline defects. Plast Reconstr Surg 1988; 81(4):561–6.
2. Taylor GI, Palmer JH. The vascular territories (angiosomes) of the body: experimental study and clinical applications. Br J Plast Surg 1987;40(2):113–41.
3. Saint-Cyr M, Wong C, Schaverien M, et al. The perforasome theory: vascular anatomy and clinical implications. Plast Reconstr Surg 2009;124(5): 1529–44.
4. Koshima I, Soeda S. Inferior epigastric artery skin flaps without rectus abdominis muscle. Br J Plast Surg 1989;42(6):645–8.
5. Offman SL, Geddes CR, Tang M, et al. The vascular basis of perforator flaps based on the source arteries of the lateral lumbar region. Plast Reconstr Surg 2005;115(6):1651–9.
6. Moon HK, Taylor GI. The vascular anatomy of rectus abdominis musculocutaneous flaps based on the deep superior epigastric system. Plast Reconstr Surg 1988;82(5):815–32.
7. Schaverien M, Saint-Cyr M, Arbique G, et al. Arterial and venous anatomies of the deep inferior epigastric perforator and superficial inferior epigastric artery flaps. Plast Reconstr Surg 2008;121(6):1909–19.
8. Wong C, Saint-Cyr M, Mojallal A, et al. Perforasomes of the DIEP flap: vascular anatomy of the lateral versus medial row perforators and clinical implications. Plast Reconstr Surg 2010;125(3):772–82.
9. Gourari A, Quignon R, Tabareau-Delalande F, et al. Thigh root reconstruction with a pedicled DIEP flap. Ann Chir Plast Esthet 2014;59(3):212–4.
10. Faramarz FK, Martin E, Paraskevas A, et al. Coverage of pelvis and thigh region by pedicled perforator flap like deep inferior epigastric perforator (DIEP). Ann Chir Plast Esthet 2005;50(6):733–8.
11. Van Landuty K, Blondeel P, Hamdi M, et al. The versatile DIEP flap: its use in lower extremity reconstruction. Br J Plast Surg 2005;58(1):2–13.
12. Ang GG, Rozen WM, Chauhan A, et al. The pedicled 'propeller' deep inferior epigastric perforator (DIEP) flap for a large abdominal wall defect. J Plast Reconstr Aesthet Surg 2011;64(1):133–5.
13. Woo KJ, Pyon JK, Lim SY, et al. Deep superior epigastric artery perforator 'propeller' flap for abdominal wall reconstruction: a case report. J Plast Reconstr Aesthet Surg 2010;63(7):1223–6.
14. Scaglioni MF, Giuseppe AD, Chang EI. Propeller flap reconstruction of abdominal defects: review of the literature and case report. Microsurgery 2015; 35(1):72–8.
15. Fang BR, Ameet H, Li XF, et al. Pedicled thinned deep inferior epigastric artery perforator flap for perineal reconstruction: a preliminary report. J Plast Reconstr Aesthet Surg 2011;64(12):1627–34.
16. Classen D. The extended deep inferior epigastric flap: a case series. Ann Plast Surg 1999;42(2): 137–41.
17. Cheng A, Saint-Cyr M. Split and thinned pedicle deep inferior epigastric perforator (DIEP) flap for vulvar reconstruction. J Reconstr Microsurg 2013; 29(4):277–82.
18. Santanelli F, Paolini G, Renzi L, et al. Preliminary experience in reconstruction of the vulva using the pedicled vertical deep inferior epigastric perforator flap. Plast Reconstr Surg 2007;120(1):182–6.
19. Muneuchi G, Ohno M, Shiota A, et al. Deep inferior epigastric perforator (DIEP) flap for vulvar reconstruction after radical vulvectomy: a less invasive and simple procedure utilizing an abdominal incision wound. Ann Plast Surg 2005;55(4):427–9.
20. Bodin F, Robert E, Dissaux C, et al. Extended vulvar immediate reconstruction using the bilateral transverse pedicled DIEP flap. J Plast Reconstr Aesthet Surg 2015;68(5):745–7.
21. Kim KS, Kim ES, Hwang JH, et al. Buttock reconstruction using a pedicled deep inferior epigastric perforator flap. Microsurgery 2011;31(3):237–40.
22. Keys KA, Louie O, Said HK, et al. Clinical utility of CT angiography in DIEP breast reconstruction. J Plast Reconstr Aesthet Surg 2013;66(3):e61–5.
23. Cheng A, Saint-Cyr M. Use of a pre-expanded "propeller" deep inferior epigastric perforator (DIEP) flap for a large abdominal wall defect. J Plast Reconstr Aesthet Surg 2013;66(6):851–4.
24. Cherry GW, Austad E, Pasyk K, et al. Increased survival and vascularity of random-pattern skin flaps elevated in controlled, expanded skin. Plast Reconstr Surg 1983;72(5):680–7.
25. Shang Z, Zhao Y, Ding H, et al. Repair of hand scars by a dilated deep inferior epigastric artery perforator flap. J Plast Surg Hand Surg 2011;45(2):102–8.
26. Song B, Jin J, Liu Y, et al. Prefabricated expanded free lower abdominal skin flap for cutaneous coverage of a forearm burn wound defect. Aesthetic Plast Surg 2013;37(5):956–9.
27. Margulis A, Adler N, Eyal G. Expanded deep inferior epigastric artery perforator flap for reconstruction of the posterior neck and the upper back in a child with giant congenital melanocytic nevus. J Plast Reconstr Aesthet Surg 2010;63(9):e703–5.
28. Grinsell D, Saravolac V, Rozen WM, et al. Pre-expanded bipedicled deep inferior epigastric artery perforator (DIEP) flap for paediatric lower limb reconstruction. J Plast Reconstr Aesthet Surg 2012;65(11):1603–5.

Pre-expanded Brachial Artery Perforator Flap

CrossMark

Yuanbo Liu, MD[a],*, Mengqing Zang, MD[a], Maolin Tang, MD[b], Shan Zhu, MD[a],
Jianhua Zhang, MD[a], Yu Zhou, MD[a]

KEYWORDS

- Perforator flap • Tissue expansion • Brachial artery • Septocutaneous perforator • Upper arm flap

KEY POINTS

- Brachial artery perforator flap is a flap based on septocutaneous perforators derived from the brachial artery, which is harvested from the medial upper arm.
- The brachial artery perforator flap is commonly used as a pedicled flap for defect reconstruction in different locations, including the head and neck, axilla, chest wall, and upper extremity.
- Many of the disadvantages of the pedicled brachial artery perforator flap can be overcome by pre-expansion of the flap.
- As there is no need to dissect the perforators through the muscle, the pre-expanded pedicled brachial artery perforator flap is quite reliable and easily to be raised.

INTRODUCTION

Early in 1597, Tagliacozzi first used the inner side of the arm as a distally based flap for nasal reconstruction. The medial upper arm flap, first described by Daniel and colleagues[1] and further investigated by Dolmans and colleagues,[2] Kaplan and Pearl,[3] and Song and colleagues,[4] has been considered a valuable reconstructive option. However, the medial arm flap has not gained popularity, and the reasons may lie in the variations in vascular anatomy, which can lead to confusion during dissection. The brachial artery and its main branches have been described as the blood supply of the medial arm flap.[1,4–6] The applications of the medial arm skin as a free flap is limited[4,6–10]; in most circumstances, it is used as a pedicled flap to reconstruct the defects on the head and neck and upper extremity.[3,10,11] At present, the medial arm flap is not conceived as a workhorse flap in the reconstructive armamentarium. Nevertheless, the medial arm skin is thin and pliable, well matched to the facial skin, and well camouflaged as a donor site, and these characteristics deserve further investigation.

The perforator flap constitutes the latest development in reconstructive surgery. When raising a perforator flap, the main source vessels and relevant muscles can be spared, minimizing donor site morbidities. Early in 1990, Carriquiry[10] demonstrated the versatility of fasciocutaneous flaps based on the medial septocutaneous vessels of the arm. By cadaveric studies and clinical observations, the authors also observed that many septocutaneous perforators from the brachial artery emerged from the medial intermuscular septum of the arm. Elevating a flap based on these perforators will not require the opening of the intermuscular septum, and the difficulty and risks of the surgery are subsequently reduced. In addition, when raising a wide and long medial arm flap, the donor site may not be closed directly and the

Disclosures: The authors have nothing to disclose.
[a] Department of Plastic and Reconstructive Surgery, Plastic Surgery Hospital, Peking Union Medical College and Chinese Academy of Medical Sciences, Ba-Da-Chu Road 33#, Beijing 100144, P.R. China; [b] Department of Anatomy, Wenzhou Medical College, Wenzhou University-Town, Wenzhou, Zhejiang 325035, P.R. China
* Corresponding author.
E-mail address: ybpumc@sina.com

Clin Plastic Surg 44 (2017) 117–128
http://dx.doi.org/10.1016/j.cps.2016.08.006

blood supply of the distal portion of the flap may be insufficient. A well-established technique, tissue expansion increases the vascularity and dimension of the flap as well as reduces donor site morbidity.[12] A significant increase in perforator artery diameter secondary to the pre-expansion procedure was demonstrated.[13] In this article, the authors demonstrated the value of pre-expanded brachial artery perforator flaps for soft tissue reconstruction and summarize their experiences in using this technique for patients with soft tissue defects of the head and neck, axilla, chest wall, and upper extremity.

TREATMENT GOALS AND PLANNED OUTCOMES

The authors applied the pre-expanded brachial artery perforator flap mainly in patients with scar, congenital melanocytic nevi, hemangioma, and neurofibroma of the head and neck, axilla, chest wall, and upper extremity to achieve excellent functional and aesthetic outcomes. This technique can provide a large, thin flap with similar color, texture, and thickness for head and neck defect reconstruction. The authors' experience with more than 50 flaps supports the claim that this technique is safe and successful in achieving superior aesthetic results. When properly planned and performed, these operations have a low complication rate and minimal donor site morbidity.

ANATOMIC BASIS OF THE BRACHIAL ARTERY PERFORATOR FLAP

The brachial artery is the continuation of the axillary artery beyond the teres major and primarily supplies the arm. The artery courses through the intermuscular septum between the biceps and the triceps. The principal tributaries of the brachial artery include the profunda brachial artery, the superior and inferior ulnar collateral arteries, and many muscular and cutaneous branches (**Fig. 1**).[14]

The authors focused on investigating the septocutaneous perforators from the brachial artery nourishing the medial skin of the arm by means of cadaveric dissection and clinical observation. They found that 1 to 3 septocutaneous perforators originating from the brachial artery along the medial septum can be identified in 1 of 3 portions of the medial arm. Meanwhile, at least one arterial perforator with visible pulsation and 2 venae comitantes can be found in the proximal, middle, and distal portions of the medial arm, respectively. The proximal and distal perforators densely distribute in the regions 3 cm distal to the central axillary fold and 5 cm proximal to the medial epicondyle, respectively (**Figs. 2 and 3**). They also found that close to the central axillary fold, the brachial artery consistently gives rise to an uppermost branch. The latter, 1 to 3 mm in diameter, not only sends muscular branches to adjacent muscles and septocutaneous perforators to the medial arm skin, but, most notably, also sends a long superficial thoracic branch. The long superficial thoracic branch, accompanied by 2 venae comitantes, 2 to 3 cm lateral and parallel to the lateral margin of the pectoralis muscle, travels within the subcutaneous fatty tissue of the lateral chest wall and terminates in the superficial fascia around the nipple-areola complex (**Fig. 4**).

PREOPERATIVE PLANNING AND PREPARATION

Before the implantation of the tissue expander, the dimension of the wound is evaluated. The authors routinely explore the location of the perforators preoperatively (**Fig. 5**). According to the location and size of the defect, one side of the medial arm is chosen as the donor area. The central axis of the flap is drawn along the medial intermuscular septum of the arm, roughly corresponding to the surface projection of the brachial artery. Two vertical lines traversing the central axillary fold and medial epicondyle of humerus are also drawn, respectively, corresponding to the superior and inferior margins of the medial arm. The lateral margins are between the midanterior and midposterior lines of the arm. The pre-expanded area can be extended to the superior or inferior margins of the medial arm, in accordance with the location of the flap pedicle (**Fig. 6**).

PATIENT POSITIONING

For the tissue expander placement and removal, the patient is positioned in the supine position with the arm abducted 90° and maximally supinated to expose the medial arm, which is completely sterilized, allowing free movement of the patient's upper extremity during the surgery. For the patient undergoing hand defect reconstruction, the bilateral upper extremities should be prepared.

PROCEDURAL APPROACH
Pre-expansion of the Brachial Artery Perforator Flap

The superior edge of the designed area is chosen as the area of incision for expander placement. An incision is made through the biceps fascia. The dissection proceeds quickly and reaches the

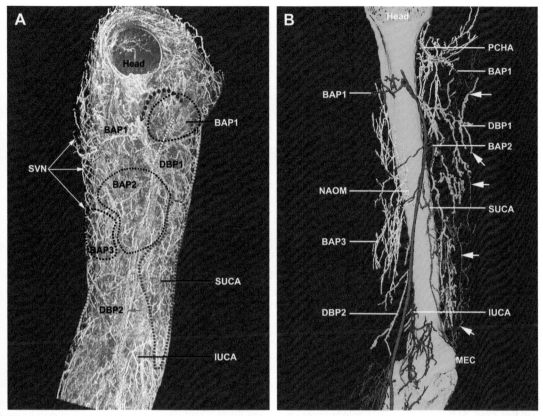

Fig. 1. Three-dimensional reconstruction of multiple tissues of the right arm. (*A*) Three-dimensional reconstruction by fast volume-rendering technique to show the subcutaneous vascular network. (*B*) Three-dimensional reconstruction by surface-rendering technique (same specimen as in *A*). (*red arrows, A*) Faintly visible trace of the brachial artery; (*white arrows; B*) An incomplete vascular chain-link along with the medial brachial cutaneous nerve and the basilic vein. BAP, brachial artery perforator; DBP, deep brachial artery perforator; IUCA, inferior ulnar collateral artery; MEC, medial epicondyle of the humerus; NAOM, nutrient artery of the muscle; PCHA, posterior circumflex humeral artery; SUCA, superior ulnar collateral artery; SVN, subcutaneous vascular network.

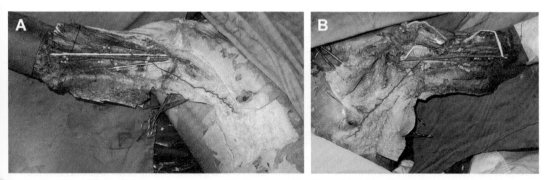

Fig. 2. The skin of the red-latex–injected arms (*A, right arm*; *B, left arm*) has been raised at the subfascial plane to expose the brachial artery and its major tributaries. Three septocutaneous perforators from the brachial artery have been illustrated on either side of the arm. Note the position of the uppermost vessel; besides sending muscular branches to the brachialis muscle and septocutaneous perforator to the medial arm skin, it also sends a notable superficial thoracic branch.

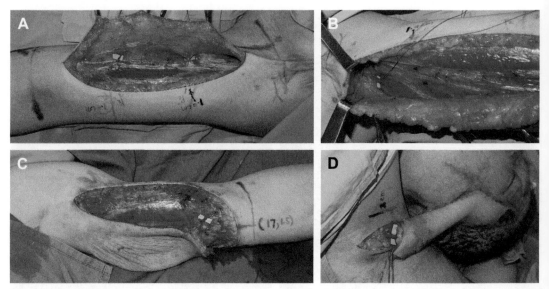

Fig. 3. (*A*) Two perforators in the middle one-third of the medial arm. (*B*) An uppermost branch from the brachial artery. (*C*) Distal perforators can be observed when raising a proximally based flap. (*D*) Proximal perforators can be explored during the pedicle division.

medial intermuscular septum of the arm. Care should be taken not to follow the fascia into the medial intermuscular septum because the ulnar and median nerves and brachial artery and vein lie in this area. At this point, many septocutaneous perforators emerging from the septum can be visualized. Perforators located in the proximal, middle, and distal portion of the medial arm are measured and recorded. If a proximally based perforator flap is designed, the dissection can be extended to the central axillary fold. If a distally based perforator flap is designed, then a skin area approximately 3 cm above the medial epicondyle should not be dissected in the first-stage operation. With this knowledge, the authors are able to incorporate the dominant perforator into the base of the flap and gain maximal vascularization. Other perforators apart from the flap pedicle are ligated and divided. The dissection continues until an adequate pocket is achieved. Then, a rectangular expander with proper size is placed into the pocket, with the filler valves routinely positioned superolaterally against the incision.

Expansion is begun 14 days later with normal saline added on a weekly basis until adequate volume has been achieved. The flap is always overexpanded to obtain more donor tissue as well as to achieve direct closure of the donor site.

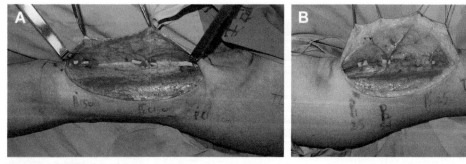

Fig. 4. (*A*) Proximal, middle, and distal septocutaneous perforators from the brachial artery are visualized. Each perforator was ramified after emerging from the medial septum and gave off many small branches distributing to the overlying flap. The longitudinal branches from the adjacent perforators formed the vascular anastomoses roughly paralleled to the medial septum. Some of these branches followed closely the medial brachial cutaneous nerve and could form a long, uninterrupted anastomotic vascular arcade. (*B*) When raising a proximally or distally based brachial artery perforator flap, the middle perforators were ligated in the main trunk, preserving the integrity of the interconnection of the secondary branches.

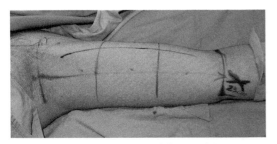

Fig. 5. Preoperative design and skin marking.

Pre-expanded Brachial Artery Perforator Flap Transfer

After the expander has been adequately inflated, the perforators are relocated using a Doppler probe. The authors prefer to resect a part of the lesion first and then design the dimension, shape, and width of the flap. The expander is removed from the previous incision corresponding to the flap superior border.

If a defect is located on the head and neck or on the hand, then a proximally or distally based brachial perforator flap is raised. The distal portion of the flap is used to reconstruct the defect, and the proximal portion is either sutured as a skin tube or overlapped with the residual lesion flap. To ensure the minimal pedicle tension and most comfortable arm position following the flap transfer, only a part of the lesion is resected. As a pedicle flap, extensive dissection of the perforators during the flap elevation is unnecessary. Capsulectomy for flap debulking is performed in some patients with relatively thick flaps (**Fig. 7**). The capsule adjacent to the pedicle can be preserved to protect the perforators and their branches. The donor site is primarily closed after drainage placement. Self-adherent bandages are used to maintain the required posture of the arm.

If a defect located on the axilla or chest wall needs to be repaired, then the flap can be raised and transferred in an island or a propeller fashion. The flap is circumferentially incised, and the perforator is retrograde dissected, even to the trunk of the brachial artery, to obtain a sufficient length of the pedicle. The flap is rotated in specific degrees to reconstruct the defect with direct closure of the donor site. Care should be taken to avoid any kinking or twisting of the pedicle.

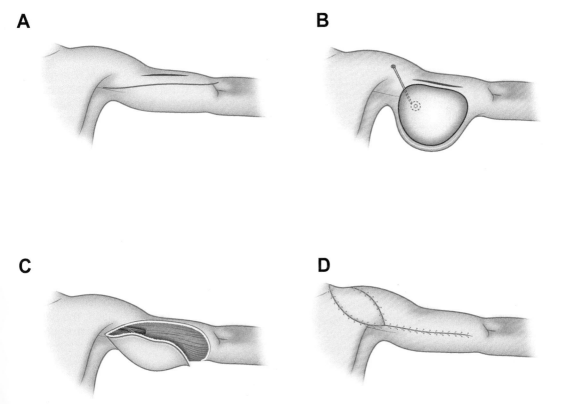

Fig. 6. Flap design and surgical technique. (*A*) Preoperative skin marking. (*B*) The expander has been adequately inflated. (*C*) The flap is raised based on the proximal septocutaneous perforator originated from the brachial artery. (*D*) Final result.

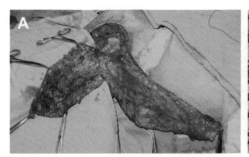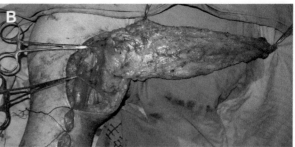

Fig. 7. (*A*) Capsulectomy for flap debulking. (*B*) The capsule has been removed.

Pedicle Division

Before cutting the flap pedicle, a tourniquet is applied to prove that the flap can survive from its recipient vascular bed. With the tourniquet in place, perfusion from the recipient site can be confirmed by capillary refilling test of the flap. The flap is divided 3 weeks after surgery. The perforators in the pedicle are recorded and ligated. The residual recipient lesion is excised and reconstructed with the proximal portion of the flap. Any extra tissue is reinserted back to the donor site.

POTENTIAL COMPLICATIONS AND MANAGEMENT
Complications Associated with the Expansion

Tissue expansion can be associated with a high rate of complication with the initial attempt. However, with more experience, the incidence of complications will decrease. The complications include, but are not limited to, hematoma, infection, implant failure, and exposure. In the authors' cases, the rate of complications associated with the expansion was low. Hematoma occurred in one patient after the surgery and required surgical re-exploration. The postoperative course was uneventful. Wound dehiscence occurred in another patient due to extensive dissection and traction during expander placement. The wound was resutured and healed.

Vascular Complications of the Flaps

There was no total flap loss in the authors' series. Partial flap necrosis and venous congestion in the distal part of the flap were rarely observed in the authors' earlier cases. Local debridement was performed if partial flap was lost. The wound was healed secondarily, closed directly, or skin grafted, depending on the size of the resultant defects.

Complications of the Donor Site

No severe complications occurred in the donor site. Although tissue expansion was used, the incisional scar in the arm tended to be wider as time

went on. The resultant donor site scar could be one of the main complaints of the patients after the surgery. None of the patients complained of shoulder stiffness or required physiotherapy after the splint had been removed.

POSTPROCEDURAL CARE

After expander implantation, the drainage and temperature of the patients need to be carefully monitored. Drains are usually taken out on postoperative day 2 or 3 when drainage decreases to 20 mL/d. Flap monitoring is performed clinically after the expanded flap is transferred. If the distal portion of the flap shows signs of venous congestion, the pedicle should be checked for twisting or kinking. A circumferential self-adherent bandage is used to immobilize the upper extremity to avoid avulsion of the pedicle.

Dressing is changed every 3 days. The patients usually get used to the gesture if the flap is used to repair the defect on the head and neck after 7 days, and the bandage can be loosened to allow limited movement of the shoulder and elbow. The vascular ingrowths of the flap are confirmed by clamping the pedicle, following a 7-day pedicle clamping training. After the pedicle division, flap monitoring is performed as mentioned above. If necessary, flap debulking or scar revision is performed 6 months after the initial surgery to further improve the aesthetic outcome.

REHABILITATION AND RECOVERY

Oral analgesics are routinely given for 2 days to alleviate the pain caused by shoulder movement after a long period of immobilization. The patients are asked to use a silicone gel sheet to prevent scar proliferation in both donor and recipient sites for 6 months.

OUTCOMES

The expanded brachial artery perforator flaps were used to resurface the wounds of the head and neck (see **Fig. 8**; **Fig. 9**), dorsum of the hand

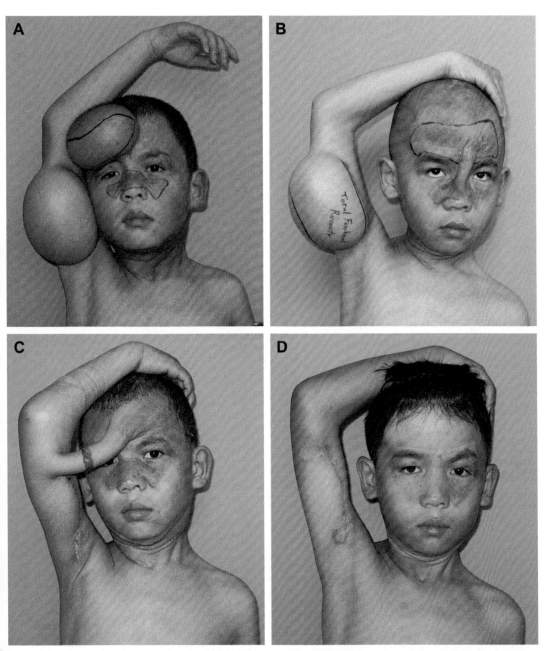

Fig. 8. (*A*) Preoperative view showing the facial and frontal scar. (*B*) Reconstruction of the nasal and facial defects using an expanded pedicle forehead flap. (*C*) After pedicle division of the forehead flap, the right pre-expanded brachial artery perforator flap was used for a total forehead reconstruction. (*D*) The appearance 1 year and 2 months after the surgery.

(**Fig. 10**), axilla (**Fig. 11**), and chest wall. The flaps were expanded over 14 to 28 weeks. The expander ranged in size from 150 to 400 mL. The dimension of the flaps ranged from 11 × 5 to 23 × 10 cm. The lateral margins of the flap can extend from the midanterior to the midposterior lines of the arm. An ipsilateral pedicle flap was used to resurface the head and neck defect, whereas a contralateral flap was used for the reconstruction of the hand defects in a cross-arm pattern. All donor sites were closed directly, including one donor site closed using a thoraco-dorsal artery perforator flap. A widening of the incisional scar was expected, and scar revision might be required in both the donor and the recipient sites.

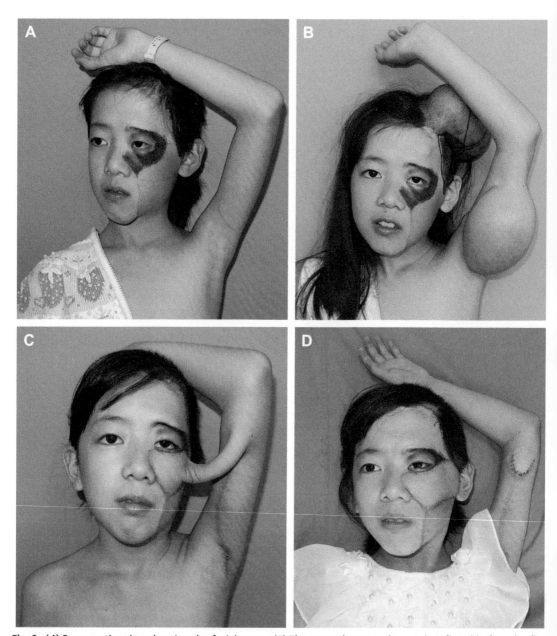

Fig. 9. (*A*) Preoperative view showing the facial nevus. (*B*) The expander was adequately inflated before the flap transfer. (*C*) A distally based brachial artery perforator flap was used to reconstruct the defect following nevus removal. (*D*) The flap survived completely.

CASE PRESENTATIONS
Case 1

A 7-year-old boy presented with a facial scar after a burn involving the parts of the forehead, nose, and cheek. In the first stage, 2 expanders measuring 200 and 150 mL were implanted in his right medial arm and residual normal forehead skin. Fourteen weeks later, the expanded forehead flap was transferred to resurface the defect after the removal of the facial and nasal defects. Three weeks later, the pedicle forehead flap was divided and inset on the recipient site. The frontal scar was completely resected and a total forehead measuring 14 × 6 cm was reconstructed using a distally based pre-expanded brachial artery perforator flap. After another 3 weeks, the pedicle of the brachial artery perforator flap was divided and inset on the forehead. The boy was satisfied with his appearance (see **Fig. 8**).

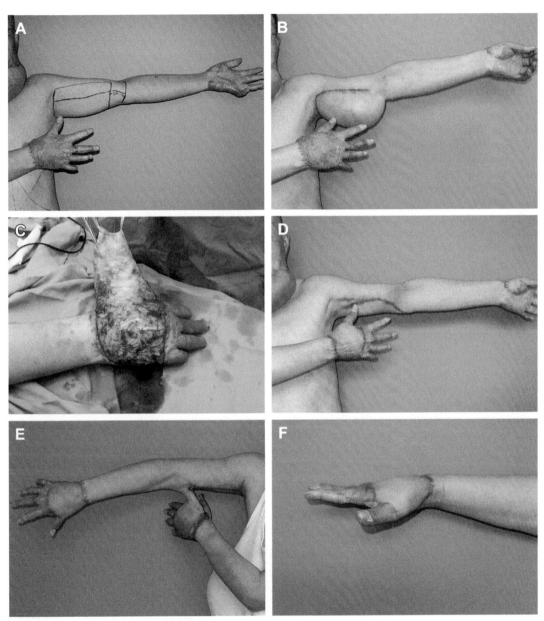

Fig. 10. (*A*) Preoperative view showing the right hand scar and flap design in the contralateral medial arm. (*B*) The expander was adequately inflated. (*C*) The scar of the dorsum of the right hand was resected and the scarred flap would be overlapping sutured with the flap. (*D*) Final appearance of the right hand and donor site of the left medial arm. (*E*) The anterior view of the right hand. The right distally based brachial artery perforator flap was still attached to the left hand. (*F*) Lateral view of the right hand.

Case 2

A 9-year-old girl was born with a large congenital nevus on her left face. She was previously treated with an expanded cervicofacial flap. The nevus was not completely resected, and severe deformation and asymmetry of the face occurred after surgery. In the first-stage operation, a 200-mL expander was implanted under the medial arm flap region. Sixteen weeks later, when the expander was adequately inflated, the residual nevus was resected, and contracture was completely released. The resultant facial defect was reconstructed using a pre-expanded distally based brachial artery perforator flap. Three weeks later, the pedicle of the flap was divided, and the flap was inset on the recipient site. The flap survived, and the girl was happy with her appearance (see **Fig. 9**).

Case 3

A 36-year old man suffered from a burn injury to his bilateral hands. The dorsal defects were covered initially with a split-thickness skin graft. After resection of the scar and skin graft, the dorsum of his hands was resurfaced with contralateral distally based pre-expanded brachial artery perforator flap. The recipient hand was positioned below the upper donor arm with a long pedicle attached to the donor site. This maneuver allowed comfortable movement of both upper extremities. The patient tolerated this position well during the 3 weeks before flap division and final inset. After surgery, the function and appearance of both hands greatly improved, and the patient ultimately returned to his original occupation (see **Fig. 10**).

Case 4

A 7-year-old boy had severe bilateral axillary scar contractures from a burn. In the first-stage operation, 2 rectangular expanders measuring 200 mL were implanted under the bilateral medial arm region. Twenty weeks later, the pre-expanded brachial artery perforator propeller flaps were raised and used to correct the bilateral axillary scar contracture. The flaps survived completely, and the range of motion of the shoulder joints was greatly improved (**Fig. 11**).

DISCUSSION

The medial site of the upper arm is an ideal donor site because of its thin, elastic, and hairless skin that allows a well-hidden scar. Although there have been various reports about the vascular supply of the skin, free medial arm flap has not gained popularity.[4,6–9,15] Many investigators stated that the superior ulnar collateral artery is the main supplier of medial arm skin.[1,2,6–9,11,15,16] Although this arterial branch sends cutaneous branches to the medial arm and may serve as the pedicle of a flap, it is intimately associated with the ulnar nerve. When raising a flap based on it, the ulnar nerve should be meticulously dissected from the intimately associated vessels. This dissection can be done, but it needs extra effort, and the nerve may be compromised when raising the flap.

The superficial brachial artery is also reported as a vascular supply for the medial arm flap.[5,6,15] Iwahira and colleagues[5] described a new flap based on this vessel but stated that it was only present in 25% of cases. Preoperative angiography is mandatory to ensure the existence of this vessel. Song and colleagues[4] described that the medial arm flap can be based on the branches of the biceps artery. Uncertainty in the position of the musculocutaneous perforators and intramuscular dissection, which may compromise the muscle function, greatly limits application of this kind of the flap. Many investigators described harvesting the medial arm flap based on the direct cutaneous branches of the brachial artery.[6,15,17]

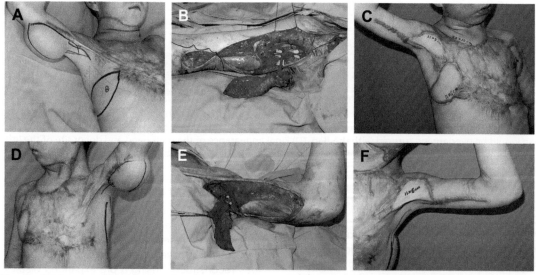

Fig. 11. (*A*) Preoperative view showing the right axillary contracture and the flap design. (*B*) The right brachial artery perforator flap measuring 11 × 5 cm was raised. (*C*) Postoperative view. (*D*) Preoperative view showing the left axillary contracture and the flap design. (*E*) The left brachial artery perforator flap measuring 11 × 6 cm was raised. (*F*) Postoperative view.

Carriquiry[10] even reported that a fasciocutaneous flap can be elevated based on the medial septocutaneous vessels of the arm. There is no need to open the medial intramuscular septum when raising a brachial artery septocutaneous perforator flap, which reduces the difficulty of the operation and minimizes donor site morbidities. When the perforator flap concept and tissue expansion technique are applied to the conventional medial arm flap, the vascularization of the flap can be subsequently enhanced with primary donor site closure.

Basically, flaps harvested in the medial upper arm can be either used to reconstruct the defects around the elbow and axilla as a pedicle flap[3,10,18] or transferred as a free flap.[4,6–9,15] However, free flap surgery requires microsurgical expertise and can be restricted by patients' comorbidities. Pedicle medial arm flaps have been used for facial defect reconstruction.[3,19] It is an easy and safe procedure and can provide large skin paddle well matched to the face skin. Extension dissection and skeletonization of the perforating vessels are not needed during the surgery. Criticism of using this flap is the passive immobilized posture that the patient must maintain before division of the pedicle. Pain, numbness, and possible stiffness of the shoulder are the major complaints. Recently, in addition to preoperative postural training, the authors intentionally included the perforator within the pedicle, thereby greatly lengthening the pedicle. This maneuver greatly improves the range of motion of the patients' shoulder and alleviates discomfort. Therefore, temporary discomfort of the shoulder will be resolved after the surgery. In the authors' experience, this technique is more suitable for the thin and young adult, particularly pediatric patients. Obese, elderly, or emotionally unstable patients should not be candidates for this procedure.

Distally based pedicle medial arm flap has been used for the reconstruction of defect around the elbow.[3,10] The authors reported the reconstruction of defects following soft tissue sarcoma resection using the freestyle perforator-based propeller flap harvested from the medial upper arm.[20] For patients undergoing elective surgery, pre-expanded brachial perforator flap might be an alternative option for elbow defect reconstruction.

The uppermost branch from the brachial artery, 1 to 3 mm in diameter, sends off muscular branches to the adjacent muscles, septocutaneous perforator to the medial skin of the upper arm, and a long superficial thoracic branch. The septocutaneous perforator travels distally within the subcutaneous fatty tissue and anastomoses with the branches of the other septocutaneous perforators from the brachial artery. A pre-expanded brachial perforator flap based on this vessel, with either pedicled or propeller designs, can be used to reconstruct the defects on the axilla and chest wall. For the reconstruction of defects in the cubital or axillary area, the vascular pedicle of the brachial artery perforator flap should be skeletonized, and an adequate length of the pedicle should also be achieved so as to avoid kinking or twisting of the pedicle. The authors have reported using nonexpanded brachial perforator flap for reconstruction of radiation ulcer of the chest wall.[21] The authors anticipate that the proximally based brachial perforator flap might be a useful option for the reconstruction of partial breast defect. The authors' limited cadaveric study revealed the existence of a superficial thoracic branch, which has a mean length of 22 cm. A lateral thoracic flap may be raised on this branch. Furthermore, this branch may serve as a superolateral pedicle for the nipple-areola complex when performing reduction mammoplasty.

SUMMARY

Considering the excellent functional and aesthetic outcomes, the authors believe the pre-expanded brachial artery perforator flap is a good option for patients who have soft tissue defects of the head and neck, upper extremity, chest wall, and breast with high demand for aesthetic outcomes, with the premise that they are willing to invest more time into the treatment.

ACKNOWLEDGMENTS

The authors express their deepest gratitude to Prof. Maolin Tang, Department of Anatomy, Wenzhou Medical College, Wenzhou University-Town, Wenzhou, Zhejiang 325035, P.R. China, for providing them the invaluable 3D vasculature reconstruction of the upper arm, as shown in **Fig. 1**.

REFERENCES

1. Daniel RK, Terzis J, Schwarz G. Neurovascular free flaps: a preliminary report. Plast Reconstr Surg 1975;56:13–20.
2. Dolmans S, Guimberteau JC, Baudet J. The upper arm flap. J Microsurg 1979;1:162.
3. Kaplan EN, Pearl RM. An arterial medial arm flap–vascular anatomy and clinical applications. Ann Plast Surg 1980;4:205–15.
4. Song RY, Song YG, Yu YS, et al. The upper arm flap. Clin Plast Surg 1982;9:27–35.
5. Iwahira Y, Maruyama Y, Hayashi A. The superficial brachial flap. Ann Plast Surg 1996;37:48–54.

6. Karamürsel S, Bağdatli D, Demir Z, et al. Use of medial arm skin as a free flap. Plast Reconstr Surg 2005;115:2025–31.

7. Newsom HT. Medical arm free flap. Plast Reconstr Surg 1981;67:63–6.

8. Breidenbach WC, Adamson W, Terzis JK. Medial arm flap revisited. Ann Plast Surg 1987;18:156–63.

9. Matloub HS, Ye Z, Yousif NJ, et al. The medial arm flap. Ann Plast Surg 1992;29:517–22.

10. Carriquiry CE. Versatile fasciocutaneous flaps based on the medial septocutaneous vessels of the arm. Plast Reconstr Surg 1990;86:103–9.

11. Bhattacharya S, Bhagia SP, Bhatnagar SK, et al. The medial upper arm fasciocutaneous flap. An alternative flap to cover palmar defects of hand and distal forearm. J Hand Surg Br 1991;16:342–5.

12. Abbase EA, Shenaq SM, Spira M, et al. Prefabricated flaps: experimental and clinical review. Plast Reconstr Surg 1995;96:1218–25.

13. Hocaoglu E, Emekli U, Cizmeci O, et al. Suprafascial pre-expansion of perforator flaps and effect of pre-expansion on perforator artery diameter. Microsurg 2014;34:188–96.

14. Thomas BP, Geddes CR, Tang ML, et al. Vascular supply of the integument of the upper extremity. In: Blondeel PN, Morris SF, Hallcok GG, et al, editors. Perforator flaps: anatomy, technique, & clinical applications. 2nd edition. St Louis (MO): Quality Medical Publishing, Inc; 2013. p. 300–27.

15. Chi Z, Gao W, Yan H, et al. Reconstruction of totally degloved fingers with a spiraled parallelogram medial arm free flap. J Hand Surg Am 2012;37:1042–50.

16. Cormack GC, Lamberty BG. Fasciocutaneous vessels in the upper arm: application to the design of new fasciocutaneous flaps. Plast Reconstr Surg 1984;74:244–50.

17. Cil Y, Kocabıyık N, Ozturk S, et al. A new perforator flap from distal medial arm: a cadaveric study. Eplasty 2010;10:541–8.

18. Maruyama Y, Onishi K, Iwahira Y. The ulnar recurrent fasciocutaneous island flap: reverse medial arm flap. Plast Reconstr Surg 1987;79:381–8.

19. Bin S, Yuanbo L, Ji J, et al. Preexpanded pedicle medial arm flap: an alternative method of massive facial defect reconstruction. Aesthetic Plast Surg 2011;35:946–52.

20. Zang M, Yu S, Xu L, et al. Freestyle perforator-based propeller flap of medial arm for medial elbow reconstruction. Microsurg 2015;35:411–4.

21. Zang M, Guo L, Liu Y. Propeller medial arm flap: a plan "B" for reconstruction of radiation ulcer of the chest wall. J Plast Reconstr Aesthet Surg 2014;67:1769–70.

Pre-expanded Anterolateral Thigh Perforator Flap for Phalloplasty

Salvatore D'Arpa, MD, PhD*, Britt Colebunders, MD,
Filip Stillaert, MD, Stan Monstrey, MD, PhD

CrossMark

KEYWORDS

- Phalloplasty • Skin expansion • ALT flap • LCFA flap • Perforator flap • Pre-expanded flap

KEY POINTS

- The anterolateral thigh (ALT) perforator flap is a valuable alternative to the radial forearm flap for patients who do not wish to have the forearm scar.
- ALT flap phalloplasty leaves visible scarring in the thighs owing to skin grafting of its donor site.
- Pre-expansion of an ALT flap allows primary donor site closure.
- Preoperative perforator location with computed tomography angiography is crucial to the success of the procedure.

INTRODUCTION

Since the first description in 2005,[1] phalloplasty with a free or pedicled anterolateral thigh (ALT) flap has gradually gained popularity for penile reconstruction[2–14] as an alternative to the standard radial forearm flap (RFF).[15]

The main advantage of the ALT flap in this indication is avoidance of the large forearm scar, which has become a recognizable sign of this operation because of the increasing attention received from the media. Very large flaps are needed for a phalloplasty and the donor site subsequently needs skin grafting. As a result, the donor site is quite noticeable because a hairless skin graft with a depression is left at the donor site. If the donor site is located in the forearm, it is not only quite visible and difficult to conceal unless long sleeves are worn, but also a recognizable sign of the operation performed (**Fig. 1**).

If an ALT flap is used for phalloplasty, the RFF donor site scars are avoided. However, a donor site scar will be present in the thigh, combined with the scars needed for skin graft harvest (**Fig. 2**). With the RFF and ALT, there is not only the flap donor site scar, but also the split thickness skin graft donor site, which is often more painful than the flap donor site itself.

There is a particular subset of patients who want to avoid both scars because, although the thigh scars can be easily concealed whit a pair of shorts while dressed, they cannot be concealed when naked and are very close to the genital area. These patients would rather avoid disfigurement of the area that is the center of their masculinity and intimacy. Pre-expansion of the ALT allows donor site scarring to be minimized in these patients (**Fig. 3**).

TREATMENT GOALS AND PLANNED OUTCOMES

Pre-expansion of a conventional ALT flap has 3 main goals:

1. Allowing primary donor site closure;
2. Improving the perforator's vascular territory;
3. Thinning of the flap.

Disclosure Statement: The authors have nothing to disclose.
Department of Plastic and Reconstructive Surgery, Ghent University Hospital, De Pintelaan, 185, K12C, Gent 9000, Belgium
* Corresponding author.
E-mail address: salvatore.darpa@uzgent.be

Clin Plastic Surg 44 (2017) 129–141
http://dx.doi.org/10.1016/j.cps.2016.08.004

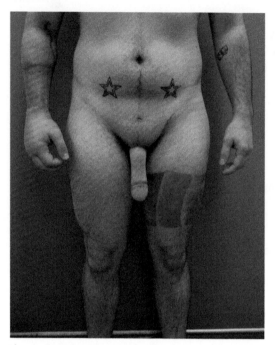

Fig. 1. Postoperative result of a radial forearm flap (RFF) phalloplasty showing the typical scar at the donor site. Because this is the only application for use of such a large RFF, this scar has become a recognizable sign of the operation, which not all patients like to have. Scars in the thigh are also present due to harvest of STSGs for coverage of the RFF donor site.

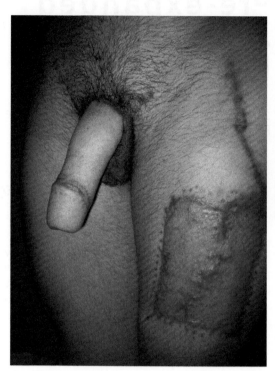

Fig. 2. Postoperative result of an anterolateral thigh (ALT) and superficial circumflex iliac perforator flaps phalloplasty. Although concealable with regular clothing, when naked the scars in the thigh, owing to both ALT and split thickness skin graft harvest, are apparent.

In this particular application, the goal of preoperative expansion of the ALT flap is achieving primary donor site closure. Improving the perforator's vascular territory is not needed in this case. The flap measures 14 × 18 cm on average and survival is not an issue. Partial flap necrosis is a very uncommon occurrence, even without prior expansion. Selection of the largest perforator with the aid of a preoperative computed tomography (CT) angiography warrants complete flap survival.

Flap thinning would be extremely desirable and was one of the goals we planned of pursuing when we first started expanding the ALT. Unfortunately, for this particular flap 2 expanders need to be placed medially and laterally to the perforator and expansion only results in a peripheral thinning of the flap with the flap's fat being squeezed toward the perforator in the middle of the flap. This kind of deformation is of little use in a phalloplasty because a lot of bulk is created in the middle of the flap, where it cannot be thinned out.

The planned outcome of preoperative ALT expansion in phalloplasty is to allow primary donor site closure, avoid the disfiguring scar and the painful skin graft donor site in the thigh.

PREOPERATIVE PLANNING AND PREPARATION

Preoperative location of the perforator is crucial to flap planning. A CT angiography is used for this purpose.[10] The CT angiography allows the most distal perforator with the largest caliber, the longest (to comfortably reach the pubis), with the best subcutaneous branching and the most convenient intramuscular or septal course, providing a preoperative navigation that cannot be obtained by simple Doppler location.

The radiologist provides distances from the anterior superior iliac spine based on an x–y axis (**Fig. 4**) drawn on the thigh and the position of the perforator is marked on the patient's skin. The flap is drawn accordingly with the perforator lying along its midline and close to its proximal margin. Then the expander's base (20 × 7 cm) is drawn outside of the flap's borders (**Fig. 5**) because, as described, placing the expanders in the flap will squeeze the fat toward the midline, which is not desirable in this case.

PATIENT POSITIONING

The patient is placed in the supine position. The ipsilateral arm can be abducted or adducted

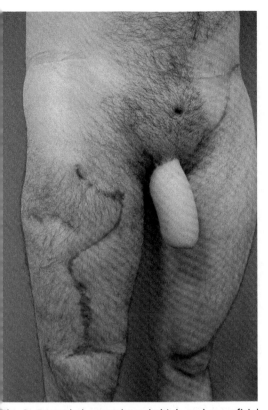

Fig. 3. Expanded anterolateral thigh and superficial circumflex iliac perforator flaps phalloplasty donor site, 5 months postoperatively. For comparison, here is an early postoperative image of a phalloplasty after expansion. The donor site has been closed with an inverted "Y" scar and no skin graft donor site is present in the thigh. The scars are still red but already much less disfiguring than those in **Fig. 2**.

based on the surgeon's preference. Abduction will provide greater room for the placement of the lateral expander because the hand, with the arm adducted, comes in close proximity to the lateral incision and pocket.

PROCEDURAL APPROACH
Expander Placement

Two remote "W" incisions[16] are performed some centimeters caudal to the inguinal ligament (see **Fig. 5**) and deepened to the deep fascia. Then the 2 pockets are dissected, bluntly or with the cautery, with the aid of a lighted retractor to obtain hemostasis. Care must be taken not to deepen the plane too much because the sensory nerves lie on top of the fascia and they must not be damaged. Once the pocket is complete, a superficial (3–5 mm of fat left on the skin flap) pocket is dissected cranially to the incision to allow for remote port placement in a position that shall be

as easily accessible as possible (**Fig. 6**). Before expander placement, two 12-F suction drains are placed in the pocket. The air is emptied from the expanders and they are partially filled with methylene blue–tinted saline, which allows easy visualization of the fluid coming out of the expanders during ambulatory postoperative expansion. Partial inflation keeps the expander distended and allows easy placement without folding (**Fig. 7**). Once the expander and ports are in position, easy accessibility of the ports is double checked before closure (**Figs. 8** and **9**).

Donor Site Closure

At the time of flap transfer (**Fig. 10**), the flap is harvested first, with the expander left in place to maintain skin stretch and inflated with extra 100 to 150 mL to obtain some intraoperative expansion.

Donor site closure begins with expander and valve removal through the easy access of the defect left by the flap. Dissection is suprafascial and then on the plane of the deep capsule of the expander, which will result in division of the capsule into a superficial and a deep part. While the deep part is not touched, the superficial is scored extensively to maximize the advancement of the skin flaps, extending the capsular incision to the superficial fascia in a way very similar to galeal scoring in the scalp (**Fig. 11**). Then the flaps are brought together and temporarily held together with skin staples. Two big dog ears will form distally that are eventually resected, resulting in inverted "Y" or "T" scars (**Figs. 12–16**). Suction drains are placed underneath the flaps.

POTENTIAL COMPLICATIONS AND THEIR MANAGEMENT

There are no specific complications of ALT flap pre-expansion; potential complications are those commonly related to tissue expansion. Like any specific body region, the anatomy accounts for some peculiarities. In the thigh, the subcutaneous fat is quite dense, fibrous, and thick, and skin perforation and exposure is very unlikely.

We have observed 2 leaks from the inflation ports that needed replacement likely owing to puncture with an exceedingly large needle. Infection can be a complication and can be prevented with appropriate technique. We have had an infection when we associated liposuction to expander placement. Infection is treated with expander removal, culture-guided antibiotic therapy and expander re-placement once the infection is cured. Placement without the aid of an CT angiography carries the risk of discontinuation of the procedure because the right perforator is missed.

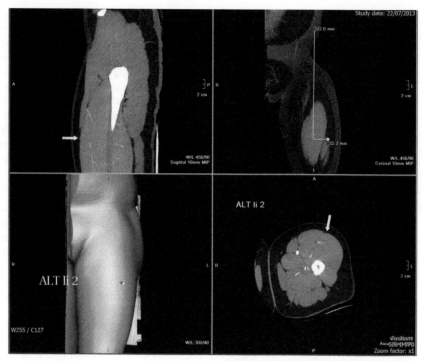

Fig. 4. An example of a preoperative computed tomography angiography. The sagittal (*upper left*), coronal (*upper right*), and axial (*lower right*) views of the perforator course together with a 3-dimensional reconstruction of the skin with the projection on the skin of the point of emergency from the fascia of the perforator (*lower left*), are provided. In the upper right coronal view, the distances measured from the anterior superior iliac spine are provided. Thus in a single image information about the course and position of the perforator are provided.

POSTPROCEDURAL CARE

Patients are immediately mobilized and discharged after drain removal. Expansions are begun after 2 weeks and are usually performed

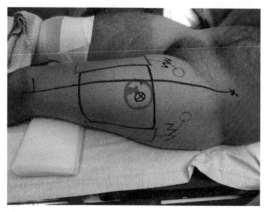

Fig. 5. Same patient as **Fig. 4**. A line is drawn connecting the anterior superior iliac spine (ASIS) to the upper lateral border of the patella. Using the angiographic computed tomography measurement in **Fig. 4**, the projection on the skin of the perforator is marked with a black, circled X, exactly 222 mm below and 32 mm laterally from the ASIS. Afterward the flap is drawn (*black rectangle*). The skin projection of the 2 expander pockets is drawn just lateral and medial to the flap to have little overlapping with the flap once the expanders are inflated. The expander base and remote ports are drawn in green. The ports are placed in an easily reachable position when the patient is lying supine. The "W" incisions (*black*) are placed in between.

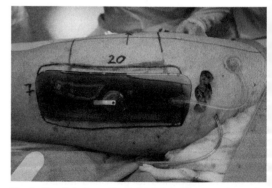

Fig. 6. Medial view of a right thigh (the knee is on the left hand side of the picture) at the time of expander placement. The pocket has already been dissected through the "W" incision, which allows wider exposure with the same length compared with a linear incision. The drain is in place. Saline (150 mL) colored with methylene blue is injected in the expander after all air has been removed. The expander is placed on the skin in the same position that it will eventually have inside the pocket.

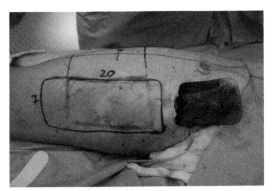

Fig. 7. Same view as in **Fig. 6**. The partial inflation of the expander facilitates insertion by keeping it distended and avoiding folding.

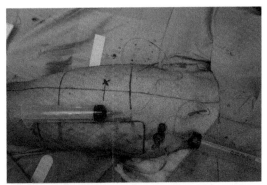

Fig. 9. Bird's eye view, knee on the left hand side. The figure shows the 2 expanders with the procedure completed for the lateral one and to be completed for the medial one, to show the 2 moments of placement of the needle in the port. The syringe on the right is connected to the medial port before closure. At this point, the port is probed to verify easy access before closure, for eventual replacement. The syringe on the right has been used for a final inflation of the expander after closure, to ensure obliteration of dead space within the pocket to avoid fluid collection.

weekly. The whole process usually takes 4 to 6 months. It is thus initiated approximately 6 months before phalloplasty.

Overexpansion is usually performed and is stopped until a circumference gain of at least 14 cm has been obtained. During this period, especially when the expanders are fully inflated, physical activity is limited because the volume of the expanders restricts movement. Sports and activities that involve lower limb movements and that are at risk for trauma to the thighs are restricted. The patients comply well and wear larger trousers to accommodate the inflated expanders.

REHABILITATION AND RECOVERY

Once the expanders are removed and the flap transferred, recovery is relatively fast and no specific rehabilitation is needed. Because of the phalloplasty, the patients stay in bed for 10 days. When

allowed to walk, no specific problems have been observed.

OUTCOMES

The charts of 91 pedicled ALT flap phalloplasties performed between 2004 and 2016 were retrospectively reviewed. Nine patients (10%) underwent pre-expansion of the ALT flap in preparation for a pedicled ALT flap phalloplasties. Seven patients

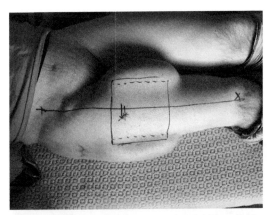

Fig. 10. Bird's eye view, knees on the right hand side. Preoperative markings of a right pre-expanded anterolateral thigh flap. The CT scan showed 2 septal perforators coming close to each other in this case. This picture shows how the expanders, although placed laterally to the flap, eventually – with inflation – do expand underneath the flap as well, causing some peripheral thinning.

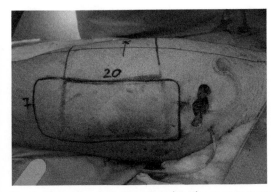

Fig. 8. Same view as in **Figs. 6** and **7**. The remote port is inserted last. The pocket for the port is dissected in a different – more superficial – plane and with a bottleneck to prevent the port from slipping back toward the incision once inserted.

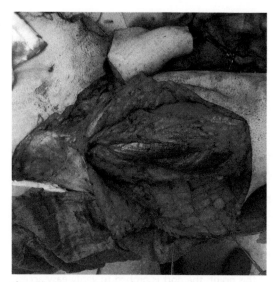

Fig. 11. Intraoperative, bird's eye view after flaps transfer. Knees on the right hand side. The anterolateral thigh flap is wrapped around the ipsilateral superficial circumflex iliac perforator flap (not visible) that has been used for urethral reconstruction and whose donor site is clearly visible. The thigh flaps for closure has been dissected and the capsular scoring is clearly visible on the lateral flap, held in the bottom of the picture by 2 skin hooks.

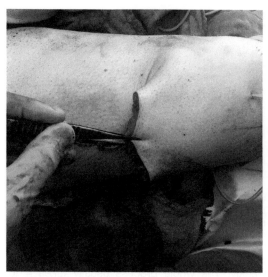

Fig. 13. Close up view of the distal dog ears. The midpoint is brought proximally with forceps to show the correction needed to eliminate the 2 dog ears.

Seven of 9 patients underwent eventual phalloplasty with an ALT flap (see **Table 1**). In 1 patient (case 2 in **Table 1**) who had no preoperative CT angiography, no suitable perforator was identified and the procedure was converted in a free RFF phalloplasty. Another patient (case 8 in **Table 1**) had an infection that eventually forced removal of the implants. Because of this delay and of a significant weight gain that caused fat thickening in the

were operated for female-to-male sex reassignment surgery, 1 for reconstruction after penile amputation, and 1 for reconstruction after bladder extrophy (**Table 1**). Six patients had a preoperative CT scan.

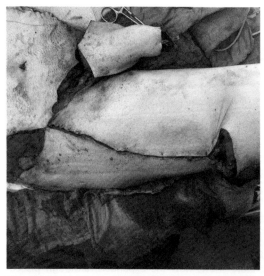

Fig. 12. Same view as in **Fig. 11**. The wound edges have been temporarily approximated with skin staples and 2 dog ears form distally.

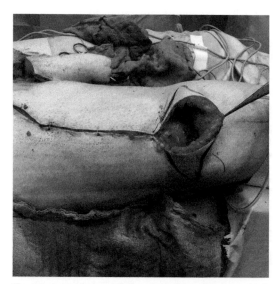

Fig. 14. Lateral view of the wound on the right thigh (*knee on the right hand side*). The skin resection is drawn in blue. Fat resection will extend further to avoid residual dog ears. The forceps are kept in the same position as **Fig. 13** to allow for comparison.

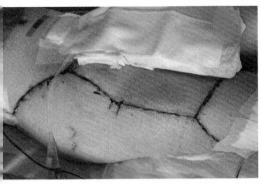

Fig. 15. Donor site after closure. The resulting scar is an inverted "Y".

thigh, we abandoned the ALT flap phalloplasty and performed an RFF phalloplasty instead.

In cases 2 and 3, there was a leak from the expander inflation ports that required their replacement. The expanders did not deflate. The leak was probably due to the use of a large needle for inflation.

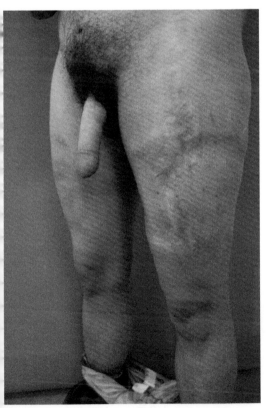

Fig. 16. Four years postoperative result. Despite some scar widening in the middle, the scar is little visible. No skin graft harvest scars are present. The inverted "T" can be seen distally above the knee.

The only infection was observed in the patient in whom we performed flap liposuction for thinning purposes in the same operation as expander placement (case 8 in **Table 1**). Because it is only 1 case, we cannot conclude that liposuction might be related to infection. More data are needed, although it seems that performing the 2 procedures simultaneously is better avoided if possible.

Donor site closure was primary with a double dog ear resection distally that resulted in an inverted "T" or "Y" appearance in 6 cases and with 2 opposed advancement flaps in 1 case. After flap harvest, all donor sites but one healed uneventfully. This case (case 6 in **Table 1**) had 2 advancement flaps for donor site closure, the medial of which had a partial necrosis with a wound dehiscence that eventually required skin grafting. We would discourage use of these 2 flaps for donor site closure and we would use 2 big rotation flaps—if flaps are needed because primary closure is not possible—instead.

There were no flap-related complications like partial or total necroses.

In 2 cases (cases 1 and 2 in **Table 1**) lipofilling was performed twice for correction of a contour deformity in the thigh.

CASE DEMONSTRATIONS
Case 1

A 36-year-old female to male transgender patient was admitted for phalloplasty with a pre-expanded ALT flap combined with a free RFF for urethral reconstruction (**Figs. 17–19**; see **Table 1**, Case 5). Two rectangular expanders of 750 mL each were implanted on the left thigh and expanded with 1000 mL until a 14-cm circumference gain was achieved, which took 11 weeks. Seven months after expander placement, phalloplasty was performed with the pre-expanded ALT flap combined with a free RFF. The RFF was anastomosed end to side to the femoral artery and end-to-end to the greater saphenous vein. The pedicled ALT flap was transferred as a pedicled flap with 2 sensory nerves that were anastomosed to 1 ilio-inguinal nerve and to one of the dorsal clitoral nerves. The ALT flap donor site was closed primarily. Coronaplasty was performed 6 weeks after the initial operation. Erectile and testicular implants were placed 3 years after the operation. One year later, a minor correction was performed to reduce the penile size. At 5 years follow-up the patient is doing fine.

Case 2

A 29-year-old female-to-male transgender patient (see **Table 1**, Case 9) was admitted for a

Table 1
Patients data

Patient	Diagnosis	First Procedure	Phalloplasty	Donor Site Closure	Complications	Date Operated (ALT Flap)	Secondary Procedures
1	FTM	Expander placement	Previous phallo + Pedicled ALT	Primary	None	10/2004	Lipofilling
2	FTM	Expander placement	Pedicled ALT	Primary	Expander leakage	08/2009	Lipofilling
3	BEX	Expander placement	RFF (no good ALT perforators	NA	Expander leakage	NA	None
4	SCC	Expander placement	Pedicled ALT + free RFF	Primary	None	06/2010	None
5	FTM	Expander placement	Pedicled ALT + free RFF	Primary	None	03/2011	None
6	FTM	Expander placement	Pedicled ALT + pedicled SCIAP	Advancement flaps	Donor wound dehiscence	11/2015	None
7	FTM	Expander placement	Pedicled ALT + pedicled SCIAP	Primary	None	12/2015	None
8	FTM	Expander placement + thinning by liposuction	Free RFF (refused ALT)	NA	Infection	NA	None
9	FTM	Expander placement	Pedicled ALT + pedicled SCIAP	Primary	None	04/2016	None

Abbreviations: ALT, anterolateral thigh; BEX, bladder extrophy; FTM, female to male; NA, not applicable; RFF, radial forearm flap; SCC, squamous cell carcinoma; SCIAP, superficial circumflex iliac perforator flap.

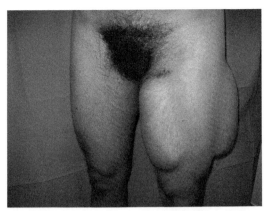

Fig. 17. Case 1 (see text for details). Three-quarters preoperative view of the expanded thigh.

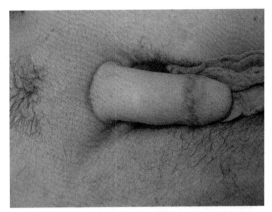

Fig. 19. Case 1 (see text for details). Postoperative view after volume reduction of the phallus by narrowing the base with a wedge resection on the ventral side.

phalloplasty with a pre-expanded ALT flap and a superficial circumflex iliac perforator flap for urethral reconstruction because he wanted no scars in his forearm (**Figs. 20–23**). Two 750-mL rectangular expanders were placed in his right thigh and inflated, over 13 weeks, with 1000 and 775 mL. Four months after the operation, the patient underwent a phalloplasty with a pedicled ALT flap combined with a pedicled superficial circumflex iliac perforator flap for urethral reconstruction. Two lateral femoral cutaneous nerve branches harvested with the ALT flap were connected to 1 ilio-inguinal nerve and 1 dorsal clitoral nerve. The procedure was uncomplicated and the donor sites were closed primarily. Coronaplasty has not yet been performed. The patient had a postoperative urinary infection that was treated with antibiotics and, 1 year after the operation, is voiding well and waiting for coronaplasty and placement of erectile and testicular implants.

Case 3

A 43-year-old patient (see **Table 1**, case 4) came to our attention for penile reconstruction after amputation for a squamous cell carcinoma (**Figs. 24–28**). Two 750-mL rectangular tissue expanders were placed in the right thigh based on perforator location with a CT angiography. Because the superficial circumflex iliac perforator flap was unavailable due to scarring from the previous groin sentinel node biopsy, a pre-expanded RFF was planned as well and another 750-mL expander placed in the left forearm. The RFF was anastomosed end to side to the femoral artery and end-to-end to the greater saphenous vein and the pedicled ALT flap wrapped around it with its cutaneous sensory nerves connected to 1 ilio-inguinal nerve and to one of the dorsal nerves of the glans. Coronaplasty was performed 1 week later. One year after the operation, an erectile implant was placed.

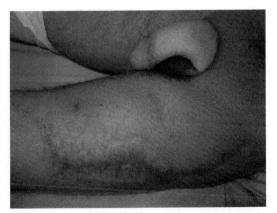

Fig. 18. Case 1 (see text for details). Postoperative view before penile correction. The linear thigh scar has widened, probably owing to some residual tension.

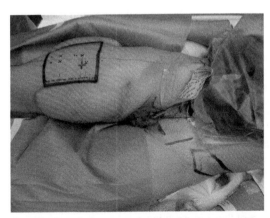

Fig. 20. Case 2 (see text for details). Intraoperative view after completion of vaginectomy and reconstruction of the fixed part of the urethra, before phalloplasty.

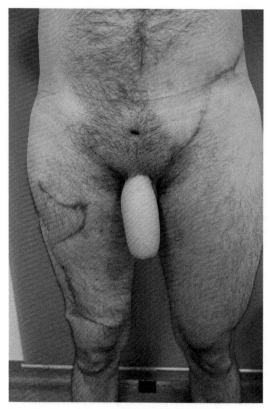

Fig. 21. Case 2 (see text for details). Postoperative frontal view showing 2 dog ears that will fade over time and the contour deformity of the right thigh.

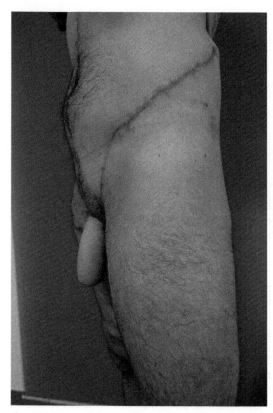

Fig. 22. Case 2 (see text for details). The left lateral view shows the linear scar of the superficial circumflex iliac perforator flap that extends far laterally to obtain an adequate pedicle length to reach the pubis.

DISCUSSION

The first case report of a pre-expanded free ALT came from Tsai,[17] who visualized the perforators through a large incision and placed a subfascial expander. Other reports followed[18–21] of its use as a free flap in burn wounds with the dual advantages of thinning the flap and closing the donor site primarily or reducing the skin graft and potentially increasing vascularity. As described above, the increase in vascularity is not needed and the usefulness of thinning the flap cannot be applied to phalloplasty. When the flap is thinned by expansion, the flap above the expander thins out but the part where the pedicle enters the flap stays thicker.

There are also some reports of pre-expanded flaps in phalloplasty surgery with the RFF,[22] the suprapubic flap,[23] or scapular flap.[24] In these cases, just a reduction of the area to be grafted and an insensate phallus are obtained, whereas a pre-expanded ALT flap always allows preservation of flap's innervation.

Over the years, we have refined our technique to optimize outcomes. A CT angiography is used routinely to accurately locate perforators and expanders are placed accordingly. This way the unfortunate occurrence observed in patient 3 of **Table 1** is avoided (**Fig. 29**). Expansion is routinely carried out until a circumference gain corresponding to the flap's width is achieved. Closure is performed directly and a dog ear usually forms distally, which is excised resulting in an inverted "T" or "Y" design. Patient are instructed on wearing large trousers to accommodate the bulk of the expanders. The flap can be farther thinned to the level of the suprascarpal fat provided that the regions were the nerves and the perforator lie are avoided. This thinning might sometimes result in a temporary venous congestion (fast capillary refill) that normally subsides within 30 minutes. The ALT flap is harvested without any fascia and is best tunneled underneath the rectus femoris and sartorius muscles, and then through a wide subcutaneous tunnel, to reach the pubic area. If an appropriate perforator is chosen based on CT angiography studies, the perforator is long enough to transfer a pedicled flap and avoid microsurgical anastomoses. The patient is kept with his thigh slightly bent to avoid any traction on the pedicle

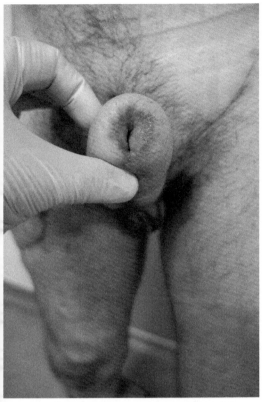

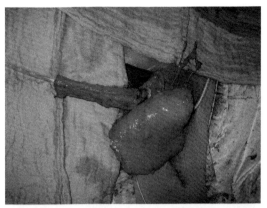

Fig. 25. Case 3 (see text for details). Left lateral intra-operative view. The belly is on the right hand side. The free radial forearm flap is wrapped around the drain placed into the bladder through the urethra and the anterolateral thigh (ALT) flap is ready to be wrapped around it. The nerves ready for coaptation can be seen coming from the ALT flap.

Fig. 23. Case 2 (see text for details). Close up view of the external urinary meatus, made of the suture of the superficial circumflex iliac perforator and the anterolateral thigh flaps.

for the first 3 days. Once the flap is tubed, any tension must be avoided. If there is any tension that might cause flap compression with postoperative edema, a skin graft is best placed ventrally to relieve this tension and avoid vascular compromise.

The presence of the expanders is cause of discomfort, especially toward expander completion, because the expanders hold a considerable volume. Patients try to partially conceal the expanders by wearing very large trousers. It is indeed a procedure for a small group of patients (10%) in our series, who accept the presence of the expanders and the additional operation and ambulatory inflations needed to reduce the donor site scarring. These patients must be very well-informed and have sufficient motivation because they have to put extra effort to go

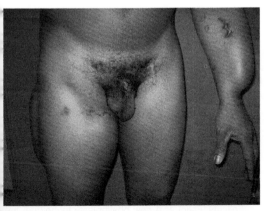

Fig. 24. Case 3 (see text for details). Preoperative view after completion of tissue expansion in the forearm and thigh.

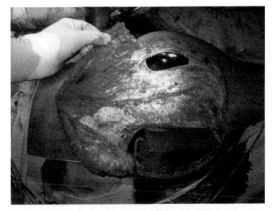

Fig. 26. Case 3 (see text for details). Intraoperative view before expander removal. The fascia has been closed.

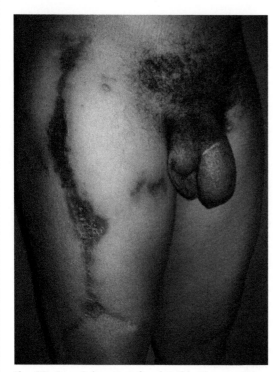

Fig. 27. Case 3 (see text for details). Three-quarters right postoperative view shows some widening and discoloration of the scar, not uncommon in people with dark skin.

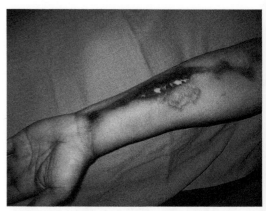

Fig. 28. Case 3 (see text for details). Widening and discoloration are observed also in the forearm skin.

SUMMARY

Preoperative expansion is a valuable tool for minimizing donor site scarring in ALT flap phalloplasty because it allows not only prevention of the unsightly donor site graft, but also scarring and pain related to a split thickness skin graft harvest. Preoperative perforator location with a CT angiography allows minimally invasive expander placement.

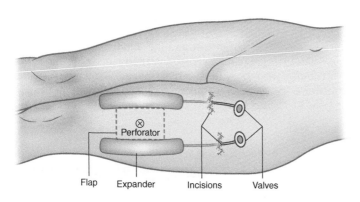

Flap   Expander   Incisions   Valves

Perforator

Fig. 29. This schematic drawing shows how incisions, expander, and valves shall be placed once the perforator is located by means of a CT scan. For more information, see **Figs. 4** and **5** and the relative legends, and the "preoperative planning and preparation" and "procedural approach: expander placement" sections.

through a longer process, additional operations, and extra costs.

Also, it has to be pointed out that in this cases reduction of scars is achieved at the expenses of contour. It has to be discussed with the patient that indeed the patch like scars due to skin grafting will be avoided. But avoidance of scars comes at the expenses of contour because the thinned expanded skin will cause a depression and a contour deformity in the thigh that will need future lipofilling sessions to be corrected.

REFERENCES

1. Ceulemans P. The Pedicled Anterolateral Thigh Flap (ALT) Perforator Flap: A New Technique for Phallic Reconstruction. Paper presented at the XIV Biennial Symposium of the Harry Benjamin International Gender Dysphoria Association (HBIGDA). Bologna, Italy, April 6–9, 2005.
2. Felici N, Felici A. A new phalloplasty technique: the free anterolateral thigh flap phalloplasty. J Plast Reconstr Aesthet Surg 2006;59:153–7.

3. Mutaf M, Isik D, Bulut Ö, et al. A true nonmicrosurgical technique for total phallic reconstruction. Ann Plast Surg 2006;57:100–6.

4. Lumen N, Monstrey S, Selvaggi G, et al. Phalloplasty: a valuable treatment for males with penile insufficiency. Urology 2008;71(2):272–6.

5. Lumen N, Monstrey S, Ceulemans P, et al. Reconstructive surgery for severe penile inadequacy: phalloplasty with a free radial forearm flap or a pedicled anterolateral thigh flap. Adv Urol 2008;704343.

6. Descamps MJ, Hayes PM, Hudson DA. Phalloplasty in complete aphallia: pedicled anterolateral thigh flap. J Plast Reconstr Aesthet Surg 2009;62(3):e51–4.

7. Lee GK, Lim AF, Bird ET. A novel single-flap technique for total penile reconstruction: the pedicled anterolateral thigh flap. Plast Reconstr Surg 2009; 124(1):163–6.

8. Rubino C, Figus A, Dessy LA, et al. Innervated island pedicled anterolateral thigh flap for neo-phallic reconstruction in female-to-male transsexuals. J Plast Reconstr Aesthet Surg 2009;62(3):e45–9.

9. Rashid M, Aslam A, Malik S, et al. Clinical applications of the pedicled anterolateral thigh flap in penile reconstruction. J Plast Reconstr Aesthet Surg 2011; 64(8):1075–81.

10. Sinove Y, Kyriopoulos E, Ceulemans P, et al. Preoperative planning of a pedicled anterolateral thigh (ALT) flap for penile reconstruction with the multidetector CT scan. Handchir Mikrochir Plast Chir 2013; 45(4):217–22.

11. Liu CY, Wei ZR, Jiang H, et al. Preconstruction of the pars pendulans urethrae for phalloplasty with digestive mucosa using a prefabricated anterolateral thigh flap in a one-arm patient. Plast Reconstr Surg Glob Open 2013;1(7):e53.

12. Holzbach T, Giunta RE, Machens HG, et al. Phalloplasty with pedicled anterolateral thigh flap ("ALT-Flap"). Handchir Mikrochir Plast Chir 2011;43(4): 227–31 [in German].

13. Hasegawa K, Namba Y, Kimata Y. Phalloplasty with an innervated island pedicled anterolateral thigh flap in a female-to-male transsexual. Acta Med Okayama 2013;67(5):325–31 [Erratum appears in Acta Med Okayama 2014;68(3):183].

14. Morrison SD, Son J, Song J, et al. Modification of the tube-in-tube pedicled anterolateral thigh flap for total phalloplasty: the mushroom flap. Ann Plast Surg 2014;72(Suppl 1):S22–6.

15. Monstrey S, Hoebeke P, Selvaggi G, et al. Penile reconstruction: is the radial forearm flap really the standard technique? Plast Reconstr Surg 2009; 124:510–8.

16. Matton GE, Tonnard PL, Monstrey SJ, et al. A universal incision for tissue expander insertion. Br J Plast Surg 1995;48(3):172–6.

17. Tsai FC. A new method: perforator-based tissue expansion for a preexpanded free cutaneous perforator flap. Burns 2003;29:845–8.

18. Hallock GG. The preexpanded anterolateral thigh free flap. Ann Plast Surg 2004;53:170–3.

19. Hallock GG. Tissue expansion techniques to minimize morbidity of the anterolateral thigh perforator flap donor site. J Reconstr Microsurg 2013;29(9):565–70.

20. Acartürk TO. Aesthetic reconstruction of the postburn neck contracture with a preexpanded anterolateral thigh free flap. J Craniofac Surg 2014;25(1):e23–6.

21. Hocaoğlu E, Arıncı A, Berköz Ö, et al. Free pre-expanded lateral circumflex femoral artery perforator flap for extensive resurfacing and reconstruction of the hand. J Plast Reconstr Aesthet Surg 2013;66(12):1788–91.

22. Solinc M, Kosutic D, Stritar A, et al. Preexpanded radial forearm free flap for one-stage total penile reconstruction in female-to-male transsexuals. J Reconstr Microsurg 2009;25(6):395–8.

23. Terrier JÉ, Courtois F, Ruffion A, et al. Surgical outcomes and patients' satisfaction with suprapubic phalloplasty. J Sex Med 2014;11(1):288–98.

24. Dong L, Dong Y, He L, et al. Penile reconstruction by preexpanded free scapular flap in severely burned patient. Ann Plast Surg 2014;73(Suppl 1):S27–30.

Pre-expanded Free Perforator Flaps

Emre Hocaoğlu, MD

KEYWORDS

- Pre-expansion • Pre-expanded perforator flap • Perforator flap • Free flap • Free tissue transfer
- Microsurgery

KEY POINTS

- All preoperative planning activities (perforator designation, perforator and source vessel tracing, and detection of neighboring perforators) should be executed on the patient in the same position as they will be lying during the flap harvest procedure.
- Exposure of the designated perforator should be avoided during the expander implantation session.
- At each inflation session, a smaller volume of saline compared with a conventional tissue expansion is administered, which causes minimal lengthening in the overall expansion period.
- Dissection of the nonexpanded side first allows the surgeon to approach the perforator through untouched tissues such that this part of the procedure becomes less complex, almost the same as a conventional perforator flap dissection.

 Video content accompanies this article at http://www.plasticsurgery.theclinics.com.

INTRODUCTION

Soon after Taylor and Palmer[1] demonstrated an average of 374 direct or indirect cutaneous perforators of greater than 0.5 mm diameter, Koshima and Soeda[2] published the first clinical use of the perforator flap technique. There has recently been rapid and great improvement in the perforator flap technique and a great variety of donor sites have been introduced to the literature.[3–9] In addition to these, pre-expansion of perforator flap donor sites provided additional support in donor tissue supplies.[10–16] All these improvements have provided great alternatives to treat most defects using local, regional, or distant pedicled pre-expanded perforator flaps. Thus, the need for free transfer of skin flaps seems to be reduced. However, there could still be some circumstances that necessitate free transfer of pre-expanded perforator flaps.

Pre-expanded perforator flaps are the most recent technical way to shape tissue for exact needs. Using this tissue as a free flap gives the surgeon a wide range of mobility. For the time being, the pre-expanded free perforator flap technique has been covered in the literature through a limited number of contributions including a case series,[17] a few case reports,[10,11,18] and cases incorporated in pre-expanded perforator flap series.[15,19,20] With the combination of the finest microsurgical skills executed during perforator flap techniques and advanced methods of tissue handling, such as tissue expansion and free tissue transfer, reconstruction with free pre-expanded perforator flaps serves as one of the highest rungs of the reconstructive ladder.

Disclosure: None.
Department of Plastic Reconstructive and Aesthetic Surgery, Istanbul Faculty of Medicine, Istanbul University, Fatih, Istanbul 34093 Turkey
E-mail address: emrehocaoglu@gmail.com

Clin Plastic Surg 44 (2017) 143–152
http://dx.doi.org/10.1016/j.cps.2016.08.011

TREATMENT GOALS AND PLANNED OUTCOMES

Adding a "pre-expansion" to the treatment plan means that a multistage (usually two) procedure is accepted by the patient. Pre-expanded free perforator flaps are preferred over free perforator flaps for four reasons: (1) broader flap (eg, one pre-expanded free perforator flap instead of two free perforator flaps), (2) thinner flap (eg, no need for extra secondary debulking procedures or no need for primary microsurgical flap thinning procedures), (3) more reliable flap (eg, one perforator is usually enough instead of multiple perforators), and (4) less donor site scarring and deformity. Although the list will surely be longer in the near future, the indications are listed in **Box 1**.

Free tissue transfer is a safe and reliable means of obtaining skin for extensive resurfacing and release procedures.[21] Furthermore, it renders multiple donor sites available for a single defect. Accordingly, free transfer of pre-expanded perforator flaps is a reliable option and especially benefits cases of donor site stringency. For instance, a diffuse scarred area with contractures can be resurfaced with a super-thin and super-wide perforator flap provided that this flap incorporates more than one perforator. Moreover, the patient and surgeon have to accept a badly scarred donor site because it will almost certainly be closed using a skin graft or sutures that are too tight. Nevertheless, for resurfacing of that same diffuse scarred area with contractures, if the patient does not have a broad enough donor site and/or if the donor site only has one suitable perforator, which would not be enough for an extensive flap, and/or if the patient has limited tolerance for donor site scar and/or if there is a need for a thin flap with good vascularity, a pre-expanded free perforator flap is a preferable alternative. Indications for free transfer of pre-expanded perforator flaps are listed in **Box 2**.

Contraindications for performing free pre-expanded perforator flaps are associated with free tissue transfer, tissue expansion, or both. These are appraised as relative contraindications but have strong influence over decision-making (**Box 3**).

PREOPERATIVE PLANNING AND PREPARATION

Everything starts with a generalized preoperative work-up for free flap surgery. During the evaluation of the patient a multisession surgical treatment plan involving lengthy operations should be kept in mind. A meticulous investigation of any comorbidities, previous surgeries and completed treatments, history about hypercoagulability, medications, and drug and smoking habits is an indispensable opening.

Subsequently it is better first to zoom in on the defect site and then on the donor site. Features and history about the defect or scar or contracture site (type of trauma, tumor, and previous treatment attempts, such as radiotherapy, failed free flaps), its neighborhood (eg, lymph node dissection, radiotherapy), and the recipient vessels (imaging, such as computed tomography angiography, magnetic resonance angiography, or color-Doppler ultrasonography) are handled.

Assessment of the donor site includes examining the tissue color, thickness, pliability and expansibility, the tissue supply, probable pedicle length, and probable morbidity. Initially, a

---

Box 1
Indications for pre-expanded perforator flaps

1. Esthetic resurfacing of extensive scarred areas on the face, neck, anterior chest wall, and breasts.

2. Release and resurfacing of severe contractures incorporated in extensive scars on the face, neck, anterior chest wall, axilla, breasts, perineum, hands, and upper and lower extremities.

3. Resurfacing giant congenital nevi.

4. Penis reconstruction (a more pliable, thinner, and broader flap facilitates reconstruction of a penis or construction of a neophallus with a more natural size and shape, especially in the tube-in-tube approach).

5. Esophageal reconstruction (a more pliable and thinner flap with better vascularity).

Box 2
Indications for free transfer of pre-expanded perforator flaps

1. Adjacent or regional perforasomes are already scarred or have limited area and/or expansibility.

2. Use of the adjacent or regional skin will cause an unacceptable additional scar and/or contracture.

3. Adjacent/regional perforasomes are not suitable for implanting an expander.

4. Providing extra vascularity to the recipient site would be an issue (eg, defect in an ischemic extremity).

Box 3
Contraindications for performing free pre-expanded perforator flaps

1. Inadequate recipient vessels of the defect site and its neighborhood.
2. The only suitable recipient vessels exist inside the vicinity of the zone of injury (in cases of chronic traumatic defects).
3. Recipient vessels in the vicinity of radiotherapy zone.
4. Unsuitable health status (ongoing significant comorbidities) for multiple-session operations or lengthy operations.
5. Drug usage, cigarette smoking, immune suppression, ongoing chemotherapy.
6. Reluctance of the patient to receive multiple operations or lengthy operations.
7. Suspicion of low compliance of the patient with multiple postoperative outpatient controls required in the expansion period.
8. Ongoing sport/physical activities that would increase the risk for extrusion of the expander.
9. Inexperienced microsurgical team.

hand-held Doppler examination is made to predict vascularity and perforasomes of the determined donor site. For detection of relevant perforators of the donor site, documenting diameters and subcutaneous, suprafascial, subfascial, and intramuscular traces of these perforators, and also documenting the source vessel and its trace,

either computed tomography angiography or color-Doppler ultrasonography are used. All imaging studies and evaluations should be performed in the same patient position as that used during the flap harvest procedure.

Preimplantation (before the expander implantation session) drawings on the donor site include the following (**Fig. 1**):

1. The chosen perforator's point of perforation through the fascia
2. Trace of the chosen perforator and the source vasculature
3. Expander pocket
4. Incision of the implantation session
5. Perforators in the neighborhood

Preoperative drawings of the flap harvest session are made on the expanded donor site and the recipient site. A flap with appropriate design, congruent to the probable defect shape, is plotted on the donor site. The boundaries of the flap design incorporate at least the chosen perforator and its subcutaneous trace at the non-expanded pole and a large portion of the expanded skin (**Fig. 2**). Usually flap size is planned as the largest dimensions that would allow primary closure of the donor site. In patients for whom the priority is resurfacing as extensively as possible, broad flaps are planned without considering primary closure of the donor site. Thus, flap size decision-making is a patient-based approach. One must always remember that although these patients are eager to get rid of as much of their scarring as possible, at the same time they are already sensitive and responsive to additional scars.

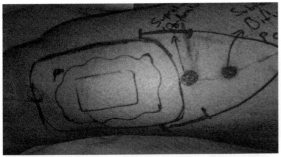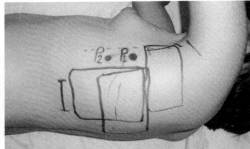

Fig. 1. Examples of donor site markings in preimplantation phase of pre-expanded perforator flap procedures. (*Left*) On the left thigh of a patient, a self-inflating rectangular tissue expander implantation site is drawn distal to a lateral circumflex femoral artery (LCFA) perforator. Color Doppler ultrasonography revealed a subfascial bifurcation (marked on the skin as the *proximal blue dot*) of a muscular branch of descending branch of the LCFA into a perforator artery and a terminal muscular artery. The *distal blue dot* marks the perforation point of the fascia by the perforator vessels. Two possible positions for the incision are drawn. (*Right*) Around these two thoracodorsal artery perforators, three possible locations for a rectangular tissue expander are marked.

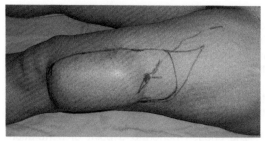

Fig. 2. Expanded donor site of a lateral circumflex femoral artery perforator (LCFAP) flap. Flap design and dimensions, perforation point, and the subcutaneous trace of LCFAP vessels and trace of the source vessel are marked on the skin.

PATIENT POSITIONING

Determining the patient position involves considering three main factors: (1) flap donor site, (2) recipient site, and (3) two team approach (simultaneous or sequential). Classic positional approaches for the harvest of particular perforator flap donor sites have stood the test of time and are the main determining factors for patient positioning. When there is an opportunity to work simultaneously in two teams, one of which harvests the flap and the other prepares the recipient site and recipient vessels, a variation of the classic position for that particular flap type may be indicated. When there is a chance to choose a particular donor site that allows a two-team approach, there is no need to look for a variation in the classic harvest position, but when perforator flap donor sites are limited and the classic harvest position of the chosen donor site does not permit a two-team approach, there are two possibilities: find an intermediate-form of patient position or not to work simultaneously, but sequentially. Another important point is that the patient position should be the same during preoperative imaging studies, expander implantation session, and the flap harvest session.

PROCEDURAL APPROACH

The procedure incorporates any general principle regarding microsurgery, free flap surgery, and perforator flap surgery.[14,15,21–23] Additionally, there are some technical details concerning free pre-expanded perforator flaps:

First Surgery (Expander Implantation)

A limited incision of the skin and subcutaneous tissue is followed by a suprafascial dissection of a pocket. The pocket is designed in accordance with the particular expander type. The emerging

point and the subcutaneous trace of the chosen perforator should already have been drawn on the skin preoperatively and with the guidance of these markings, the dissection proceeds elaborately, taking care not to expose the chosen perforator, and is stopped within 1 cm to 2 cm of the perforator (see **Figs. 1** and **2**). A closed suction drain is usually placed on the floor of the pocket and the expander is placed on the drain. The expander is inflated to about one-tenth of its total volume just before wound closure.

First Postoperative Period (Tissue Expansion Period)

Inflation starts 3 weeks after the implantation and continues once or twice a week thereafter. Smaller volumes of saline (less than one-tenth of the total volume) compared with a conventional tissue expansion are administered at each inflation session. This approach causes minimal lengthening in the overall expansion period. During the inflation period, repeated monitoring of perforator artery flow, at least with a hand-held Doppler device, is a requisite (if possible, during each inflation session). The pressure of the expander should not block the flow through the perforator artery. About an extra month following the last inflation session is usually required for optimal tissue expansion.

Second Surgery (Flap Harvest)

The location and course of the perforator is marked on the skin and the surgery begins with suprafascial dissection and perforator exploration. Dissection begins from the nonexpanded side of the flap (**Fig. 3**). Dissecting the nonexpanded side first allows the surgeon to approach the perforator through untouched tissues. Usually the capsule around the expander comes close to

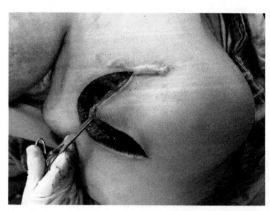

Fig. 3. Pre-expanded perforator flap harvest begins from the nonexpanded side (the patient in **Fig. 1**, *right*).

the perforator by as near as a few millimeters. If additional perforators are encountered, they are also conserved until the chosen perforator is dissected successfully up to the source vessels.

Perforator dissection through the fascia and muscle is almost always the same as a conventional perforator flap harvest (**Figs. 4** and **5**, Video 1). Very rarely, foreign body reaction involves peri-perforator tissue and renders the tissue more fragile and as such the dissection becomes more challenging.

In the event of an opportunity of a simultaneous two-team approach, the recipient site team releases the contractures using incisions without scar resections and prepares the recipient vasculature. Scar resection is postponed until successful harvest of the flap is guaranteed. Our approach in deciding flap dimensions is mentioned in the "preoperative planning" section.

Flaps are harvested under loupe magnification (×3.5–4.5), anastomoses are performed using an operating surgical microscope under higher magnification (×10–40). Surgery is performed under hypotensive anesthesia (lower limit of systolic blood pressure is usually kept at 90 mm Hg) until arterial anastomoses are completed. For optimizing the flap inflow, hypotension is preferably treated via fluid administration. Heparin is routinely used intraoperatively but never postoperatively. Just before clamping the recipient vasculature, 80 IU/kg of heparin is administered systemically. During and after performance of the anastomoses, the operating room is kept warm. Regarding pediatric patients, the principles of free flap surgery are similar to adults but it is technically more challenging, especially in free perforator flap surgery because of the miniaturized structures.

In cases of flaps with huge surface areas, which raises suspicion of vascular insufficiency, an extra surgical session for delay phenomenon may be

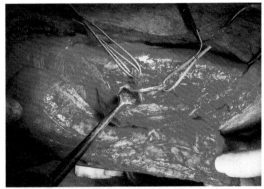

Fig. 5. Completed intramuscular dissection of a lateral circumflex femoral artery perforator (identified by *two blue vascular loops*) and its relationship with the femoral nerve branches (identified by *one blue vascular loop*). The vascular loops lie on the rectus femoris muscle, and the vastus lateralis muscle is retracted by a Langenbeck retractor.

added to the procedure. It is performed via skin, subcutaneous tissue, and the periexpander capsule incision all around the planned flap except on one side (usually sparing the side of the perforator) (**Fig. 6**). This extra session can be executed under sedation and ends with primary dermal suturation of the incisions. The delay procedure lasts 2 weeks.

In cases of suspicion of vascular insufficiency after the flap harvest, just before the division of pedicles, intraoperative indocyanine green fluorescence angiography is a valuable tool in imaging nonperfused flap regions[24] and making recipient site resections accordingly.

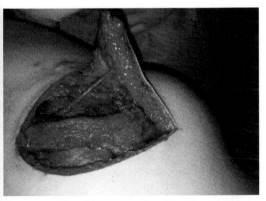

Fig. 4. Completed intramuscular dissection of a thoracodorsal artery perforator.

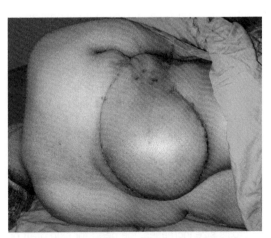

Fig. 6. After 2 weeks of delay period a huge pre-expanded thoracodorsal artery perforator flap is ready to be harvested.

POTENTIAL COMPLICATIONS AND THEIR MANAGEMENT

1. Hematoma and/or seroma: During pocket preparation, careful ligation of the extra perforators located in the dissection zone and meticulous hemostasis before expander implantation almost always prevents such complications. We use closed suction drains in both surgical procedures.
2. Expander failure: Deflation, puncture, and persistent pain necessitate change of the expander and sometimes the donor site.
3. Expander extrusion: Infection may cause expander exposure, purulent drainage, and expander extrusion. Copious irrigation and antibiotics seldom works. Donor site skin is damaged in various amounts, which may necessitate a change in the donor site. However, the procedure could be completed successfully with some loss in flap area if expander exposure is seen in the late period of tissue expansion because of necrosis. Local wound care gives enough time for reasonable expansion (**Fig. 7**).
4. Pedicle strain or rupture, accidental perforator sectioning during flap harvest: If it is not an avulsion, flap can be transferred with a short and small diameter pedicle. This necessitates supramicrosurgery experience. In cases of avulsion injury, there is usually not much one can do about salvaging the flap unless there is another suitable perforator.
5. Erroneous planning of the shape and/or dimensions of the flap: Scar resection should be performed in concordance with flap size. If the flap is larger than the chosen perforator can feed, partial necrosis is unavoidable. In such circumstances, keeping the secondary perforators intact (if possible) and making additional anastomoses if necessary or resecting the nonperfused regions detected through intraoperative indocyanine green fluorescence angiography may be performed.
6. Pedicle kinking and rotation: Probably one of the most dangerous but preventable complications in the free transfer procedure is unnoticed rotation of the perforator segment of the pedicle. Rotation of the source vessel is easily recognized, thus it rarely remains rotated but the most dangerous part lies between the source vessel and the subcutaneous tissue.
7. Partial necrosis: Minor loss is resolved by advancement of the remaining part. As the necrosis size increases, the need for skin graft or another flap also increases. After 6 to 12 months, the remaining flap is re-expanded

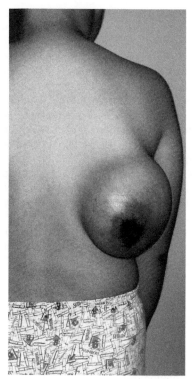

Fig. 7. Necrosis that happens toward the end of the expansion period causes no change in the surgical procedure except some loss of the gained tissues. Simple wound care and terminating the inflation provides enough time for preparation of the second surgery.

and additional resurfacing including the grafted site may be achieved.

8. Total necrosis: Split thickness skin graft is used for closure of the wound formed after debridement, and secondary flap procedures are planned for the remaining deformity.

POSTPROCEDURAL CARE

- Just before the patient awakens from general anesthesia, diluted bupivacaine is locally injected around the recipient site sutures and the donor site suture line (maximum dose, 1 mg/kg).
- It is important to maintain a pain-free postoperative period. Intravenous patient-controlled analgesia is the preferred method for adult and pediatric patients.
- The patient's room is kept warm and quiet.
- Urine output of at least 1 mL/kg/hour is targeted and systolic blood pressure is kept above 100 mm Hg.
- Flap monitoring is carried out via clinical observation (color, capillarity, temperature,

turgor, bleeding pattern) and hand-held Doppler signals.

- In the postoperative period, systemic low-molecular-weight heparin is administered in a prophylactic dosage for the first week.

REHABILITATION AND RECOVERY

Rehabilitation is planned according to the specific needs of the patient. Physical rehabilitation is especially important in pediatric patients with contracture and young adults in whom postural changes have occurred secondary to contractures. After a successful surgical management, for instance a contracture release and an extended scar resection, intensive physical therapy enables recovery of the losses.

OUTCOMES

In pre-expansion of free perforator flaps, we have used rectangular and round tissue expanders sizes ranging from 400 mL to 700 mL. Average expansion period was 19 weeks. Single expander was used in all free flap cases but our experience about pedicled pre-expanded perforator flaps leads to a conclusion that double expanders for a single perforator is a way of optimizing pre-expansion process. With this technique we were able to resurface and release extended scars and contractures of the anterior chest wall, neck, and upper extremity by thin, pliable, and extended flaps. Moreover these flaps have sustained compatibility with the recipient sites of pediatric patients in terms of rapid growth and morphology. No secondary thinning procedures were needed for the transferred tissues. Donor sites where tight closure had been performed needed revision, especially in case of pediatric patients.[14,15]

Case 1

A 17-year-old girl presented with burn sequelae on her right hand. Scars, contractures, and traumatic syndactylysations caused severe functional and esthetic problems (**Fig. 8**).[11] Lateral circumflex femoral artery perforator (LCFAP) flap donor site

was prepared by a 400 mL tissue expander, which was overfilled to 600 mL, in 22 weeks. Resection of scars and release of the contractures of the metacarpophalangeal joints resulted in a defect about 18 cm × 8 cm. Coverage of this defect with a thin and pliable skin flap resulted in a functional and esthetic reconstruction with minimal donor site morbidity (**Figs. 9** and **10**, Video 2).

Case 2

A 10-year-old girl presented with broad scars and contractures of the axilla, anterior chest wall, and breasts (**Fig. 11**).[14] After an expansion period of 14 weeks, a 400-mL expander was overfilled to 700 mL without any complications. Pre-expanded intercostal artery perforator (ICAP) flap was successfully harvested and transferred to the defect formed by substantial resection of the scars and release of the contractures of the axilla and breast. Follow-up during the rapid growth phase of this patient enabled us to observe the great contribution of ICAP flap to the healthy rapid development of the breasts (**Figs. 12–14**, Video 3). Hence, this was perfect timing for treatment in this specific case.

DISCUSSION

Free transfer of pre-expanded thoracodorsal artery perforator (TDAP) flap,[14,15,17] pre-expanded LCFAP flap,[10,11,18,19] pre-expanded internal mammary artery perforator flap,[20] pre-expanded ICAP flap,[14] and pre-expanded lumbar artery perforator flap[14] has been handled in the literature. Almost all of these flaps have been used in the treatment of thick and rigid broad scar tissues and contractures of different sites of the body. These extensive, thin, pliable skin flaps were mostly used for resurfacing visible regions of the body, such as the face, neck, anterior chest wall, axilla, hands, and breasts where esthetics in reconstruction are important.

In literature pre-expanded free LCFAP flap was used for contractures of hand[11] and cervical region.[10,18,19] Most important advantage of this flap is to enable a simultaneous two-team

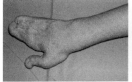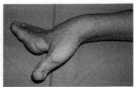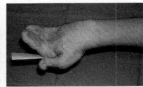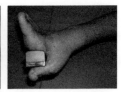

Fig. 8. Severe functional and esthetic problems of the hand before treatment. (The first and third photographs have been *adapted from* Hocaoğlu E, Arıncı A, Berköz O, et al. Free pre-expanded lateral circumflex femoral artery perforator flap for extensive resurfacing and reconstruction of the hand. J Plast Reconstr Aesthet Surg 2013;66:1789; with permission).

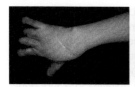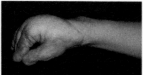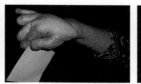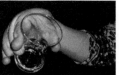

Fig. 9. Five years after reconstruction with free pre-expanded lateral circumflex femoral artery perforator flap and minor revision procedures.

approach. Other advantages are LCFAP flap's familiar harvest technique because it is one of the workhorse perforator flaps and its well-concealed donor site. Color mismatch is the main disadvantage when used for cervicofacial reconstruction.

Wang and colleagues[17] used pre-expanded free TDAP flaps for releasing contractures and resurfacing scars of the cervicofacial region. The average flap size was 22 cm × 14 cm and pedicle length was 14.4 cm. Besides the fact that dorsal trunk skin color does not ideally match with the cervicofacial region, this series clearly demonstrates that free pre-expanded TDAP flap is a versatile option for extended resurfacings and functional contracture releases.

Zan and colleagues[20] used pre-expanded free internal mammary artery perforator flaps for extended middle and upper facial resurfacings. In their series, average flap size was 18 cm × 9 cm and there was no partial or total flap necrosis. The authors draw attention to the limited area of this flap (as much as two facial aesthetic units) and probable deformation of the breasts in female patients.

Almost all relevant authors prefer to place the expander over the fascia. When compared with deeper planes, such as under the fascia or muscle, suprafascial expansion results in a more effective tissue expansion, thinner flap, and less donor site morbidity.[15]

The most important disadvantage of pre-expanded perforator flaps is absolutely pertinent for free transfer: that is the peripheral location of the pedicle, which is a potential threat for partial necrosis. As we handled this issue in our previous articles, we recently place two expanders around

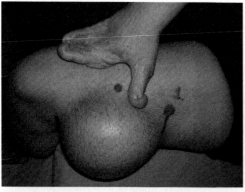
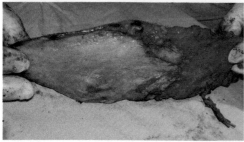
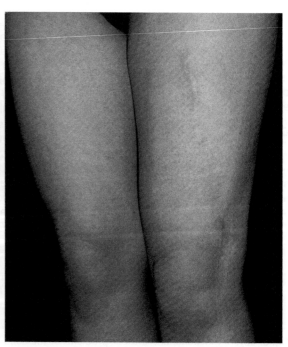

Fig. 10. Before the flap harvest surgery, donor site evaluation with handheld Doppler device and color Doppler ultrasonography revealed three perforators around the expanded tissue. Flap was harvested on the most proximal perforator. Five-year-old donor site scar is not bothersome.

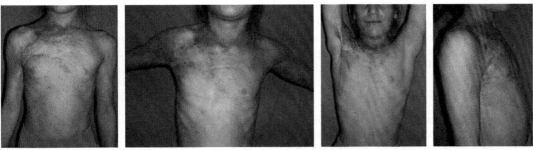

Fig. 11. Scars and contractures of the axilla, anterior chest wall, and breasts causing deplacement of the nipple areola complex during arm movement. (The first, second and third photographs have been *adapted from* Hocaoğlu E, Aydin H. Preexpanded perforator flaps of the dorsolateral trunk in pediatric patients. Plast Reconstr Surg 2013;131:1077–86; with permission).

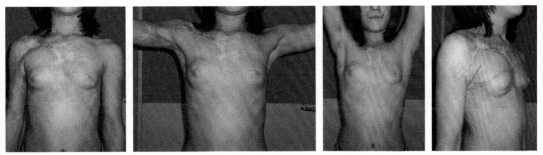

Fig. 12. One year after reconstruction with free pre-expanded intercostal artery perforator flap (patient is 11 years old). Flap keeps up with the growing body and the growing breasts.

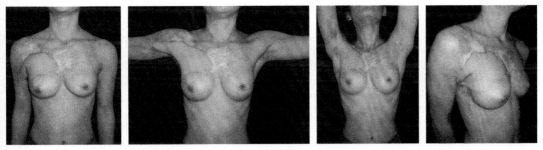

Fig. 13. Five years after the flap transfer, there is a remarkable concordance between the flap and the recipient region.

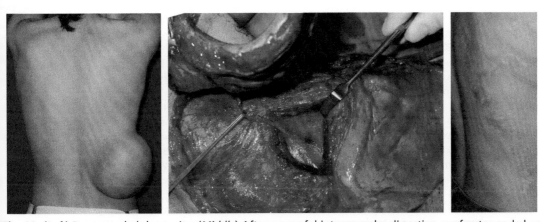

Fig. 14. (*Left*) Pre-expanded donor site. (*Middle*) After successful intramuscular dissection, perforator ended on the intercostals space. (*Right*) Donor site scar after 5 years of postoperative follow-up.

the perforator so that we centralize the pedicle on the flap. This approach, called "periperforator circumferential expansion," seems to be a good solution and more feasible for the pre-expanded free perforator flaps.[14,15]

SUMMARY

The three main concepts that reconstructive surgeons use in their practice are replacing like with like,[25] in vivo tissue engineering, and the indisputably growing value of gaining and preserving esthetics in reconstruction. The three main tools used for these issues are tissue expansion, free tissue transfer, and perforator flaps. As one of the latest generation tools, free pre-expanded perforator flaps offer useful, effective, ingenious but demanding solutions for the management of dreadful deformities. But this tool is still in need of technical development.

SUPPLEMENTARY DATA

Supplementary data related to this article can be found online at 10.1016/j.cps.2016.08.011.

REFERENCES

1. Taylor GI, Palmer JH. The vascular territories (angiosomes) of the body: experimental study and clinical applications. Br J Plast Surg 1987;40:113–41.
2. Koshima I, Soeda S. Inferior epigastric artery skin flaps without rectus abdominis muscle. Br J Plast Surg 1989;42:645–8.
3. Maciel-Miranda A, Morris SF, Hallock GG. Local flaps, including pedicled perforator flaps: anatomy, technique, and applications. Plast Reconstr Surg 2013;131:896e–911e.
4. Gir P, Cheng A, Oni G, et al. Pedicled-perforator (propeller) flaps in lower extremity defects: a systematic review. J Reconstr Microsurg 2012;28:595–601.
5. Hamdi M, Rasheed MZ. Advances in autologous breast reconstruction with pedicled perforator flaps. Clin Plast Surg 2012;39:477–90.
6. Hofer SO, Mureau MA. Pedicled perforator flaps in the head and neck. Clin Plast Surg 2010;37:627–40.
7. Teo TC. The propeller flap concept. Clin Plast Surg 2010;37:615–26.
8. Wallace CG, Kao HK, Jeng SF, et al. Free-style flaps: a further step forward for perforator flap surgery. Plast Reconstr Surg 2009;124(6 Suppl):e419–26.
9. Geddes CR, Morris SF, Neligan PC. Perforator flaps: evolution, classification, and applications. Ann Plast Surg 2003;50:90–9.
10. Tsai FC. A new method: perforator-based tissue expansion for a preexpanded free cutaneous perforator flap. Burns 2003;29:845–8.
11. Hocaoğlu E, Arıncı A, Berköz Ö, et al. Free pre-expanded lateral circumflex femoral artery perforator flap for extensive resurfacing and reconstruction of the hand. J Plast Reconstr Aesthet Surg 2013;66:1788–91.
12. Saint-Cyr M, Schaverien M, Rohrich RJ. Preexpanded second intercostal space internal mammary artery pedicle perforator flap: case report and anatomical study. Plast Reconstr Surg 2009;123:1659–64.
13. Kulahci Y, Sever C, Uygur F, et al. Pre-expanded pedicled thoracodorsal artery perforator flap for postburn axillary contracture reconstruction. Microsurgery 2011;31:26–31.
14. Hocaoğlu E, Aydin H. Preexpanded perforator flaps of the dorsolateral trunk in pediatric patients. Plast Reconstr Surg 2013;131:1077–86.
15. Hocaoğlu E, Emeklı U, Çızmecı O, et al. Suprafascial pre-expansion of perforator flaps and the effect of pre-expansion on perforator artery diameter. Microsurgery 2014;34:188–96.
16. Lu F, Gao JH, Ogawa R, et al. Preexpanded distant "super-thin" intercostal perforator flaps for facial reconstruction without the need for microsurgery. J Plast Reconstr Aesthet Surg 2006;59:1203–8.
17. Wang AW, Zhang WF, Liang F, et al. Pre-expanded thoracodorsal artery perforator-based flaps for repair of severe scarring in cervicofacial regions. J Reconstr Microsurg 2014;30:539–46.
18. Acartürk TO. Aesthetic reconstruction of the postburn neck contracture with a preexpanded anterolateral thigh free flap. J Craniofac Surg 2014;25:e23–6.
19. Tsai FC, Mardini S, Chen DJ, et al. The classification and treatment algorithm for post-burn cervical contractures reconstructed with free flaps. Burns 2006;32:626–33.
20. Zan T, Li H, Du Z, et al. Reconstruction of the face and neck with different types of pre-expanded anterior chest flaps: a comprehensive strategy for multiple techniques. J Plast Reconstr Aesthet Surg 2013;66:1074–81.
21. Saint-Cyr M, Wong C, Buchel EW, et al. Free tissue transfers and replantation. Plast Reconstr Surg 2012;130:858e–78e.
22. Vyas K, Wong L. Intraoperative management of free flaps: current practice. Ann Plast Surg 2014;72:S220–3.
23. Zhang B, Wan JH, Wan HF, et al. Free perforator flap transfer for reconstruction of skull base defects after resection of advanced recurrent tumor. Microsurgery 2014;34:623–8.
24. Liu DZ, Mathes DW, Zenn MR, et al. The application of indocyanine green fluorescence angiography in plastic surgery. J Reconstr Microsurg 2011;27:355–64.
25. Gillies HD, Millard DR Jr. The principles and art of plastic surgery. 1st edition. Boston: Little, Brown & Co; 1957.

Pre-expanded Bipedicled Supratrochlear Perforator Flap for Simultaneous Reconstruction of the Nasal and Upper Lip Defects

Shaoqing Feng, MD, PhD[a,1], Zheng Zhang, MD[a,1], Wenjing Xi, MD[a,1], Davide Lazzeri, MD[b], Yong Fang, MD, PhD[a,*], Yi Xin Zhang, MD, PhD[a,*]

KEYWORDS

- Supratrochlear perforator forehead flap • Nasal reconstruction • Upper lip reconstruction
- Tissue expansion

KEY POINTS

- The supratrochlear perforator vessels come in pairs in the forehead, which permit 2 flaps to be harvested at the same time.
- The forehead is an excellent source of skin and soft tissue for most nasal reconstruction. Because the upper lip is adjacent to the nose, the forehead should be a possible donor site for upper lip reconstruction.
- The pre-expanded, bipedicled supratrochlear perforator flap technique allows the reconstruction of the nose and the upper lip, 2 independent units, with 2 flaps from 1 donor site.
- The pre-expansion technique can provide abundant tissue so that the donor site can be closed directly after the 2 flaps are harvested. Meanwhile, the pre-expansion is a flap delay procedure that can enhance the blood perfusion of the flaps, especially in their distal parts.

INTRODUCTION

The nose and upper lip are 2 adjacent units in the middle of the face that have prominent aesthetic status for humans. Defects in these 2 units are extremely conspicuous. The nose and upper lip are 2 projecting structures in the face, hence are prone to be damaged in trauma, or flame or chemical burns and also can be violated by tumor and infections. On the other hand, they tend to be destroyed together because of their adjacent positions. Simultaneous reconstruction of the 2 central facial units is a complex and challenging issue for plastic surgeons.

The principles of replacing "like with like" and achieving a unit or subunit reconstruction is well established. In 1956, Gonzalez-Ulloa[1] described the regional aesthetic "units" of the face, based on skin thickness, to emphasize the need for restoring facial skin units in complete regions as

The authors have nothing to disclose.
^a Department of Plastic and Reconstructive Surgery, Shanghai Ninth People's Hospital, Shanghai Jiao Tong University School of Medicine, 639 Zhi Zao Ju Road, Shanghai 200011, P.R. China; ^b Plastic Reconstructive and Aesthetic Surgery Unit, Villa Salaria Clinic, Via Filippo Antonio Gualterio 127, Rome 00139, Italy
¹ The first 3 authors equally contributed.
* Corresponding author.
E-mail addresses: fangyong1020@hotmail.com; zhangyixin6688@hotmail.com

plasticsurgery.theclinics.com

opposed to patch work. Burget and Menick[2] developed the facial "units" principle and also divided the nose into "subunits" based on skin quality, border outline, and 3-dimensional contour. They looked at facial surfaces as convex and concave regions that allow for different light reflection. Burget and Menick[2] emphasized that if a graft or a suture line is matched to the shape of a subunit, the natural appearance of facial light and shadows can be restored. Indeed, following the "units" and "subunits" concept, an optimal reconstructive result can be achieved because the scars are hidden within the joints between units or subunits and perceived as normal facial topography. More importantly, myofibroblasts lie in the recipient site under the transferred flap. They will contract, causing the transposed skin flap to rise above the level of adjacent skin. The flap will appear as a distracting patch if the defect is filled without regard to the subunit outline. When an entire subunit is resurfaced, the pincushioned flap shrinkwraps could augment, rather than distort, the contour of a subunit. The authors summarize these concepts and put forward the concept of the double "S" principle (similarity and subunit) for the facial reconstruction. The first "S" stands for the "similarity" of the donor site to the defect area and the second "S" means the reconstruction should be based on the different "subunits" of the face. Performing facial reconstruction according to this principle can dramatically improve the final appearance of facial scars and surgical outcomes.[3]

Many techniques have been described in the literature for the reconstruction of nose and upper lip defects. The easiest approach to resurfacing facial soft tissue defects is skin grafting. However, this method should generally be avoided because of the hyperpigmentation, secondary contracture, and poor texture. Free flaps can act as workhorse flaps in reconstruction for acute wounds and defects after trauma or tumor resection,[4–6] but their poor color and texture matching are the main reasons and patients very often need a second or third or even more revisions to improve cosmetic outcome. Most of the reports are focused on the forehead flap for the reconstruction of nose and local flaps for the reconstruction of the upper lip.[7,8] However, multiple donor sites are required and local flaps can resurface only small defects. Moreover, patients with composite nasal tissue losses often have facial injuries around the defect, reducing the availability of the donor site. Thus, it may be difficult to find an appropriate local flap for upper lip reconstruction. Yoshihiro and colleagues[9] reported their technique of using the split-scalping forehead flap for the reconstruction

of defects of the nose and upper lip. This technique reduced the number of donor sites but the cosmetic of hemi-forehead donor site was unpleasant and required skin grafting. Because the forehead area is an excellent source of skin and soft tissue for most nasal reconstructions in clinical practice,[10] and it also has the superior color and texture match to the facial skin, the forehead area should be a possible donor site for both nose and upper lip reconstruction. Based on the work of pioneers and the anatomic features of the facial vessels, which come in pairs, we present our experience with the pre-expanded, bipedicled supratrochlear perforator flaps for simultaneous nasal and upper lip resurfacing. This novel approach allows the reconstruction of multiple facial subunits with tissue of similar color and texture to the recipient site from a single donor site.

TREATMENT GOALS AND PLANNED OUTCOMES

To improve the final appearance of facial scars and surgical outcomes, we put forward a concept of double "S" principle (similarity and subunit) for the facial reconstruction. The first "S" stands for the "similarity" of the donor site to the defect area and it is a selection criteria of the best donor site in reconstructive surgery. The forehead region should be the optimal choice owing to the neighborhood relationship and similar color and texture to the nose and upper lip. The second "S" means the reconstruction should be based on the different "subunits" of the face so as to restore facial skin unit or subunit with the same tissue and hide the scars within the joints between units or subunits. The nose and upper lip should be restored separately because they belong to different units of the face.

Based on the double "S" principle and with the help of tissue expansion technique, we applied the pre-expanded bipedicled supratrochlear perforator flap for simultaneous reconstruction of the nasal and upper lip defects from a single donor site. With the experience of more than 30 cases, we think that this technique is simple and safe in achieving excellent aesthetic results in nasal and upper lip reconstruction. When properly planned and performed, this operation can also obtain a low complication rate and minimal donor site morbidity.

PREOPERATIVE PLANNING AND PREPARATION

Patients with burn scar contractures of the nose and upper lip were operated on with the pre-expanded, bipedicled supratrochlear flap in our

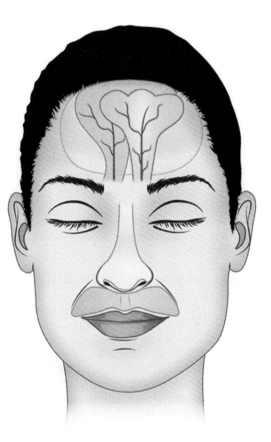

Fig. 1. The design of the pre-expanded bipedicled supratrochlear perforator flaps to resurface the nasal and upper lip defects at the same time.

department (**Fig. 1**). All operations were performed by the senior author (YXZ) under general anesthesia. A detailed informed consent about the operative technique, surgical risks, and potential complications were signed by the patients. The preoperatively photograph included full-face and both frontal and lateral views. Facial radiographs, computed tomography scans, or MRI are occasionally needed to clarify bony and soft tissue defects to the midface. The patients were asked to take a bath before the operation and a usual prophylactic antibiotic administration was done preoperatively.

PATIENT POSITIONING

All patients are placed in a supine position during the operation.

PROCEDURAL APPROACH

The operation is performed under general anesthesia, avoiding the distortion created by local anesthesia or the chemical blanching of epinephrine.

Stage 1: Expander Placement

A silicone tissue expander is inserted into the subgaleal plane of the forehead. The access incision is placed 1 to 2 cm within the hairline with the pocket extended from the hairline to the supraorbital rims bilaterally. Both the subgaleal pocket and the tissue expander are irrigated with antibiotic solution. The rectangular expander size ranges from 100 to 200 mL with the remote injection port embedded in the scalp. Twenty percent of the expander volume is inflated through the injection at the time of the expander placement so as to maintain some tension on the newly created pocket. A closed suction drainage is used for 1 to 2 days.

The expansion process begins 2 weeks postoperatively. Using saline solution and a 23-gauge hypodermic needle, 10% to 20% of the expander volume is injected twice a week until a final volume of 2.5 times the expander capacity is reached. A full expansion can be achieved usually in 3 months.

Stage 2: Flap Transfer

All the important landmarks and reference points are identified and marked before the first incision. The hairline, eyebrows, the outline of the nasal and upper lip units or subunits, and the margin of the scar are all marked with ink. The entire scar tissue around the nose and upper lip is removed. The release of the scars is considered complete only when all the landmarks return in their normal anatomic position. Until then, the exact sizes of defects of nose and upper lip could be measured. The reconstruction should follow the principle of unit/subunit, so not only the scar itself but also healthy tissue in the same unit/subunit is removed. Two templates are designed based on the size of the nose and upper lip defects.

Two independent supratrochlear artery perforator flaps are then marked side by side on the expanded forehead tissue. The 2 flaps have an axial pattern blood flow of which the supratrochlear vessels are the primary supply, and the anastomoses of the dorsal nasal, supraorbital, and angular arteries are the secondary supply[11] (**Fig. 2**). This secondary nourishment increases the flap's consistent blood supply and the proximal two-thirds of the pedicle may be quite narrow while the remaining part of the flap is extended to incorporate all the previously expanded skin area. The robust blood supply of the forehead area frees us from the concerns about the survival of the distal portion of the flap, so more attention can be paid to the reconstruction of defects. The bases of the 2 flaps are at the orbital margin, near the medial end of the eyebrow. The 2 pedicles should lie side by side in the glabella area and be marked

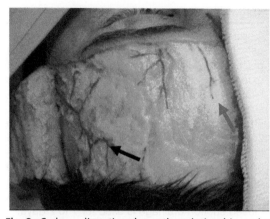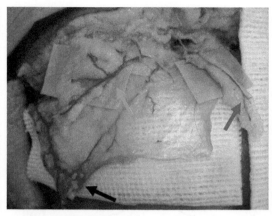

Fig. 2. Cadaver dissection shows the relationship and anastomoses of the supratrochlear vessels (*red arrow*), supraorbital vessels (*green arrow*), and superficial temporal vessels (*black arrow*).

1.2 to 1.5 cm in width to allow an arc of rotation of 180° to cover the nasal or upper lip defect without any torsion or kinking of the vessels. One flap is designed in a trilobed fashion and is used for nasal defect resurfacing. Another flap, based on the contralateral supratrochlear vessels, is marked longer than the first one and with an "L" shape to ease the placement of the pedicle beside the nose when it rotates to cover the defect of the upper lip. In addition, a curved distal edge is incorporated in the flap component to reflect the convexity of the upper lip. The dimensions of the flaps are planned accurately by the use of the templates. The flap sizes are approximately increased by 0.5 cm on each side to prevent the distortion of tissues at the time of contracture during the healing process. The length of the flap depends on the distance from the pivot point of the orbital margin to the recipient site. If a longer pedicle is needed,

the pivot point of the flap could be lowered toward the medial canthus and closer to the defect. Another way to achieve a longer pedicle is to place the flap more distally within the hairline, although a small amount of hair at the distal end of the flap is included. In female patients, hair could be removed later with laser or other procedures, whereas in male patients the hair on the flap can simulate the moustache. Attention should be paid that excessive tension (the flap is too short or too small, the pedicle is too wide or twisted) can devascularize the flap and cause ischemia.

A silicone nasal prosthesis is used as a support to the flap avoiding its contracture when a vascularized intranasal lining is already present or restored (**Fig. 3**). Cartilage grafts are not performed at this stage of reconstruction in case that the potential infection will damage it because the wound cannot be closed entirely at the pedicle

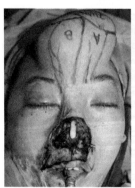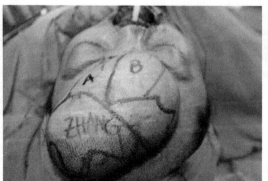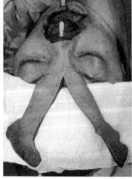

Fig. 3. The scars and residual normal skin are removed within the subunits of nose and upper lip and all the landmarks are returned to their normal anatomic position. Two independent supratrochlear perforator flaps are then marked side by side on the expanded forehead tissue. One flap is designed in a trilobed fashion and is used for nasal defect resurfacing. Another flap with an "L" shape is marked longer than the first one and is used for upper lip defect resurfacing. In addition, a curved distal edge is incorporated in the flap component to reflect the convexity of the upper lip. The flap sizes are increased by approximately 0.5 cm on each side to prevent the contracture during the healing process. Note a silicone nasal prosthesis is used as a support of the flap avoiding its contracture secondary.

site. The forehead donor site is sutured directly without tension in almost all cases. Alternatively, a secondary healing without skin graft is chosen. The raw surfaces of the pedicles are left to heal by secondary intention or covered by a full-thickness skin graft at the same stage (**Fig. 4**).

Stage 3: Unilateral Pedicle Division and Thinning

Both the components of the supratrochlear perforator flaps require 3 weeks to heal successfully. Then the pedicle of the flap designed for the upper lip defect resurfacing is cut as the flap can survive with the blood supply from the recipient site. The site of pedicle division is marked to ensure an adequate amount of tissue to resurface the recipient site. The proximal side of the pedicle is thinned with the trimming of fat and frontalis muscle and is inset medially to the eyebrow to resurface the scar and fill the defect of the harvesting procedure. The nasal flap is raised upward from its lower margin

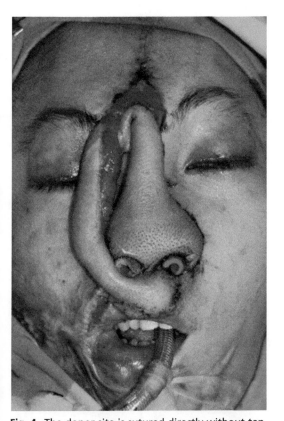

Fig. 4. The donor site is sutured directly without tension. The raw surfaces of the pedicles are left to heal by secondary intention. The exudation of the raw surface would cease when the granulation tissue has grown 1 week later. Note the suitable size drainages are left into the nostrils to decompress the intranasal pressure.

and is thinned and shaped to enhance the nasal reconstruction. Most frequently, it is completely re-elevated off the nose along the ideal nostril margin without any significant vascular risk because of the safety of the distal supply of the flap achieved with the delay at the time of its transfer. The ideal nasal flap should carry no more than 2 to 3 mm of fat layer to achieve an optimal and supple "skin only" flap to resurface the nose. The underlying excess of soft tissues, including scar, frontalis muscle, and subcutaneous tissue that healed into a rigid structure are excised to carve an ideal 3-dimensional subsurface architecture (**Fig. 5**). At this stage, the silicone nasal prosthesis is replaced with cartilage grafts having the right size for the optimal support and reshaping of the nostril margins and to avoid alar rim retraction and airway collapse postoperatively (**Fig. 6**). The importance of the rigid, 3-dimensional support framework cannot be overvalued for an ideal nasal contour. Once soft tissues are contracted by scar, secondary placement of cartilage grafts is less effective. Finally, the forehead flap is repositioned on the recontoured recipient bed with quilting sutures to close the dead space and to remodel the concave regions of nose. Peripherally, the flap is sutured with a single layer of fine sutures.

Stage 4: Second Pedicle Division

Three weeks after stage 3 (6 weeks after the flap transfer), the second pedicle could be divided. Further refinements are also performed at this stage. After the division of the pedicle, the part of the flap over the upper aspect of the defect is raised and distinct dorsal lines, flat sidewalls, and alar creases are created with an accurate soft tissue excision. The inset procedure is completed with quilting sutures and peripheral sutures. The proximal stump of the pedicle is trimmed, thinned, and inset as a small inverted "V" medially to the eyebrow to achieve a satisfactory eyebrow separation. The scar is in this way hidden into the normal frown lines.

In some cases, a later revision 3 to 6 months postoperatively may be required to enhance the cosmetic result. In particular, further definition of the alar crease, thinning of a thick nostril margin, and modifying the cartilage support grafts may be necessary for the nasal flap and thinning the flap, reshaping of the philtrum, revision of the upper lip bow may be required for the upper lip flap. Pressure therapy to the revised upper lip flap, especially in the philtrum region is essential to achieve a better cosmetic outcome. Such revisions are not considered a failure but a beneficial supplement of the reconstructive surgery.

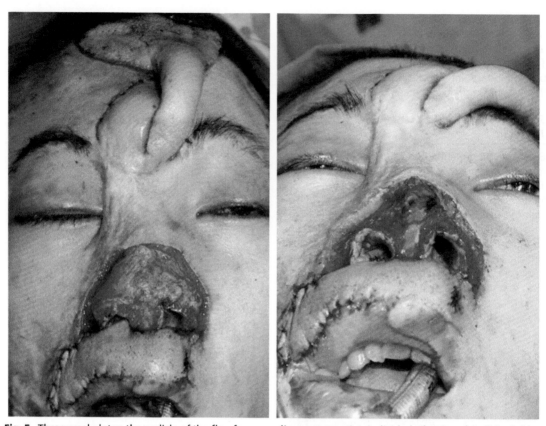

Fig. 5. Three weeks later, the pedicle of the flap for upper lip reconstruction is divided. The site of pedicle division is designed to ensure an adequate amount of tissue to resurface the recipient site according to the subunit principle. The nasal flap is re-elevated off the nose along the ideal nostril margin carrying only 2 to 3 mm of fat layer to achieve an optimal and supple "skin only" flap. The underlying excess of soft tissues, including scar, frontalis muscle, and subcutaneous tissue are excised to carve an ideal 3-dimensional subsurface architecture that would be visible through the overlying thin conforming forehead cover skin and would have the shape of a nose.

POTENTIAL COMPLICATIONS AND THEIR MANAGEMENT

Complications of the pre-expanded bipedicled supratrochlear perforator forehead flap are similar to the conventional forehead flap for nasal reconstruction and tissue expansion surgery. These include bleeding, infection, scarring, visible cartilage grafts, asymmetries, asymmetric nostrils, and nasal obstruction, as well as implant failure,

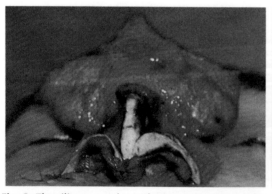

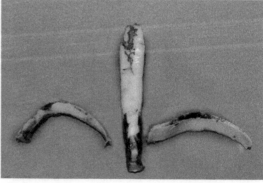

Fig. 6. The silicone nasal prosthesis is replaced and the costal cartilage is used to reconstruct a dorsal graft and carve as alar margin battens to restore a skeletal framework.

infection, and implant exposure. Postoperative complications of distal flap necrosis are rare, except in smokers. Long-term cigarette smoking affects the arterial circulation of the forehead skin. The pre-expansion has a benefit for smokers by enhancing the vascular safety of the flap through the delay phenomenon. Costal cartilage harvesting complications include pain, bleeding, infection, hypertrophic scarring, pneumothorax, and cartilage wrapping.

The overall complication rates are related to the surgery planning, flap design, and the experience of the individual surgeon. Most of the complications that occur during these operations are minor complications and do not interfere with successful outcome of the multistage procedure.

POSTOPERATIVE CARE

On the first postoperative day after the bipedicle flap transfer stage, the medication is changed and both pedicles are cleaned. The dressing is changed every day during the first week postoperation if the raw surface of the pedicles is not skin grafted. We prefer this approach because the exudation will cease when the granulation tissue covers the raw surface 1 week later, and the choice of avoiding skin graft decreases donor site morbidity.

If the donor site cannot be closed with direct sutures because of the large sizes of the harvested flaps, skin grafts or local flaps are not needed. It will close biologically by the process of wound contraction. No contraction occurs in the open defect for the first 3 weeks. Then, the wound will rapidly contract, cure, and produce a satisfactory result. A revision of the scar on forehead may be needed in these cases because of color mismatch.

REHABILITATION AND RECOVERY

Silicone gel or sheets are used to treat and prevent postoperative hypertrophic scarring. The suitable size drainages are left into the nostrils for at least 3 months to decompress the intranasal pressure. Pressure therapy is used onto the already thinned upper lip flap and onto the reshaped philtrum region to accomplish better cosmetic results.

OUTCOMES

With our approach, we successfully harvest forehead tissue for simultaneous total nasal and upper lip resurfacing from one single donor site. No microsurgical transfer is necessary and in most of the cases, the donor site is sutured directly with an aesthetically pleasing scar. Although the expansion stage does represent a drawback of

the procedure because it adds operative time and costs and reduces patient compliance, we believe that the pre-expansion stage is worthwhile given the excellent results that can be achieved with minimal donor site morbidity.

Case 1

A 40-year-old woman sustained severe chemical burn to her face 5 years ago. Scars extended from the lower half of her right face through the mental region, upper lip to the nose. The right nasal ala, half of the nasal dorsum, the columella, tip, and the upper lip were affected by the contracted scar. The pre-expanded bipedicled supratrochlear perforator flaps were designed to resurface the resultant nasal and upper lip defects following the scar excision. Another neck expanded flap prefabricated with the superficial temporal vessels was used for facial and mental region resurfacing. A 4-stage operation was performed as planned during 4.5 months. Another fine adjustment operation to the final result was performed 3 months postoperatively. The patient was followed for 1 year, good aesthetic results were achieved, and no complications were encountered. The donor site was closed primarily with aesthetically pleasing well-concealed linear scars (**Fig. 7**).

Case 2

A 32-year-old man presented with facial scars 3 years after sustaining flame burns to the face. Treatment of hypertrophic scars on the nose and upper lip was the target of the patient who came to our department. The pre-expanded bipedicled supratrochlear perforator flaps were designed to resurface the resultant nasal and upper lip defects following the scar excision. A 4-stage operation was performed as planned during 4.5 months. No later revision operation was performed. The patient was followed for 6 months; the color and texture match of the reconstructed nose and upper lip were good. The donor site scar was not conspicuous (**Fig. 8**).

DISCUSSION

The nose and upper lip are 2 prominent units in the middle face and tend to be damaged together in trauma, burns, and infections because of their adjacent positions. Simultaneous reconstruction of the 2 central facial units is a challenging task for plastic surgeons.

In the reconstruction of facial units, matching color and texture is the main consideration for aesthetic result. Therefore, the local and adjacent

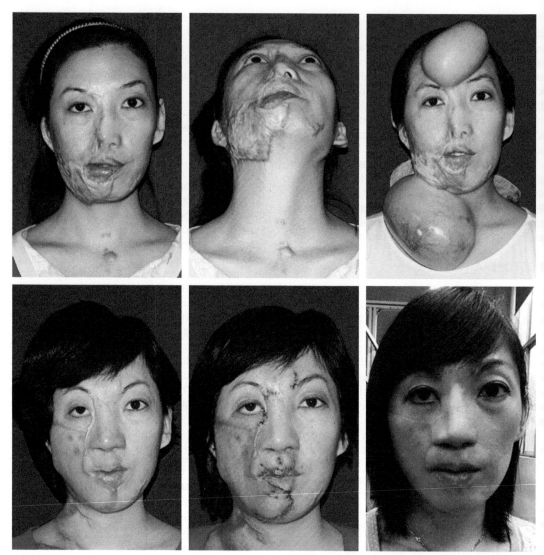

Fig. 7. (*Above left and middle*) Preoperative photograph of a 40-year-old woman suffering from chemical burn. Note the scars of nose, upper lip, mental region, and lower half of right face. (*Above, right*) One tissue expander, sized 100 mL, was embedded in the forehead region with final inflation volume of 250 mL. This expanded flap was planned to design as bipedicled supratrochlear perforator flaps used for the reconstruction of nose and upper lip. Another neck expanded flap prefabricated with the superficial temporal vessels was used for facial and mental region resurfacing, with 450 mL tissue expander inside, with final inflation volume of 1130 mL. (*Below, left*) Three months after the nasal and upper lip defect reconstruction using bipedicled supratrochlear perforator flaps and the facial and mental defect resurfacing using prefabricated neck expanded flap. (*Below, middle*) Revision of the scars at margin of the flap. Thinning of the upper lip flap, reshaping of the philtrum, and revision of the upper lip bow were processed in 3 months postoperatively. (*Below, right*) The result 1 year after the finial operation.

normal tissue should be considered as the primary donor site.[12] Reliable and simple surgical techniques are other factors to be considered. At present, the forehead is an excellent source of skin and soft tissue for most nasal reconstruction in clinical practice[10] and has been considered the gold standard of nasal reconstruction.[13] The color and texture of the forehead are also well matched to the other regions of the face and some reports about the clinical applications of forehead flaps in facial defect reconstruction have been published.[14,15] The robust blood supply of forehead and the anatomic features of the facial vessels, which come in pairs, make various types of forehead flaps able to be harvested safely. Zelken and colleagues[16] and Furuta and colleagues[17]

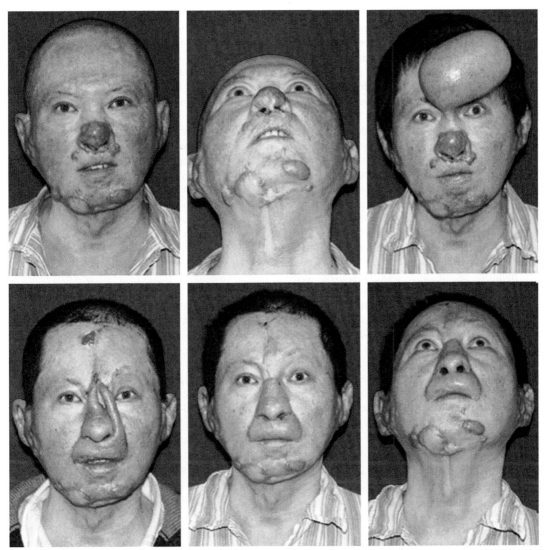

Fig. 8. (*Above*) A 32-year-old man who sustained facial scars from flame burn. Note the hypertrophic scars of nose, upper lip, and mental region of the face. (*Center, left*) One tissue expander sized 100 mL was placed under the frontalis muscle with final inflation volume of 300 mL. (*Center, right*) Bipedicled supratrochlear perforator flaps harvested side by side from the expanded forehead area were used for the reconstruction of nose and upper lip. The donor site was closed directly with only a small defect left to heal by secondary intention. (*Below*) The result 6 months after the final operation and no later revision operation was performed. A good cosmetic result was obtained.

respectively reported double forehead flaps used for the reconstruction of composite nasal defects with one flap working as nasal lining and another as nasal covering. Under the inspiration of the new idea, we assume the bipedicled supratrochlear perforator flaps technique is an ideal candidate for simultaneous nasal and upper lip resurfacing.

Expansion technique can increase the skin surface area for harvest of the 2 flaps and achieve successful primary donor site closure, and reduce the soft tissue thickness to express the deep tissues contours. Moreover, the pre-expansion is a delay procedure that enhances the perfusion of the distal part of the flap.[18] The pre-expanded, bipedicled supratrochlear perforator flap technique has the advantages of the expansion method to keep the characteristics of the forehead flap, which is an easy operation for harvest and transfer. The authors believe it is a useful option for the simultaneous reconstruction of the nose and upper lip.

Our method has several advantages. First, the pre-expanded bipedicled supratrochlear perforator flap technique allows the harvesting of sufficient and thin soft tissue for the successful simultaneous resurfacing of nasal and upper lip units separately from one single donor site. The donor site can be closed directly, resulting in minimal donor site morbidity. Second, the 2 components of the bipedicled supratrochlear perforator flaps each have an independent blood supply and the relationship between them is flexible, allowing for the resurfacing of different units independently. The procedure is technically effective and based on a common flap already familiar to reconstructive surgeons. Third, the expansion process enhances the consistency of the blood supply of the flaps, especially in their distal parts, and gives excellent results that can be achieved with minimal donor site morbidity. The pre-expansion also prevents distal flap necrosis, which is useful in smokers and in reconstructive surgery in which a large and thin skin paddle is required. Finally, in male patients, the hair-bearing distal part of the flap used to resurface the upper lip can simulate the moustache. Although this method has drawbacks associated with prolonged healing and hospitalization time, we believe the excellent final result of the whole reconstruction is worth all the discomforts that the patients endure.

SUMMARY

The pre-expanded bipedicled supratrochlear perforator flaps based on both supratrochlear vessels for the simultaneous resurfacing of total nasal and upper lip defects represent an excellent option that can achieve optimal aesthetic results from one single donor site with minimal donor site morbidity.

REFERENCES

1. Gonzalez-Ulloa M. Restoration of the face covering by means of selected skin in regional aesthetic units. Br J Plast Surg 1956;9:212–21.
2. Burget GC, Menick FJ. The subunit principle in nasal reconstruction. Plast Reconstr Surg 1985;76:239–47.
3. Fattahi TT. An overview of facial aesthetic units. J Oral Maxillofac Surg 2003;61:1207–11.
4. Cinpolat A, Bektas G, Coskunfirat OK. Complex partial nasal reconstruction using free prelaminated temporoparietal fascial flap. Microsurgery 2013;33: 156–9.

5. Jallali N, Malata CM. Reconstruction of concomitant total loss of the upper and lower lips with a free vertical rectus abdominis flap. Microsurgery 2005;25: 118–20.
6. Zhou W, He M, Liao Y, et al. Reconstructing a complex central facial defect with a multiple-folding radial forearm flap. J Oral Maxillofac Surg 2014;72: 836.e1-4.
7. De Figueiredo JC, Naufal RR, Zampar AG, et al. Expanded median forehead flap and abbe flap for nasal and upper lip reconstruction after complications of polymethylmethacrylate. Aesthetic Plast Surg 2010;34:385–7.
8. Urushidate S, Yokoi K, Higuma Y, et al. Nose and upper lip reconstruction for purpura fulminans. J Plast Reconstr Aesthet Surg 2012;65:252–5.
9. Yoshihiro S, Kenichi N, Toshiaki N. Reconstruction of larger nasal defects together with the nasal lining and the upper lip using the Split-Scalping forehead flap: a new technique. J Plast Reconstr Aesthet Surg 2011;64:1108–10.
10. Menick FJ. A 10-year experience in nasal reconstruction with the three-stage forehead flap. Plast Reconstr Surg 2002;109:1839–55 [discussion: 56–61].
11. Menick FJ. Nasal reconstruction with a forehead flap. Clin Plast Surg 2009;36:443–59.
12. Menick FJ. Facial reconstruction with local and distant tissue: the interface of aesthetic and reconstructive surgery. Plast Reconstr Surg 1998;102: 1424–33.
13. Correa BJ, Weathers WM, Wolfswinkel EM, et al. The forehead flap: the gold standard of nasal soft tissue reconstruction. Semin Plast Surg 2013;27:96–103.
14. Wang Q, Song W, Hou D, et al. Expanded forehead flaps for reconstruction of different faciocervical units: selection of flap types based on 143 cases. Plast Reconstr Surg 2015;135:1461–71.
15. Wang L, Xu F, Fan GK, et al. Forehead flap for simultaneous reconstruction after head and neck malignant tumor resection. Ann Plast Surg 2014. [Epub ahead of print].
16. Zelken JA, Chang CS, Reddy SK, et al. Double forehead flap reconstruction of composite nasal defects. J Plast Reconstr Aesthet Surg 2016;69:1280–4.
17. Furuta S, Hayashi M, Shinohara H. Nasal reconstruction with an expanded dual forehead flap. Br J Plast Surg 2000;53:261–4.
18. Callegari PR, Taylor GI, Caddy CM, et al. An anatomic review of the delay phenomenon: I. Experimental studies. Plast Reconstr Surg 1992;89:397–407 [discussion: 17–8].

Pre-expanded, Prefabricated Monoblock Perforator Flap for Total Facial Resurfacing

Tao Zan, MD, PhD[1], Yashan Gao, MD[1], Haizhou Li, MD,
Bin Gu, MD, Feng Xie, MD, PhD, Qingfeng Li, MD, PhD*

KEYWORDS

- Total facial resurfacing • Prefabricated flap • Pre-expanded flap • Cervicothoracic flap
- Stem cell transplantation

KEY POINTS

- The pre-expanded, prefabricated supercharged cervicothoracic monoblock perforator flap can be used for total and subtotal facial resurfacing.
- This flap has similar color, thickness, and texture as the face, maintains facial contour and mediates facial expression, and is large enough to cover the total face.
- Our approach includes preoperative evaluation, flap prefabrication, tissue overexpansion assisted by stem cell transplantation, flap transfer for total facial resurfacing, and multistep flap revisions.

INTRODUCTION

The resurfacing of total facial defects resulting from burn injuries, trauma, and tumor ablation remains one of the biggest challenges in reconstructive surgery.[1,2] Various reconstructive techniques exist for the treatment of total facial defects, among which skin grafting is the simplest method. However, the often complicated graft contraction and severe mismatched skin color and texture make it difficult to obtain ideal aesthetic and functional results.[3] Conventional local/regional flaps or free flaps are also used for total facial resurfacing, but the flap thickness obscures the ideal facial contours and expression. Also, conventional flaps always have problems, such as insufficient donor site and limited vascular territory.[4,5] In the past

decade, face allotransplantation has been performed for severely disfigured patients and seems to have a satisfactory risk to benefit ratio. However, this facial repair procedure could be only offered in rare and selected cases owing to its technical challenges, ethical concerns, and adverse reactions from immunosuppressive therapy.[6,7]

We have proposed the pre-expanded, prefabricated, supercharged cervicothoracic monoblock perforator flap for total facial resurfacing, which has similar color, texture, and thickness as the face and is large enough to cover total facial defects.[8] This technique could provide good functional and aesthetic outcomes for patients who have extensive facial skin and subcutaneous

Disclosure: The authors have no commercial associations or financial disclosure to the report.
Department of Plastic and Reconstructive Surgery, Shanghai Ninth People's Hospital, Shanghai Jiao Tong University School of Medicine, 639 Zhizaoju Road, Shanghai 200011, P.R. China
[1] T. Zan and Y. Gao contributed equally to this work and should be viewed as co-first authors.
* Corresponding author. Department of Plastic and Reconstructive Surgery, The Ninth Hospital, Medical School of Shanghai Jiao Tong University, Shanghai 200011, P.R. China.
E-mail address: dr.liqingfeng@yahoo.com

Clin Plastic Surg 44 (2017) 163–170
http://dx.doi.org/10.1016/j.cps.2016.08.007

deformities with undamaged muscles and deep structures.

TREATMENT GOALS AND PLANNED OUTCOMES

The goals of total facial resurfacing are to restore normal organ function (breathing, eating, vision, etc) and facial expression and to obtain a perceived normal face with normal facial outline and natural 3-dimensional structure. We have proposed a evaluation system to score the aesthetic and functional outcomes of facial resurfacing[9] (**Table 1**).

To obtain ideal aesthetic and functional outcomes, we have proposed the principle of "matching, large size, and thinner thickness" (MLT) for facial resurfacing.[10] "Matching" requires a donor site that has matched skin color and texture (soft and elastic) with the face. "Large size and thinner thickness" imply sufficient flap size to cover the whole defect and adequately thin thickness to form facial contour and expression. In addition to the matched, large and thin coverage of the defects, the formation of fine and delicate features of the central face are also very important to reflect the 3-dimensional structure of the face and to obtain a "perceived normal" face.

PREOPERATIVE PLANNING AND PREPARATION
Indications for Total Face Resurfacing

Pre-expanded, prefabricated cervicothoracic flaps are recommended for those patients identified as type III and type IV deformities according to our classification[9] and without severe destruction of the muscle.

Donor Site Selection

According to the matching principle, the anterior chest can be regarded as the ideal donor sites for facial resurfacing,[11] thus the pre-expanded, prefabricated internal mammary artery perforator (IMAP) supercharged cervicothoracic flap was our first choice for total facial resurfacing. In case of scarred anterior chest skin, the bipedicled perforator flaps from the lateral chest, back, and abdomen could be used for total facial resurfacing.

Vascular Carrier Selection

The descending branch of the lateral circumflex femoral vessels with the surrounding fascia were ideal vascular carrier for flap prefabrication based on their anatomic characters.[10] Color duplex ultrasonography was used preoperatively to evaluate the peak systolic velocity, caliber, and length of the vessels of the 2 sides and to choose the vascular carrier with better quality. Besides, the superficial temporal vessels and the thoracodorsal vessels could be used as vascular carriers.

Preoperative Evaluation with 3-Dimensional Digital Technology

Three-dimensional computed tomography and computer-aided design techniques were performed preoperatively to better evaluate and simulate the sizes and 3-dimensional structures of defects and donor site.

Table 1
Appearance and function status score

	Appearance and Function Status	Score
Aesthetic status	Nearly normal appearance	3
	Nearly normal facial outline and organs; flat, ill-defined, normally pigmented scar	2
	Mild deformation of facial outline and organs or protuberant, hard, well-defined, and hypopigmented or hyperpigmented scar	1
	Nearly normal facial outline and organs; flat, ill-defined, normally pigmented scar	0
Functional status	Nearly normal organ function and facial expression	3
	Essentially normal organ function, slightly limited or unnatural facial expression	2
	Mouth opening limited to approximately 2 finger breadths, mildly restricted nasal ventilation or expiration with a feeling of resistance, impaired eye closing or opening, obviously limited facial expression	1
	Impaired mouth closing or severely restricted mouth opening, blocked nasal ventilation, absent eye closing or opening, severely limited facial expression	0

Overall Reconstruction Planning and Communication with Patients

Total facial resurfacing requires that the patient undergo multiple procedures and their various potential complications. Therefore, an overall plan for surgical reconstruction, postprocedural care and rehabilitation is essential. This is not only helpful to the surgeon to better plan operations and to obtain improved functional and aesthetic outcomes, but also to provide the patient with understanding of the process and more positive psychological outcomes.

PATIENT POSITIONING

All producers were performed with the patient in a supine position.

PROCEDURAL APPROACH: THE PRE-EXPANDED, PREFABRICATED CERVICOTHORACIC FLAP

The entire procedures were described as follows (**Fig. 1**).

Flap Prefabrication: Fascial Flap Harvest and Transfer

The descending branch of the lateral circumflex femoral artery was designated as the vascular carrier. The full lengths of the descending branch of the lateral circumflex femoral vessels with the surrounding intramuscular septum were dissected from the rectus femoris and vastus lateralis muscles. The motor nerve to the vastus lateralis was preserved during harvest of the fascial flap. The vessels were anastomosed to the superior thyroid artery or the facial artery and their venae comitantes. A subcutaneous pocket of the cervicothoracic area was created, and the second or third IMAP was preserved carefully.[12] The flattened vascular carrier was then inset into the subcutaneous pocket and sutured with the overlying tissue. The vascular carrier could be placed superficially to reduce the flap thickness. Finally, a rectangular tissue expander ranging 400 to 600 mL was placed beneath the vascular carrier.

Tissue Overexpansion Assisted by Stem Cell Transplantation

After confirmation of pulsation in the pedicle by color duplex ultrasonography, tissue expansion began 1 week after its implantation and is performed twice a week. The skin thickness was measured by ultrasound routinely. For those patients whose expanded dermal layer was less than 1 mm thick in the middle stage of expansion,

the transplantation of bone marrow aspirate mononuclear cells (BM-MNCs) was performed as described previously as part of a clinical trial (ClinicalTrials.gov NCT01209611).[8] In brief, approximately 200 mL of bone marrow was aspirated from the anterior superior iliac spine and isolated by Ficoll density separation. The cell suspension was adjusted to a final volume of 10 to 15 mL with saline (approximately 0.5×10^6 cells/cm^2) and was injected into the expanded skin intradermally. The patients continued with the tissue expansion procedure 24 hours after injection.

Flap Transfer for Total Facial Resurfacing

When the expanded skin area was estimated to be greater than 120% of the facial defect, expansion was stopped and the flap transfer was planned. After confirmation of the pulsation in the prefabricated pedicle and the existence of IMAP, tracheotomy was performed with the assistance of an otolaryngologist before flap transfer. The prefabricated skin flap was then elevated and transferred to cover the whole facial defects, and the second or third IMAP was traced into the pectoralis major and ligated for anastomosis with the superficial temporal artery and its venae comitantes. The palpebral fissures, the labial fissures, and the nostrils were closed temporarily. An orogastric tube was inserted through a hole to provide enteral nutrition.

Flap Revision

The palpebral fissures and the labial fissure were opened 10 to 14 days after flap transfer. The revision of periocular region and the nasal reconstruction were performed 3 weeks after flap transfer. The revision of the perioral region and the pedicle division were performed 3 weeks or longer after rhinoplasty, and the debulking producers for cheeks and forehead were performed 3 months after flap transfer. Delay of these procedures might cause more retraction of the flap.

POTENTIAL COMPLICATIONS AND THEIR MANAGEMENT

The major complications related to tissue expansion are infection, deflation of the expander, and exposure of expander.[13] Mild infection could be cured with conservative treatment. Severe infection and deflation of the expander usually require removal and change of the expander. If the infection occurs at the end of expansion, earlier flap transfer could be performed. The skin thickness was measured by ultrasound routinely to avoid the

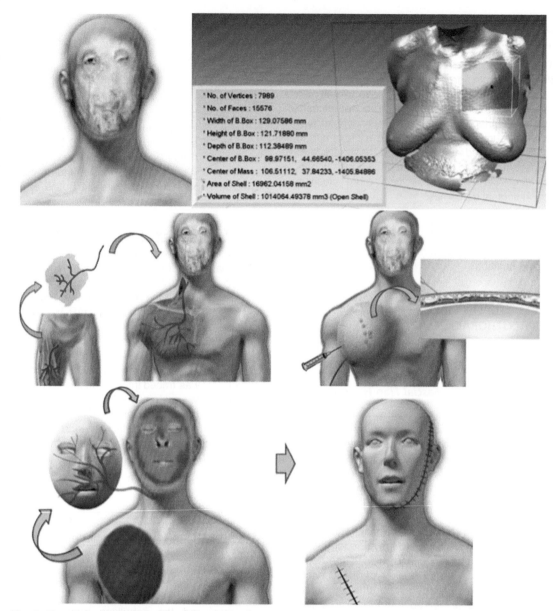

Fig. 1. The entire producers of total facial resurfacing. The patient has extensive facial deformities (*top left*). Three-dimensional computed tomography and computer-aided design technique were performed preoperatively to evaluate the sizes and 3-dimensional structures of the defect and donor site (*top right*). In the first stage, the descending branch of the lateral circumflex femoral artery, vein, and surrounding fascia were harvested as the vascular carrier and anastomosed to the superior thyroid artery and its venae comitant (*middle left*). A rectangular tissue expander was placed beneath the vascular carrier. Tissue overexpansion was performed and assisted by stem cell transplantation to obtain a larger flap (*middle right*). In the second stage, the prefabricated flap was elevated and transferred to cover the total facial defect (*bottom*).

exposure of tissue expander resulting from thinning of the skin, and BM-MNC injection was performed if necessary, as mentioned. All patients had increased skin thickness after BM-MNC injection.

During flap transfer, the second or third IMAP was preserved to ensure the blood supply reliability of the extensive resurfacing flap. After flap transfer, slight flap retractions that caused lip or lower eyelids ectropion could be corrected with full-thickness skin graft or local flap transfer.

POSTPROCEDURAL CARE, REHABILITATION, AND RECOVERY

Patients were observed at the intensive care unit for 3 days and then transferred to the ward. Airway nursing care and enteral nutrition were performed under the guidance of specialists. After the opening of labial fissure, the gastric tube was removed and the patient began to take solid food. The removal of the tracheostomy tube was conducted after rhinoplasty. A compression mask was used for at least 3 months to minimize the recurrence of facial contracture and the development of hypertrophic scarring. The rehabilitation program involving training in passive and active facial exercises was started after flap revisions. Psychological support was provided once a month or at the patient's request.

OUTCOMES

From September 2005 to September 2014, 42 patients underwent total facial resurfacing with pre-expanded, prefabricated perforator flaps in our institution, of which 40 were performed with prefabricated cervicothoracic flaps and 2 were performed with lateral thoracic flap prefabricated with thoracodorsal vessels. The aesthetic and functional status were scored before and at least 12 months after treatment based on the clinical data and photographs,[9] as mentioned. Statistically significant differences before and after treatment were evaluated using Wilcoxon matched pairs test (GraphPad Prism 5, San Diego, CA) with statistical significance established at $P<.05$.

Functional Outcomes

Facial organ function and expression were improved progressively. At 1 year of follow-up, the patients' mouth closing and opening, eyes closing and opening, nasal ventilation, and emotion expression were satisfactory. Functional status scores before and after treatment were 0.88 and 2.40, respectively. The difference of the score was statistically significant ($P<.001$).

Aesthetic and Psychological Outcomes

The aesthetic status scores before and after treatment were 1.14 and 2.26, respectively. The difference of the score was statistically significant ($P<.001$). **Figs. 2** and **3** show the preoperative and postoperative views of 2 patients who underwent facial resurfacing with a prefabricated cervicothoracic flap. The patients have not undergone formal psychological testing. However, the patients were satisfied with the aesthetic and functional results and successfully reintegrated into society.

CASE DEMONSTRATIONS
Case 1

A 41-year-old man had a totally disfigured face and severe restriction of expression after a welding injury 1 year before his first procedure. With the assistance of stem cell transplantation, a 32×30 cm^2 IMAP supercharged pre-expanded, prefabricated cervicothoracic flap was obtained and transferred to resurface the entire face. After flap transfer, the patient underwent several multistage revision surgeries including palpebral and labial opening, periocular revision, nasal reconstruction, flap debunking, and pedicle division. The follow-up at 2 years showed satisfactory aesthetic result with improved functional restoration of the face and the patient was satisfied with his "new face" (see **Fig. 2**).[8,14]

Case 2

A 30-year-old woman had chemical burns of her entire face and was not satisfied with the results of skin grafts performed 2 years before. In the first stage, the descending branch of the lateral circumflex femoral vessels and surrounding fascia was implanted to the cervicothoracic area and a 550-mL expander was placed underneath. In the second stage, a 28×26 cm^2 IMAP supercharged pre-expanded, prefabricated cervicothoracic flap was obtained and transferred to resurface the entire face. The donor site was covered by pre-expanded lateral thoracic flap. After flap transfer, the patient underwent several multistage revision operations. The follow-up at 4 years showed satisfactory aesthetic and functional outcomes (see **Fig. 3**).[14]

DISCUSSION

The reconstruction of postburn full facial deformities is a continuing challenge for plastic surgeons. Full-thickness skin grafting remains one of the most widely used technique for total face resurfacing, but is often complicated by graft retraction and mismatch of color and texture, especially in the Asian population.[15] In 1997, Angrigiani and Grilli[16] reported total face reconstruction using a bilateral scapular–parascapular free flap. However, the tissue was too bulky to allow the reconstruction of natural facial contour and expression. More recently, Spence[17] suggested reconstructing the peripheral and the central face by expanded anterior chest transposition flaps and full-thickness skin grafts, but a "patchwork face" is inevitable with this technique. In addition, the full-thickness skin grafts cannot support additional framework implantation, which

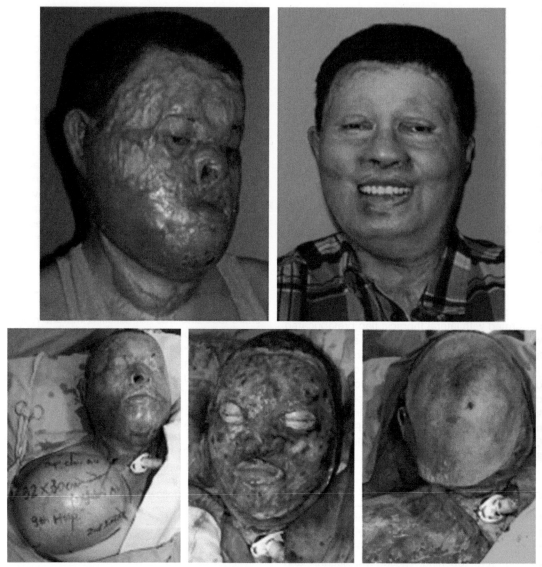

Fig. 2. A 41-year-old man suffered a totally disfigured face and severe restriction of expressions after a welding injury (*top left*). With the assistance of stem cell transplantation, a 32 × 30 cm² pre-expanded, prefabricated cervicothoracic flap was obtained and transferred to resurface the entire face (*bottom*).[8] The follow-up at 2 years showed satisfactory aesthetic result with improved functional restoration of the face (*top right*).[14]

obscures the fine facial features of the central face. In this article, we present our work of full facial resurfacing using pre-expanded, prefabricated monoblock perforator flap integrated with multi-stage revision surgeries, which not only resurfaces the entire face with uniform, pliable, color and texture matched skin, but also be able to restore the 3-dimensional structure of the face.

A primary problem of total facial resurfacing is deficiency of well-matched donor skin. Prolonged soft tissue expansion combined with transplantation of BM-MNCs could help to ameliorate with this problem. During the expansion period, routine visits were performed and the skin thickness was measured by ultrasonography. In case of skin thickness of less than 1 mm, the transplantation of BM-MNC to the expanded skin was performed. Then, after 4 weeks of inflation, the expanded skin thickness was maintained or even increased. The reliability of the blood supply is another major problem of this monoblock flap. The venous congestion and arterial insufficiency might be prevented by flap delay and/or supercharging procedures. In most patients, at least 1 IMAP and concomitant vein were preserved for additional microvascular augmentation.

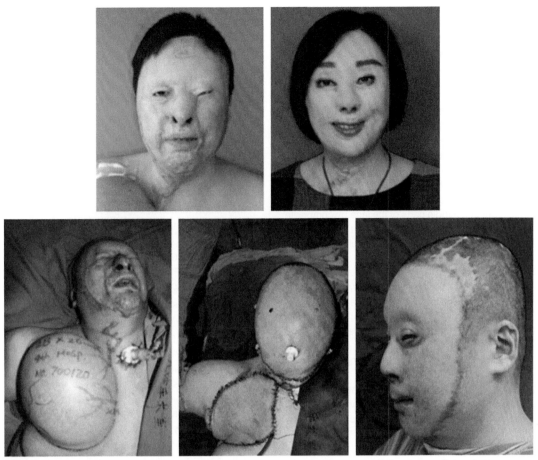

Fig. 3. A 30-year-old woman had chemical burns of her entire face (*top left*). A 28 × 26 cm² internal mammary artery perforator supercharged pre-expanded, prefabricated cervicothoracic flap was obtained and transferred to resurface the entire face. The donor site was covered by pre-expanded lateral thoracic flap (*bottom*).[14] Follow-up at 4 years showed satisfactory aesthetic and functional outcomes (*top right*).

Ten years after the first facial vascularized composite allotransplantation, there have been 37 face allotransplantations performed to date.[18] Most recently, Dr Eduardo Rodriguez and colleagues present their remarkable face allotransplantation case and described some innovative technique key points contributing to restore the normal facial anatomy and to get better aesthetic and functional outcomes, including nerve coaptation, eyelid consideration, and the transplantation of bone insert. However, although the initial question of the feasibility of performing such a complex procedure are long gone, its technical challenges, long-term consequences of immunosuppressive treatment and complications such as acute and chronic rejection continue to limit its use to strictly elective patients.[19–21] Thus, for the patients who have extensive facial skin and subcutaneous deformities with undamaged muscles and deep structures, the pre-expanded, prefabricated monoblock perforator flap may have its own advantages and could provide good functional and aesthetic outcomes to the patients with minor complications.

SUMMARY

Our 10 years of experience in this series demonstrate that the pre-expanded, prefabricated cervicothoracic skin perforator flap can be a reliable option for resurfacing total and subtotal facial defects. Our approach may replace a conventional "skin only" face allotransplantation in selected patients with good aesthetic and functional outcomes but acceptable complications.

REFERENCES

1. Oster C, Willebrand M, Ekselius L. Health-related quality of life 2 years to 7 years after burn injury. J Trauma 2011;71:1435–41.

2. Fauerbach JA, Heinberg LJ, Lawrence JW, et al. Effect of early body image dissatisfaction on subsequent psychological and physical adjustment after disfiguring injury. Psychosom Med 2000;62:576–82.

3. Latifoğlu O, Ayhan S, Atabay K. Total face reconstruction: skin graft versus free flap. Plast Reconstr Surg 1999;103:1076–8.

4. Parrett BM, Pomahac B, Orgill DP, et al. The role of free tissue transfer for head and neck burn reconstruction. Plast Reconstr Surg 2007;120:1871–8.

5. Sakurai H, Takeuchi M, Fujiwara O, et al. Total face reconstruction with one expanded free flap. Surg Technol Int 2005;14:329–33.

6. Lantieri L, Meningaud JP, Grimbert P, et al. Repair of the lower and middle parts of the face by composite tissue allotransplantation in a patient with massive plexiform neurofibroma: a 1-year follow-up study. Lancet 2008;372:639–45.

7. Lantieri L, Hivelin M, Audard V, et al. Feasibility, reproducibility, risks and benefits of face transplantation: a prospective study of outcomes. Am J Transplant 2011;11:367–78.

8. Li Q, Zan T, Li H, et al. Flap prefabrication and stem cell-assisted tissue expansion: how we acquire a monoblock flap for full face resurfacing. J Craniofac Surg 2014;25:21–5.

9. Zan T, Li H, Gu B, et al. Surgical treatment of facial soft-tissue deformities in postburn patients: a proposed classification based on a retrospective study. Plast Reconstr Surg 2013;132:1001e–14e.

10. Li Q, Zan T, Gu B, et al. Face resurfacing using a cervicothoracic skin flap prefabricated by lateral thigh fascial flap and tissue expander. Microsurgery 2009;29:515–23.

11. Edgerton MT, Hansen FC. Matching facial color with split thickness skin grafts from adjacent areas. Plast Reconstr Surg Transplant Bull 1960;25:455–64.

12. Li GS, Zan T, Li QF, et al. Internal mammary artery perforator -supercharged prefabricated cervicothoracic flap for face and neck reconstruction. Ann Plast Surg 2015;75:29–33.

13. Zan T, Li H, Du Z, et al. Reconstruction of the face and neck with different types of pre-expanded anterior chest flaps: a comprehensive strategy for multiple techniques. J Plast Reconstr Aesthet Surg 2013;66:1074–81.

14. Li Q, Zan T, Li H, et al. Reconstruction of postburn full facial deformities with an integrated method. J Craniofac Surg 2016;27:1175–80.

15. Ozmen S, Uygur S, Eryilmaz T, et al. Facial resurfacing with a monoblock full-thickness skin graft after multiple malignant melanomas excision in xeroderma pigmentosum. J Craniofac Surg 2012;23:1542–3.

16. Angrigiani C, Grilli D. Total face reconstruction with one free flap. Plast Reconstr Surg 1997;99:1566–75.

17. Spence RJ. Expanded transposition flap technique for total and subtotal resurfacing of the face and neck. J Burns Wounds 2007;6:e8.

18. Sosin M, Rodriguez ED. The face transplantation update: 2016. Plast Reconstr Surg 2016;137:1841–50.

19. Sosin M, Ceradini DJ, Levine JP, et al. Total face, eyelids, ears, scalp, and skeletal subunit transplant: a reconstructive solution for the full face and total scalp burn. Plast Reconstr Surg 2016;138:205–19.

20. Lantieri LA. Discussion: Total face, eyelids, ears, scalp, and skeletal subunit transplant: a reconstructive solution for the full face and total scalp burn. Plast Reconstr Surg 2016;138(1):220–1.

21. Meningaud JP. Discussion: Total face, eyelids, ears, scalp, and skeletal subunit transplant: a reconstructive solution for the full face and total scalp burn. Plast Reconstr Surg 2016;138(1):222–3.

Pre-expanded and Prefabricated Abdominal Superthin Skin Perforator Flap for Total Hand Resurfacing

Chunmei Wang, MD, PhD[a], Junyi Zhang, MD[b],
Sifen Yang, MD[a], Ping Song, MD[c], Lun Yang, MD[a],
Lee L.Q. Pu, MD, PhD[c],*

KEYWORDS

- Pre-expansion • Superthin perforator flap • Hand reconstruction • Finger reconstruction
- Prefabricated abdominal flap

KEY POINTS

- The blood supply of the abdominal superthin perforator flap is based on the subdermal vascular network (subdermal plexus) formed from the superficial inferior epigastric artery, deep inferior epigastric artery, and superficial circumflex iliac artery.
- The expander is implanted under the subdermal vascular network and in the cross-area between several perforators to obtain thinner and larger prefabricated superthin skin perforator flaps.
- The flap's capsule is left in place to protect the blood supply, no step is needed to thin the flap. There is no need to dissect the trunk of each perforator, and the donor site can be closed simultaneously. All of these factors make the operation more simple and safe.
- Pre-expanded and prefabricated abdominal superthin perforator flaps can establish blood supply quickly within the recipient bed, and therefore the flap pedicle can be divided in 9 to 14 days after transfer. The flap can also be used safely to provide concurrent coverage for the fingers.
- This type of flap combines the advantages of perforator flaps and tissue expansion to provide a functional reconstruction of the entire dorsal hand and fingers concurrently.

INTRODUCTION

The dorsum of the hand and fingers is difficult to reconstruct simultaneously. Skin grafting and conventional flaps cannot meet the cosmetic and functional requirements entirely. By definition, a superthin flap is distinct in that its subdermal vascular network can be seen through the nominal fat layer. This flap can also be called a subdermal vascular network flap. These superthin flaps have evolved immensely and can be used to reconstruct the hand and fingers.

The superthin perforator flap was first described in 1994 by Hyakusoku and colleagues,[1] who used a superthin perforator flap for reconstruction of the hand and fingers. Of

Disclosures: The authors have nothing to disclose.
[a] Department of Plastic and Aesthetic Surgery, Dongguan Kanghua Hospital, Dongguan, Guangdong Province, P.R. China; [b] Department of Plastic and Cosmetic Surgery, Beijing Tongren Hospital, Capital Medical University, Beijing, P.R. China; [c] Division of Plastic Surgery, University of California Davis Medical Center, 2221 Stockton Boulevard, Suite 2123, Sacramento, CA 95817, USA
* Corresponding author.
E-mail address: llpu@ucdavis.edu

Clin Plastic Surg 44 (2017) 171–177
http://dx.doi.org/10.1016/j.cps.2016.09.003
0094-1298/17/© 2016 Elsevier Inc. All rights reserved.

note, the pedicle region was kept thick to avoid injuring the perforator, and microvascular anastomosis was needed to increase the area of this flap. Subsequent modification with bipedicled superthin abdominal perforator flaps made the operation easier, but still could not provide concurrent durable coverage to fully reconstruct the fingers.[2]

The authors have found that it is difficult to resurface the whole hand and fingers because of insufficient donor skin flap, especially with regard to the fingers; it is difficult to simultaneously use the flap to cover the dorsal hand and finger defects because of the disproportionate length/width ratio of the fingers. This difficulty is challenging even with the use of axial-based flaps.

In order to enlarge the flap, the authors apply tissue expansion to the skin perforator flap. During expansion, not only does the perforator flap enlarge and thin out but the flap also becomes supercharged. Since 2006, we have used the pre-expanded and prefabricated abdominal superthin skin perforator flap to resurface extensive postburn defects of the hand after scar excision with good to excellent functional and cosmetic outcomes after reconstruction.

TREATMENT GOALS AND PLANNED OUTCOMES

The dorsum of the hand and digits is difficult to reconstruct simultaneously. We apply a pre-expanded superthin skin perforator flap to reconstruct the postburn hand and fingers for better function and appearance. This method is simple and safe, and can achieve sufficient coverage with such a superthin skin flap to the dorsum of the hand and fingers, while minimizing donor site morbidity.

PREOPERATIVE PLANNING AND PREPARATION

The sequence of operations begins with expander implantation. We usually design the flap with expander placement on the ipsilateral abdominal donor site, with direction congruent to the burned hand and slightly larger in area than the burned hand. The expander should be placed in the area with blood supply between the superficial inferior epigastric artery (SIEA), deep inferior epigastric artery (DIEA), and superficial circumflex iliac artery (SCIA) (**Fig. 1**). The size of the expander used ranges from 400 to 600 mL for adults and 200 to 300 mL for children.

The use of Doppler can help to confirm the position of perforators. Make sure to dissect the

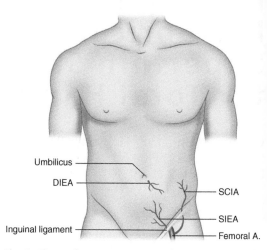

Fig. 1. The perforator anatomy in the abdominal wall.

expander pocket just under the subdermal layer, leaving a narrow layer of fat below the flap, and 2 to 4 cm away from the emerging points of adjacent perforators.

At the second stage, we plan 2 separate operations to transfer the flap onto the hand with subsequent flap division. This stage requires the upper limb to be fixated adjacent to the donor site for 9 to 14 days. Preoperative planning for stable fixation with the creation of a suitable device can achieve this task easily.

PATIENT POSITIONING

The semilateral position with cushioning to prop up the patients' buttock makes the operative procedure more convenient. However, for patients who require bilateral hand scar revisions, the supine position is ideal.

PROCEDURAL APPROACH

1. The first stage is to place the expander in the area supplied by the abdominal perforators, mainly from the SIEA, DIEA, and SCIA (**Fig. 2**). The skin flap is usually thinned with scissors to ensure adequate removal of subcutaneous fat so that a true skin-only flap is created. Attention should be paid to avoid a direct injury to the subdermal vascular network. Attention should also be paid to all the cutaneous perforators around the flap, with expander placement approximately 2 to 4 cm away from each perforator point as detected by Doppler. Cylindrical expanders are used. The volumes of expanders ranges from 400 mL to 600 mL according to the area of

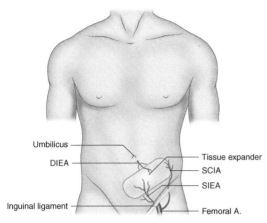

Fig. 2. The placement of a tissue expander during the first-stage procedure for pre-expansion of the superthin skin perforator flap based on the ipsilateral abdomen.

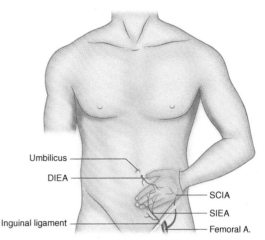

Fig. 3. The placement of a patient's hand during the second-stage procedure for prefabrication of the superthin skin perforator flap, which provides complete coverage of the hand, including fingers.

scar. For children, we use 200-mL to 300-mL expanders. The pre-expanded flaps are primarily thinned to the layer where the subdermal vascular network (subdermal plexus) can be seen through the minimal fat layer. Expanders are filled to 30% volume with saline intraoperatively, with the first fill at 3 to 5 days postoperatively after removal of the drain tube. Subsequent fills occur at regular intervals. The process of filling depends on the pressure in the expanders. When the flaps achieve sufficient dimensions with suitable geometry to cover the defect, the expanders are removed.

2. After appropriate expansion is completed, the second stage involves explanting the expander and rotation of the flap to cover the dorsal hand defect (**Fig. 3**). Our expanded flaps measure, on average, 8 × 10 to 12 × 18 cm. The flaps are large enough to cover the dorsum of the hand and fingers. After the expander is removed, the affected hand is immediately placed into the bipedicled superthin flap on the abdomen. The interdigital web spaces and some points of the flap should be fixated to the recipient base (**Fig. 4**). The affected limb is secured into position with our constructed splint for 9 to 14 days, after which the pedicle is divided.

3. In the final stage, we divide the pedicle from the abdominal wall and shape the flap for coverage over the fingers simultaneously (**Figs. 5** and **6**). Because of the pre-expansion of the flap, there is sufficient area to cover the hand and finger defects as well as to allow for abdominal donor site closure.

POTENTIAL COMPLICATIONS AND MANAGEMENT

Routine use of antibiotics in the perioperative period is necessary to prevent infection after implanting the expander. The authors usually leave a negative pressure drainage tube for 3 to 5 days postoperatively to prevent hematomas or subcutaneous seroma formation. We inject with normal saline and begin the filling process at an early stage, even while the drain is still in place, and at frequent intervals in order to prevent capsular contracture. However, the frequency must be

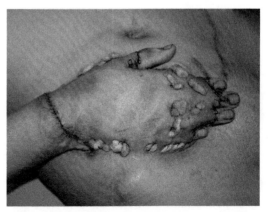

Fig. 4. After the second-stage procedure, a prefabricated superthin skin perforator flap with bipedicle connections covers the entire hand based on the previous pre-expanded flap from the abdomen.

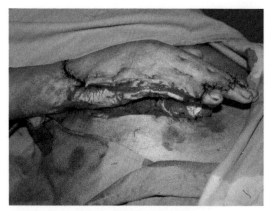

Fig. 5. Intraoperative view after the third-stage procedure (lateral view) showing the superthin skin flap for the coverage of the entire hand after division of its bipedicles.

decreased in the later phase to avoid hemodynamic compromise of the superthin flap.

Because bipedicled perforator flaps have a robust blood supply, the flaps survive well, with minimal complications such as blisters or necrosis as long as the limbs are firmly attached and the flap is well designed between the perforators. Compression dressing helps to protect the flap from venous congestion once the expanded superthin abdominal flap is transferred to reconstruct the dorsal hand defect.

POSTPROCEDURAL CARE

In the first stage, postoperatively, the indwelling negative pressure drainage tube is left for 3 to

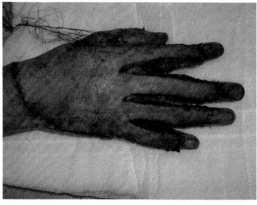

Fig. 6. Intraoperative view after the third-stage procedure showing successful separations of the distal superthin skin flap for the coverage of all 5 fingers with optimal quality of skin and adequate blood supply to each finger.

5 days. Perform routine dressing changes and observe the flap on alternate days, with careful attention to signs of hematoma, seroma, and so forth. In the second stage, after dividing and transferring the flap to the recipient site, it is important to use compression bandages to facilitate the expanded prefabricated abdominal superthin perforator flap in establishing the new blood supply quickly within the recipient bed. This new blood supply can avoid cutaneous color change and necrosis caused by the early ischemia period relative to subdermal vascular network skin graft. The surgeon must also pay close attention to the pedicle, to avoid compression on the blood supply.

REHABILITATION AND RECOVERY

Physical therapy and hand-specific therapy is necessary for optimal functional rehabilitation of the hands. The patients are asked to use silicone gel sheeting on both donor and recipient sites to avoid hypertrophic scar for 3 to 6 months. The authors have found that elastic gloves can assist in postoperative recovery of the hand.

OUTCOMES

In the early stages, the blood supply to the pre-expanded and prefabricated superthin skin perforator flap relies mainly on the pedicle. The local environment favors neovascularization and formation of increased perfusion between the flap and recipient site. Subsequently, the pedicle becomes less important as the flap develops new blood supply from the base. According to our clinical experience, this type of pre-expanded superthin skin perforator flap can tolerate the initial ischemia of flap elevation and transfer to the recipient site very well. Therefore, such a flap can be used to reconstruct the dorsal skin of the hand and fingers, offering improved color match in addition to the thinner nature of the flap.

The size of the flaps ranged from 8 × 10 cm to 12 × 18 cm in the first author's case series of 8 patients (12 flaps). Eleven flaps survived completely and only 1 flap experienced bullous epidermal necrosis at the distal aspect measuring 1 × 2 cm. This flap went on to heal without further operative procedures. The hands had good functional results with satisfactory appearance. On the abdominal donor site only a linear scar was left.

All of our patients have been followed for at least 3 years. The flaps did not shrink or discolor after the operation. Hand contractures did not recur. The youngest patient has been followed for 10 years; the flaps on her hands have grown with her.

Case 1

A 5-year-old girl had flame burns to the dorsum of both hands 1.5 years earlier, and developed hypertrophic scar over her bilateral hands (Case 1A). The authors prefabricated an abdominal skin perforator pass-bridge superthin flap via tissue expansion in 3 stages (Case 1B). First, the expander was implanted at the donor site (Case 1C). Then the bilateral dorsal hand scars were excised (Case 1D), the expander was removed, and the bipedicled flap was raised and shaped to resurface the wound (Case 1E). In addition, we divided the pedicle and formed the web spaces of the fingers (Case 1F). The donor site had no hypertrophic scar left (Case 1G a, b). The patient had satisfactory outcome for both the contour and function of the hands (Case 1H). In addition, this kind of flap reconstruction also accommodated the child's growth with good long-term outcome (Case 1I a, b).

Case 2

A 9-year-old boy had flame burns to his right hand and developed hypertrophic scars causing a claw-hand deformity 2 years after his initial injury (Case 2A a, b). The authors treated his right hand in a 3-stage procedure by designing and implanting the expander under the subdermal vascular network layer of the abdomen (Case 2B). After the expansion was complete, the dorsal scars of the right hand were excised, and we placed the hand under the pre-expanded and prefabricated abdomen skin perforator flap (Case 2C a, b). In the third stage, we released all interphalangeal joint contractures and simultaneously covered the dorsal fingers with our flap. All fingers were fixed with pins for 4 weeks. The flap survived completely and his right hand had good functional outcome and satisfactory appearance (Case 2D a–c).

DISCUSSION

It is challenging for plastic surgeons to reconstruct extensive skin defect over the dorsum of the hands and fingers. Traditionally, skin grafting was used, but the grafted skin used to shrink considerably and allowed contracture malformation to recur. The color and texture of the grafted skin were also different from the surrounding skin. In the 1970s, a new era of reconstructive

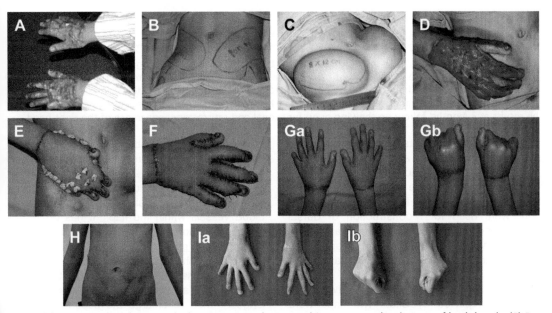

Case 1. (A) Preoperative photograph showing severe hypertrophic scars over the dorsum of both hands. (B) Preoperative design for the first-stage procedure outlining the places for placement of 2 tissue expanders for both hands in the abdomen. (C) Postoperative view showing fully expanded tissue expanders in the abdomen before the second-stage procedure. (D) Intraoperative view showing the complete excision of scars in his right hand during the second-stage procedure. (E) Postoperative view showing the total coverage of his right hand with the pre-expanded and prefabricated superthin flap after the second-stage procedure. (F) Immediate postoperative view showing complete coverage of his right hand and all 5 fingers after the third-procedure. (G a, b) The early results at 1 month postoperatively after completion of all 3-stage procedures. (H) The donor site appearance at 8 years postoperatively showing no hypertrophic scar. (I a, b) The final results at 10 years postoperatively showing satisfactory contour and function of both hands.

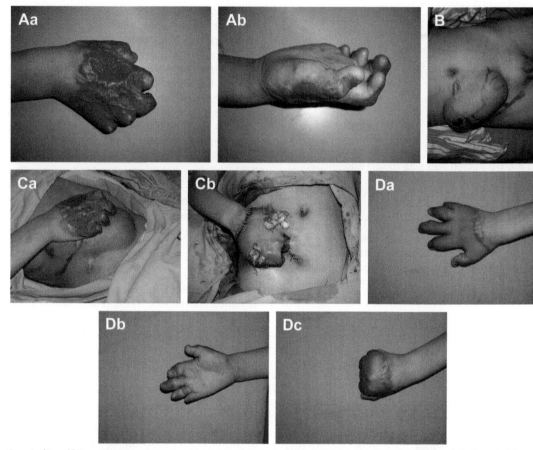

Case 2. (*A a, b*) Preoperative views showing claw deformity with hypertrophic scarring of the right hand. (*B*) Postoperative view showing the completion of tissue expansion after the first-stage procedure. (*C*) Intraoperative view showing the plan for the second-stage procedure (*C a*) and the completion of the second-stage procedure with total coverage of the hand and all 5 fingers under the pre-expanded flap after release of scars (*C b*). (*D a–c*) The results at 3 months' follow-up showing good functional and satisfactory appearance of the right hand.

surgery began with reports describing the use of island skin flaps from the abdomen and groin region. These pedicled abdominal flaps were used for coverage of soft tissue defects of the extremities. With refinement of these flaps, more and more were used for reconstruction of dorsal hand wounds. However, because flaps were usually harvested above the deep fascia, their thickness resulted in reconstructed hands was bulky.

In 1986, the subdermal vascular network flap was firstly reported by Situ.[3] The flaps were much thinner, which decreased donor site morbidity and required no sacrifice of muscle function. The texture and color of the flap are more similar to the normal skin, which improved aesthetic outcome. As these subdermal vascular network flaps became widely applied in reconstructive surgery, they were named as superthin flaps. A superthin flap is primarily thinned to the layer where the subdermal vascular network

(subdermal plexus) can be seen through the minimal fat layer during the first-stage procedure. Such a flap is likely to receive adequate blood supply because of a well-developed subdermal vascular plexus after pre-expansion and prefabrication of blood vessels within the flap.[4] It has proved to be the ideal choice to reconstruct hands for which functional and aesthetic outcomes are necessary. Furthermore, the superthin flap has been widely applied, whether free or pedicled, but the size of the superthin flap was limited. Hyakusoku and colleagues[1] tried to enlarge the superthin flap by microsurgically augmenting the blood supply of the flap. However, the free perforator flap increased the surgical difficulty. Subsequently bipedicled superthin abdominal perforator flaps made the operation easier but still could not fully provide coverage to reconstruct the fingers simultaneously.[2]

The perforator usually originated from the named artery. Multiple efforts were made to clarify the vascular anatomy and identify the proper recipient vessels.[5] The design of the flap should be according to the perforator distribution. Angiography studies have discovered more and more perforators and their related flaps.

The authors attempted to apply perforator flaps to their clinical practice. The perforator of the flap originates from overlying skin perforators, as long as the perforator can be detected by Doppler on the abdominal skin. Since 2006 we have used soft tissue expansion to enlarge the flap. The blood supply of the flap originates from the skin perforators and the subdermal vascular network (subdermal plexus), where the skin perforators flow into the subdermal vascular network. Our flap consisted of several skin perforators, such as the SIEA, DIEA, and SCIA. Every skin perforator can flow into 1 territory of the flap. Adjacent perforators are connected by indirect linking vessels.[6] The indirect linking vessels are equivalent to Taylor choke vessels, the flow in which is uncertain. During skin expansion a new network of vessel patterns develops, which has been shown by histologic studies.[7] The indirect linking vessels grow into direct linking vessels and hyperperfusion of the perforator occurs. Each perforator feeds its own vascular territory, called a perforasome, introduced by Saint-Cyr and colleagues.[8] Therefore, one perforator can perfuse its own territory and also its adjacent perforators' territories through the growth of direct linking vessels. Ultimately, blood flow in expanded tissue is redistributed and augmented, allowing these flaps to gain improved ability to survive.

A nominal layer of fat tissue is left underneath the flap, which expedites the subdermal vascular network's attachment and integration to the wound surface directly. The remodeled vascularization is similar to a full-thickness skin graft. Reports describe that the anastomotic connections between the interface of the flap and recipient site can be found as early as within the first 24 hours postoperatively.[9] After 5 to 7 days, the quantity of arterial flow returned to near normal.[10] In our second-stage operation, the flap between each finger must therefore be divided and sutured to the lateral aspect of the digit at several points, inhibiting potential blood flow of the flap between the fingers. The flap overlying the finger then remodels its vascularization within the finger wound. When we divide the abdominal flap pedicle, we also longitudinally cut the flap between the fingers to form each finger separately.

However, we still delay pedicle division until 14 days. The main reason is that the superthin flap does not have a concomitant venous plexus.[11] So far we still have not ascertained how the venous circulation develops after the pedicle of the flap is divided. Future studies will address how to establish the venous circulation.

SUMMARY

The pre-expansion and prefabrication of a superthin skin perforator flap can be an innovative option for total hand resurfacing. Our 3-statge procedures are relatively easy and safe, with minimal donor site morbidity. Pre-expansion may provide a favorable superthin skin perforator flap that can be used effectively to reconstruct a large area after scar release of the whole hand and fingers with good cosmetic and functional outcomes.

REFERENCES

1. Hyakusoku H, Pennington DG, Gao JH. Microvascular augmentation of the super-thin occipito-cervico-dorsal flap. Br J Plast Surg 1994;47:465–9.
2. Oki K, Murakami M, Tanuma K, et al. Anatomical study of pectoral intercostal perforators and clinical study of the pectoral intercostal perforator flap for hand reconstruction. Plast Reconstr Surg 2009; 123(6):1789–800.
3. Situ P. Pedicled flap with subdermal vascular network. Acad J First Med Coll PLA (Chinese) 1986;6:60–3.
4. Wang CM, Zhang JY, Yang SF, et al. The clinical application of pre-expanded and pre-fabricated super-thin skin perforator flap for reconstruction of post-burn neck contracture. Ann Plast Surg 2016; 77(Suppl 1):S49–52.
5. Hong JP, Sun SH, Ben-Nakhi M. Modified superficial circumflex iliac artery perforator flap and supermicrosurgery technique for lower extremity reconstruction. Ann Plast Surg 2013;71:380–3.
6. Saint-Cyr M, Wong C, Schaverien M, et al. Perforasome theory: vascular anatomy and clinical implications. Plast Reconstr Surg 2009;124:1529.
7. Zhang J, Gui L, Mei J, et al. A radioanatomic study of minipig skin flap model. Chin J Clin Anat 2007; 5:502–6.
8. Saint-Cyr M, Schaverien M, Arbique G, et al. Three- and four-dimensional computed tomographic angiography and venography for the investigation of the vascular anatomy and perfusion of perforator flaps. Plast Reconstr Surg 2008;121:772–80.
9. Xiao NK, Zhong DC. Biological characteristics of fibronectin and its role in wound healing. Zhonghua Zheng Xing Shao Shang Wai Ke Za Zhi 1992;8(3):228–30.
10. Liang Z, Zhou X, et al. The stereology of vessel density of super thin skin flap. Chin J Reparative Reconstr Surg 1994;8(2):76–80.
11. Ma FS. Experimental study of circulation of skin flap with subdermal vascular network. Zhonghua Zheng Xing Shao Shang Wai Ke Za Zhi 1993;9(5):344–6.

Future Perspectives of Pre-expanded Perforator Flaps

Lee L.Q. Pu, MD, PhD[a],*, Chunmei Wang, MD, PhD[b]

KEYWORDS

- Pre-expansion • Prefabrication • Pre-expanded perforator flaps • Perforator flaps • Skin flaps
- Future perspectives

KEY POINTS

- Future perspectives of pre-expanded perforator flap from 2 editors are summarized in this review.
- Pre-expanded perforator flaps will be acknowledged and used more by worldwide plastic surgeons to reconstruct large skin defects.
- Pre-expander super-thin perforator flap may become a work horse for resurfacing if surgeons can improve and master the technique of performing these 2-staged reconstructions.
- With a better understanding of the improved blood supply to the flap and prefabrication of blood supply within the flap, pre-expanded perforator flap will play a more important role in reconstructive surgery.

INTRODUCTION

Although it may still not be fully understood how blood supply to the flap can be enhanced by pre-expansion of a perforator flap, the readers can see from this special issue that the pre-expanded perforator flap has been innovatively used by many reconstructive surgeons worldwide to solve some of the most difficult and challenging problems in our specialty. Although the clinical application of a pre-expanded perforator flap is primarily focused on head and neck reconstructions such a flap has also been used to reconstruct defects in the trunk, extremities or hands. There are considerable good clinical experiences presented in this special issue; therefore, pre-expanded perforator flaps can be used to reconstruct relatively large skin and soft tissue defects with improved functional and cosmetic outcomes.

ADVANTAGES AND DISADVANTAGES OF PRE-EXPANDED PERFORATOR FLAP

The advantages of a pre-expanded perforator flap are started with the concept that such a technique combines the application of a perforator flap with tissue expansion so that more flap tissue with improved blood supply can be available for reconstruction.[1] A pre-expanded perforator flap, in general, may be more reliable than a nonexpanded conventional perforator flap because of the prefabricated blood supply within the flap during targeted tissue expansion based on perforator flaps. Such a flap can provide "like-for-like tissue" for resurfacing large skin and soft tissue defects in any area of the body. It is especially true that such a flap can also provide not only large, but also a relatively thin flap to reconstructing large skin defects, especially in the face, neck, hand, or foot

[a] Division of Plastic Surgery, University of California Davis Medical Center, 2221 Stockton Boulevard, Suite 2123, Sacramento, CA 95817, USA; [b] Department of Plastic and Aesthetic Surgery, Dongguan Kanghua Hospital, 1000 Dongguan Avenue, Dongguan 523080, Guangdong Province, P.R. China
* Corresponding author.
E-mail address: llpu@ucdavis.edu

Clin Plastic Surg 44 (2017) 179–183
http://dx.doi.org/10.1016/j.cps.2016.08.009

and other parts of the body with essentially no donor site morbidity but without the need for a subsequent skin graft or additional flap for donor site closure.[2–4] Such a flap can be performed primarily as a pedicled flap without the need for more complex microsurgical procedures.

The disadvantages of pre-expanded perforator flap include inherent problems associated with the use of a tissue expander such as infection or expander extrusion. Such a reconstruction would require staged and multiple procedures for completion. It obviously may require prolonged hospital stay for the patient and, as with any other flaps, distal ischemia of the flap may still occur and would compromise the overall outcome of the reconstruction. In addition, owing to variations of perforator anatomy in each patient, some expertise would be required for preoperative mapping of the perforators so that during a preoperative design the expanders can be accurately placed for maximum effect of the prefabricated blood supply within the flap.[5]

UNDERSTANDING OF IMPROVED BLOOD SUPPLY TO PRE-EXPANDED PERFORATOR FLAP

Although the current understanding on how the vascular supply to the flap can be improved after pre-expansion of a perforator flap has been focused on the delayed phenomena, it is very true that the overall mechanisms on prefabrication of blood supply within a pre-expanded perforator flap would be more than just a delayed phenomenon but still less clearly understood. However, static 3-dimensional computed tomographic (CT) and dynamic 4-dimensional CT angiographies have been introduced to plastic surgery by Saint-Cyr and colleagues[6] to investigate vascular anatomy and perfusion of a perforator flap. The static 3-dimensional CT angiography can assess vascular anatomy in the coronal axial and sagittal planes and the dynamic 4-dimensional CT angiography can evaluate the perfusion of a perforator flap by visualizing the actual filling of flap circulation over a short time interval in 3 dimensions.[6] With these 3-dimensional or 4-dimensional CT angiographies, we are confident that prefabrication of blood supply within a pre-expanded perforator flap can be assessed live in patients that can provide extremely valuable information on what has happened in terms of how the blood supply within the flap could be enhanced after pre-expansion. In addition, large animal studies can also be performed with the use of these innovative techniques to determine and understand how the prefabrication of blood supply within

pre-expanded perforator flaps. With a better understanding of the mechanism on prefabrication of blood supply to a pre-expanded perforator flap, plastic surgeons will be able to have much clever use of such a flap for various reconstructions and to minimize complications through a better preoperative design for such a flap reconstruction.

IMPROVEMENT OF TISSUE EXPANSION AND ITS RELATED ISSUES

Because the creation of a pre-expanded perforator flap requires the placement of a tissue expander, any improvement of the tissue expander and its expansion process would definitely improve the outcome of such a flap reconstruction. This would include designing a different size, shape, or contoured expander similar to expanders used in breast reconstruction. Surgical techniques to minimize the trauma of expander placement such as endoscopic placement of expander may also improve the outcome of such a flap reconstruction. Could the expander be controlled by the patient for subsequent tissue expansion with a newly designed gas generated expansion used in breast reconstruction?[7] Any of these refinements or innovations could definitely improve the overall outcome of tissue expansion for creation of a pre-expanded perforator flap.

Improvement of the expansion process may also contribute to the final outcome of a pre-expanded perforator flap. Can the expansion process be performed in a more speedy fashion but minimizing the complication rate of flap ischemia or expander extrusion? Some of the innovative therapies such as the application of the patient's own stem cells could enhance the tissue regeneration and improve ischemia during the tissue expansion that may essentially speed the expansion process and have more and better flap tissue available for reconstruction.[8] In addition, topical administration of an angiogenic growth factor may also improve or minimize flap ischemia during tissue expansion for a pre-expanded perforator flap.[9]

MORE ACCURATE PRE-EXPANSION OR POST-EXPANSION PERFORATOR MAPPING

More accurate mapping of the perforator(s) before or after expansion of a pre-expanded perforator flap can be critical for the success of such a flap reconstruction. Because multidetector row computed tomography angiography is a novel imaging technology that can acquire both static and dynamic 3-dimensional or even 4-dimensional images of macrovascular and microvascular anatomy of a perforator flap, we believe this new image method can provide fairly accurate information about the location, type, size, and course of perforator(s) in any given area of the body and can potentially be quite valuable in the preoperative planning of a perforator flap, especially a freestyle type of perforator flap.[5] With aid of this type of technology, identification of the perforator(s) in the flap donor site can be very useful to ensure the accurate placement of the tissue expander and its effect on enhancement of blood supply within the pre-expanded perforator flap via prefabrication of its blood supply.[10]

With wide application of perforator flap for reconstruction, some plastic surgeons prefer a relatively simple technique to map perforators during the design of a perforator flap. This is especially true by using color duplex imaging for the identification of perforators in a given region of the body before the placement of an expander in a selected donor site because perforators can be mapped with a color duplex scanner.[11] Such a method can also be reasonably accurate to identify the perforator anatomy and has been used frequently by one of the authors for preoperative planning of many commonly used perforator flaps such as anterolateral thigh perforator flaps, deep inferior epigastric perforator flaps, or even freestyle perforator flaps with good success. However, such technology is very much operator dependent and cannot assess the profusion of each identified perforator within the perforator flap.

STANDARDIZED PROTOCOL OF HOW TO PERFORM PRE-EXPANDED PERFORATOR FLAPS

Although pre-expanded perforator flaps have been used by a number of plastic surgeons worldwide to perform reconstruction primarily for the face and neck region, the standard protocol on how to perform this 2-staged pre-expanded perforator flaps are quite variable and have not been standardized. Just like any other procedures in plastic surgery, a more standardized way to perform a pre-expanded perforator flap would definitely ensure better clinical result with more reproducible outcome by many other surgeons. Therefore, pre-expanded perforator flaps should also be standardized in terms of patient selection, preoperative perforator mapping, selection and placement of a tissue expander, expansion process and the subsequent second-stage reconstruction by removal of the tissue expander, and subsequent definitive reconstruction and possible future revision surgeries. In this way,

pre-expanded perforator flaps can be adapted and learned by more plastic surgeons worldwide to better serve their unique group of reconstructive patients with improved but consistent clinical outcome.

IMPROVEMENT OF OUTCOME AND MINIMIZING COMPLICATIONS

Like any other reconstructive surgery, refinement of reconstructive procedures is always necessary to improve the final outcome. Because this kind of reconstruction commonly occurs in the face and neck region, the cosmetic appearance after such a reconstruction can be quite critical. When combined with some of the cosmetic surgical techniques for facial and neck rejuvenation, the reconstruction outcome after pre-expanded perforator flap reconstruction for resurfacing of the face and neck can definitely be improved. In addition, fat grafting may also play a role to improve the overall cosmetic result after such a reconstruction in flap donor and recipient sites, because fat grafting may not only serve as fillers but also have regenerative potential to improve tissue condition.[12] In addition, the donor site's scar management would definitely improve overall satisfaction of patients. With advanced laser technology or other techniques, donor site scarring could be minimized with modern approach to the scar of the donor site.[13]

Just like any other flaps, distal ischemia of the flap may occur after pre-expanded perforator flap reconstruction. Therefore, the more accurate preoperative planning with placement of expander under identified perforators in the flap donor site, ischemic complications of the pre-expanded perforator flap can be minimized. In addition, the flap's super-charge can also be considered to improve the distal flap ischemia, although microsurgical technique should be required to provide such super-charge to the flap.[14,15] Additionally, the role of stem cells or angiogenic growth factors may be used to improve the distal flap ischemia.[8,9]

EXPANDED INDICATIONS OF PRE-EXPANDED PERFORATOR FLAPS

There is no doubt in our mind that pre-expander thin perforator flaps will continue to be used to reconstruct large face or neck skin defect if the time would be allowed for delayed reconstruction after release of burn scar contracture. Because pre-expanded perforator flaps have been used to reconstruct relatively large skin defects with improved functional and cosmetic outcomes, the pre-expander super thin perforator flap may become a work horse for resurfacing of a large face, neck, or other body area of skin defect if surgeons can master the technique to perform these 2-staged reconstructions for their patients. Such a flap can also be used for resurfacing of the dorsal hand or foot or even an extremity with better tissue match if a large area of reconstruction is needed. Such a reconstruction may provide good to excellent functional and cosmetic outcome but avoid a skin graft for closure of the donor site. Pre-expanded perforator flaps can also be used in organ reconstruction such as penile reconstruction with the flap tissue from the anterior–lateral thigh region or vaginal reconstruction with the flap tissue from the abdomen. This kind of reconstruction can really minimize donor site complications and provide more freedom to plastic surgeons for flap inset so that reconstructive and cosmetic outcome can greatly be improved.

Pre-expander free perforator flap can be a new option for plastic surgeons. The pre-expanded perforator free flap can be more reliable to reconstruct even for a larger area of soft tissue defect but to avoid a skin graft to the donor site. Pre-expanded perforator flap in combination with microsurgical technique are an innovative approach for soft tissue reconstruction with more tissue can be transferred but with minimized donor site morbidities.

It is our opinion that a pre-expanded perforator flap may be able to replace a "skin-only" total facial allotransplantation with "like-for-like" flap tissue for reconstruction but without the need of postoperative immunosuppression for patients and with possibly equivalent functional and cosmetic outcome compared with facial allotransplantation.[15]

SUMMARY

The pre-expanded perforator flap is an innovative reconstructive option for selected patients. It has distinct advantages to simplify the reconstructive surgery and be able to provide good to excellent outcomes after reconstruction. Although it still has some disadvantages and is only indicated for delayed reconstruction, such a reconstructive approach can be a safe, reliable option for carefully selected patients. With a better understanding of the improved blood supply to the flap as well as the mechanism on prefabrication of blood supply within the flap, pre-expanded perforator flap will definitely play an increased role in reconstructive surgery. With a standardized protocol for flap surgery, preoperative evaluation and postoperative care, it can be performed for indicated patients by many plastic surgeons worldwide with

improved reconstructive and cosmetic outcomes. This is another exciting field of reconstructive plastic surgery because it combines perforator flap surgery with tissue expansion technique and such an approach will have its distinguished role in plastic surgery. We are looking forward to greater use and development of pre-expanded perforator flap surgery in the future.

REFERENCES

1. Tsai F-C. A new method: perforator-based tissue expansion for a preexpanded free cutaneous perforator flap. Burns 2003;29:845–8.
2. Wang C, Zhang J, Yang S, et al. The clinical application of preexpanded and prefabricated super-thin skin perforator flap for reconstruction of post-burn neck contracture. Ann Plast Surg 2016;77(Suppl 1):S49–52.
3. Zan T, Li H, Du Z, et al. Reconstruction of the face and neck with different types of pre-expanded anterior chest flaps: a comprehensive strategy for multiple techniques. J Plast Reconstr Aesthet Surg 2013; 66:1074–81.
4. Zang M, Zhu S, Song B, et al. Reconstruction of extensive upper extremity defects using pre-expanded oblique perforator-based paraumbilical flaps. Burns 2012;38:917–23.
5. Yang S, Wang CM, Ono S, et al. The value of multidetector row computed tomography angiography for preoperative planning of freestyle pedicled perforator flaps. Ann Plast Surg 2016. [Epub ahead of print].
6. Saint-Cyr M, Schaverien M, Arbique G, et al. Three- and four-dimensional computed tomographic angiography and venography for the investigation of the vascular anatomy and perfusion of perforator flaps. Plast Reconstr Surg 2008;121:772–80.
7. Connell TF. Patient-activated controlled expansion for breast reconstruction using controlled carbon dioxide inflation: confirmation of a feasibility study. Plast Reconstr Surg 2014;134:503e–11e.
8. Yang M, Li Q, Sheng L, et al. Bone marrow-derived mesenchymal stem cells transplantation accelerates tissue expansion by promoting skin regeneration during expansion. Ann Surg 2011; 253:202–9.
9. Mittermayr R, Slezak P, Haffner N, et al. Controlled release of fibrin matrix-conjugated platelet derived growth factor improves ischemic tissue regeneration by functional angiogenesis. Acta Biomater 2016;29: 11–20.
10. Wang C, Yang S, Fan J, et al. Clinical application of prefabricated super-thin perforator flaps after expansion in the reconstruction of facial and cervical scar. Zhonghua Zheng Xing Wai Ke Za Zhi 2015;31: 5–10 [in Chinese].

11. Dorfman D, Pu LL. The value of color duplex imaging for planning and performing a free anterolateral thigh perforator flap. Ann Plast Surg 2014;72(Suppl 5):S6–8.

12. Coleman SR, Katzel EB. Fat grafting for facial filling and regeneration. Clin Plast Surg 2015;42:289–300.

13. Commander SJ, Chamata E, Cox J, et al. Update on postsurgical scar management. Semin Plast Surg 2016;30:122–8.

14. Ono S, Chung KC, Takami Y, et al. Perforator-supercharged occipitocervicopectoral flaps for lower face and neck reconstruction. Plast Reconstr Surg 2012; 129:879–87.

15. Li Q, Zan T, Li H, et al. Flap prefabrication and stem cell-assisted tissue expansion: how we acquire a monoblock flap for full face resurfacing. J Craniofac Surg 2014;25:21–5.

Index

Note: Page numbers of article titles are in **boldface** type.

A

Abdominal superthin skin perforator flap,
pre-expanded prefabricated, for total hand
resurfacing, **171–177**
  complications and management of,
    173–174
  outcomes of, 174–175, 176
  postprocedural care in, 174
  preoperative planning for, 172
  procedural approach for, 172–173
  rehabilitation and recovery following, 174
  treatment goals and outcomes, 172
Acoustic Doppler sonography, handheld, for
perforator identification, 24–26, 27

B

Brachial artery perforator flap, pre-expanded,
117–128
  anatomic basis of, 118, 119, 120, 121
  case demonstrations of, 135–138
  complications and management of, 122
  flap transfer in, 121–122
  outcomes of, 133–135
  patient positioning for, 118
  postprocedural care in, 122
  preoperative planning and preparation for,
    118, 121
  procedural approach in, 118–122
  treatment goals and planned outcomes, 118
  pre-expansion of, 118–121

C

Color duplex sonography, for perforator
identification, 26–27
Computed tomographic angiography, for perforator
identification, 28

D

Deep inferior epigastric artary flap. See *Paraumbilical
perforator flap.*

E

Epigastric perforator flap, pre-expanded deep
inferior, **109–115**
  anatomy of, 109–110, 111
  clinical results of, 114
  complications and management of, 112

  expansion process for, 111–112
  flap harvest/inset of, 112
  outcomes of, 112–113
  patient positioning for, 111
  postprocedural care for, 112
  preoperative planning and preparation for,
    110–111
  procedural approach for, 111–112
  treatment goals and planned outcomes, 110

F

Fat layer in body, different distributions of, 7, 8–9

H

Hand resurfacing, abdominal superthin skin
perforator flap for. See *Abdominal superthin
perforator flap, pre-expanded prefabricated.*

M

Magnetic resonance angiography, for perforator
identification, 28–29
Mammary artery perforator flap, internal pre-
expanded, **65–72**
  anatomy of, 66–67
  complications and management of, 68
  expander placement and expansion process
    for, 67–68
  flap harvest/inset for, 68
  linking vessels for, 66–67
  literature reports on, 71
  outcomes of, 69, 70–71
  patient positioning for, 67
  postprocedural care in, 68–69
  preoperative planning and preparation for, 67
  procedural approach for, 67–68
  rehabilitation and recovery following, 69
  treatment goals and planned outcomes of, 67
Monoblock perforator flap, pre-expanded
prefabricated, for total facial resurfacing, **163–170**
  appearance and function status score, 164
  case demonstrations of, 167–169
  cervicothoracic flap for, 165
  complications and management of,
    165–166
  outcomes of, 167
  postprocedural care in, 165–166

Monoblock (*continued*)
  preoperative planning and preparation for,
    164–165
  procedural approach for, 165
  rehabilitation and recovery following,
    166–167
  treatment goals and planned outcomes,
    164

N

Nose and upper lip, simultaneous reconstruction of,
  pre-expanded supratrochlear perforator flap for.
  See *Supratrochlear perforator flap.*

P

Paraumbilical perforator flap, pre-expanded, **99–108**
  case demonstrations of, 103–107
  donor site complications, 103
  expansion complications, 102
  outcomes of, 103
  patient positioning for, 100
  postprocedural care following, 103
  preoperative planning and preparation for, 100
  procedural approach for, 100–102
  rehabilitation and recovery following, 103
  treatment goals and planned outcomes, 100
  vascular complications, 102
Perforator flaps. See also specific flaps.
  assessment of course of, 23–24, 25
  computed tomography design for, 22, 23, 24
  design of, 24, 25, 26
  harvest of, step-by-step approach to, 22–24,
    25, 26
  pre-expanded, advantages and disadvantages of,
    179–180
    angiosomes in, 2, 4
    classifications of, 6–9
    clinical applications of, **13–20**
    contemporary concepts of, 3–5
    cross-area of blood supply in, 5–6, 7
    current concepts of, **1–11**
    donor site selection for, 14
    expanded indications for, 181–182
    expander placement for, 15
    expansion phase of, 15
    fabricated flap, 18
    fat layer layer of body and, 7, 8–9
    flap extension and flap delay compared for, 5
    flap selection in, 16–17
    formed capsule and, 5
    future perspectives of, **179–183**
    how to perform mapping of, standardized
      protocol of, 181
    improved blood supply to, understanding
      of, 180

  incision for, 15
  mapping of, more accurate, 180–181
  outcome of, improvement of, 181
  pedicled, 15
  perforator location for, 15
  pocket creation for, 15
  postoperative management of, 18–19
  preoperative evaluation for, 14–15
  previously published works on, 14
  recipient site evaluation for, 14–15
  studies on, 5
  super-thin flap, 18
  tissue expansion for, improvement of, 180
    methods of, 5
  two-stage, procedural algorithm for, 15, 18
  types of anastomosis in, 2, 3
  updated knowledge on, 2–3
  pre-expanded free, 18, **143–152**
    complications and management of, 148–149
    contraindications to, 144, 145
    indications for, 144
    outcomes of, case demonstrations of, 149–152
    patient positioning for, 146
    postprocedural care in, 148–149
    preoperative planning and preparation for,
      144–145
    procedural approach for, 146–147
    treatment goals and planned outcomes of, 144
  preoperative assessment of, 21–22
    tools for, 27
  preoperative planning of, case presentation of,
    22, 23
    imaging studies for, **21–30**
  rotation and inset of, 24, 26
  selection of, 22–23

S

Super-thin skin perforator flaps, pre-expanded,
  31–40
    case demonstrations of, 36–38
    complications and mnaagement of, 35
    outcomes of, 35
    patient positioning for, 33
    postprocedural care in, 35
    preoperative planning and preparation of,
      32–33, 34
    procedural approach for, 33–35
    rehabilitation and recovery following, 35
    tissue expander for, placement of, 39
    treatment goals using, and planned
      outcomes, 32
  pre-expanded intercostal, **73–89**
    clinical anatomy and, 74, 75
    clinical case demonstrations, 80–87
    complications and management of, 78–79
    expander placement for, 76

expander removal/flap transposition for, 76–78
expander selection for, 75
hematoma in, 79
infection in, 79
outcomes of, 80
patient positioning for, 75–76
pedicle division in, 78
postprocedural care in, 79–80
preoperative planning and preparation for,
    74–75
procedural approach for, 76–78
rehabilitation and recovery following, 80
surgical planning for, 74–75
treatment goals and planned outcomes of, 74
Supraclavicular artery perforator flap(s), in
    literature, 60
pre-expanded, **49–63**
    outcomes of, 56, 57–58, 59–60
    postprocedural care, rehabilitation, and
        recovery following, 54–56
    preoperative planning, preparation, and patient
        positioning for, 50
    procedural approach for, 50–52, 53, 54
    treatment goals and planned outcomes of, 50
Supratrochlear perforator flap, expanded bipedicled,
    for nasal/upper lip reconstruction, **153–162**
        case demonstrations of, 159, 160, 161
        complications and management of, 159
        outcomes of, 159
        postoperative care in, 159

preoperative planning for, 154–155
procedural approach for, 155–157
rehabilitation and recovery following, 159
treatment goals and planned outcomes,
    154
pre-expanded bipedicled, for nasal/upper lip
    defects, 154

T

Thoracodorsal artery perforator flap, pre-expanded,
    91–97
        complications and management of, 92–93
        outcomes of, 93, 94, 95
        patient positioning and surgical technique for,
            92, 93
        postprocedural care in, 93
        preoperative planning and preparation for, 92
        rehabilitation and recovery following, 93
Transverse cervical artery perforator flap, pre-
    expanded, **41–47**
        case demonstrations of, 44, 45, 46
        complications and management of, 42
        outcomes of, 43
        patient positioning for, 42
        postprocedural care in, 43
        preoperative planning and preparation for, 42
        procedural approach for, 42, 43
        rehabilitation and recovery following, 43
        treatment goals and planned outcomes of, 42

Moving?

Make sure your subscription moves with you!

To notify us of your new address, find your **Clinics Account Number** (located on your mailing label above your name), and contact customer service at:

Email: journalscustomerservice-usa@elsevier.com

800-654-2452 (subscribers in the U.S. & Canada)
314-447-8871 (subscribers outside of the U.S. & Canada)

Fax number: 314-447-8029

Elsevier Health Sciences Division
Subscription Customer Service
3251 Riverport Lane
Maryland Heights, MO 63043

*To ensure uninterrupted delivery of your subscription, please notify us at least 4 weeks in advance of move.

Printed and bound by CPI Group (UK) Ltd, Croydon, CR0 4YY

08/05/2025

01864696-0015